The Laryngeal Mask Airway

A Review and Practical Guide

We dedicate this book to our families and friends with gratitude for their support and encouragement.

The Laryngeal Mask Airway

A Review and Practical Guide

J R Brimacombe MB ChB FRCA MD
Clinical Associate Professor
University of Queensland
Cairns Base Hospital
Cairns
Queensland
Australia

A I J Brain LMSSA FFARCSI
Honorary Consultant Anesthesiologist
Royal Berkshire Hospital
Reading
UK

Honorary Research Fellow
Institute of Laryngology
University of London
UK

A M Berry MB ChB FRCA
Associate author
Clinical Senior Lecturer
University of Queensland
Nambour General Hospital
Nambour
Australia

W. B. Saunders Company Ltd
London Philadelphia Toronto Sydney Tokyo

W. B. Saunders Company Ltd 24–28 Oval Road
London NW1 7DX

The Curtis Center
Independence Square West
Philadelphia, PA 19106-3399, USA

Harcourt Brace & Company
55 Horner Avenue
Toronto, Ontario, M8Z 4X6, Canada

Harcourt Brace & Company, Australia
30–52 Smidmore Street
Marrickville
NSW 2204, Australia

Harcourt Brace & Company, Japan
Ichibancho Central Building
22-1 Ichibancho
Chiyoda-ku, Tokyo 102, Japan

This book is printed on acid-free paper

A catalogue record for this book is available from the British Library

ISBN 0-7020-2321-3

Typeset by Phoenix Photosetting, Lordswood, Chatham, Kent
Printed and bound in Great Britain by The University Press, Cambridge

Contents

Foreword

The publication of the first book on a relatively new, but extremely valuable airway device, the laryngeal mask airway (LMA), written by two of the most knowledgeable and prominent authors in the field, one of whom is the inventor, is an important event. The LMA is the most significant advance in airway management since the introduction of the oropharyngeal airway and the tracheal tube several decades ago. In terms of functional and clinical significance, the LMA fills in the large gap between the variably effective, nonsealed, easy-to-insert oropharyngeal airway, and the almost invariably effective, sealed, but relatively difficult-to-insert invasive tracheal tube. Consequently, and as a result of this functional and clinical significance, the LMA has become, in a remarkably short period of time, as frequently used in many developed countries for routine elective situations as the oropharyngeal airway or the tracheal tube. Furthermore, in many difficult airway situations, the LMA may succeed when the other two fundamental approaches to the airway fail.

The authors of this book are most appropriate. Dr Joseph Brimacombe's increasing prominence as an LMA expert has paralleled, and has therefore been as explosive as, the increasing acceptance of the LMA. In my experience, no one has written and published more high quality communications in this field than has Dr Joseph Brimacombe; not surprisingly, his research papers are based on an enormous personal clinical experience of the LMA. I have shared several reviews of submitted articles with, and have had my own articles reviewed by, Dr Joseph Brimacombe, and I am confident that Dr Brimacombe has the entire world's literature on the subject at his immediate command.

Dr Archie I J Brain is the sole inventor of the LMA and he has almost single-handedly introduced the device to the world. The development of the LMA from 1981 to 1988 and its introduction from 1983, when the first paper was published, until the present represent many years of devoted work. As the knowledge that constitutes the contents of this book was accumulated, Dr Brain maintained the highest degree of intellectual integrity and enthusiastically promoted, and stayed abreast of, the research necessary to accumulate that knowledge. Furthermore, his creative mind is relentlessly productive and many improvements in the LMA are under study/development. My strong impression of Dr Brain and the LMA is that what is before the anesthesia community now is just the beginning rather than the end of highly effective and functional supraglottic airway devices.

In summary, one can be certain, based on the authorship, that this books brings all the world's literature into one clinically relevant practical guide. In brief, the message of the Foreword is simple: the first book on a very useful device, by extraordinarily qualified and gifted authors and teachers, is an important event. I am delighted to have played a small part in the process.

Jonathan L Benumof, MD
Professor of Anesthesia, University of California, San Diego UCSD Medical Center

Preface

The laryngeal mask airway (LMA) was introduced into the USA in 1991 and is gradually gaining popularity as a general purpose airway for anesthesia practice and for management of the difficult airway. Most anesthesiologists will have had some exposure to the device and will be on the early part of the learning curve. Others will have acquired sufficient skill and understanding to attempt more advanced uses. However, as elsewhere in the world, the acquisition of skill and knowledge has been hindered by a variety of misconceptions and a lack of appropriate training.

The main impetus for writing this book was the need to provide a single tome containing all the scattered literature on the LMA which would also function as a complete practical guide. This should be of assistance to established practitioners who are having difficulties with the LMA or wish to use it in more advanced areas, to trainees preparing to learn the technique, and to researchers requiring a reference resource. As such, the book brings together over 1000 publications and interrelates them in a useful and comprehensive way. In doing so it deals with the concepts behind LMA design and its history, provides complete practical guidance for users and describes the anatomical, physiological and pathophysiological implications. The indications, contraindications and problems associated with its use are analyzed in the context of clinical practice. Training issues, basic and advanced uses are described and discussed with special emphasis on its use in the difficult airway and during resuscitation outside the operating room. Finally, the future direction of LMA design and development is discussed.

J R Brimacombe
A I J Brain
October 1996

Acknowledgments

We would like to thank: Alison Berry and Chandi Verghese for their remarkable contributions to research and teaching in the field; Robert Gaines-Cooper for making the LMA a reality; John Nunn, Michael Rosen and Jonathan Benumof for realizing its clinical importance; Jane Gaines-Cooper for keeping us on the right track; and Neil Shorney for his early inspiration. We would also like to thank our anesthetic and surgical colleagues, the Cairns Base, Royal Berkshire, Dunedin and Berkshire Independent Hospitals for their tireless support. Finally, the staff of Gensia (San Diego) should be credited for the responsible manner in which they have introduced the LMA into the USA.

1 Introduction

Concept

Airway management for most of the twentieth century has been dominated by the face mask and tracheal tube. However, from an engineering viewpoint, the way these artificial airways are connected to the respiratory tract is less than ideal. When a face mask is used, the gap between the base of the tongue and the glottis is not bypassed. This may cause obstruction during anesthesia when upper airway muscle tone decreases[1] and gravity approximates the pharyngeal tissues[2] – a problem only partly solved by manipulation of the head, neck and jaw and the insertion of a Guedel oropharyngeal airway[3]. Tracheal intubation bypasses this problem, but involves positioning a tube within a tube and inflating a sealing balloon in a highly sensitive area where capillary flow is easily interrupted and epithelial damage common[4,5]. In addition, intubation is usually a direct vision technique which requires the use of a laryngoscope and muscle relaxants with their associated complications[6–8].

For over 200 years the pharynx has been considered a possible location for an airway device and there have been several designs in which the distal end of the airway fitted into the oro- or laryngopharynx. These include: Curry's silver tracheal cannula (1792), O'Dwyer's tube (1890s)[9], Hewitt's airway (1908)[10], Guedel's airway (1933)[11], Shipway's airway (1935)[12], Leech's 'Pharyngeal bulb gasway' (1937)[13] and Fink's Vallecular airway (1957)[14]. Some of these devices attempted to form an airtight seal with the respiratory tract by forming a plug in the upper pharynx[13,15], but none obtained widespread clinical acceptance since they were difficult to place, occasionally traumatic or formed an unreliable seal. The conceptual innovation of the laryngeal mask airway (LMA) was that it formed an airtight seal around the glottis rather than plugging the pharynx and by following the path of deglutition was simple and atraumatic to insert. Recently two new oropharyngeal airways have been described and are currently undergoing evaluation: Mehta's supraglottic oropharyngeal airway (1990)[16] and Greenberg's cuffed oropharyngeal airway (1991)[17–22]. Both devices form an airtight plug in the proximal pharynx and are atraumatic and easy to insert, but are likely to require a degree of manual manipulation for successful use and may not form an effective seal.

A history of oropharyngeal and nasopharyngeal airways (1880–1995) has been written by McIntyre with a view to determining if the objectives of the LMA were described collectively with reference to earlier airways[23]. The author considered that 'the LMA represents a perception of the need for a device with multiple qualities in our contemporary anaesthetic practice'. It is a 'fortunate co-incidence of increasing needs for clinical perfection, manufacture capability, drugs to suit the occasion, and one individual's recognition of the situation and motivation to meet the challenge'. The anatomical, physiological and pathophysiological changes that occur in the airway during general anesthesia have been recently reviewed by Burwell and Jones[24,25].

History

An account of the invention, early clinical trials and experimental work from which the LMA evolved has been published[26]. Key historical events are listed in Table 1.1. In brief, the LMA was designed in 1981 by Archie Brain, a British anesthesiologist working at the Royal London Hospital, UK, as part of a specific search for an airway that was more practical than the face mask and less invasive than a tracheal tube. The inventor applied principles of bioengineering to the functional anatomy of the pharynx both in terms of anatomical fit and methods of placement. In considering possible options, he was struck by the similarity between the contour of the elliptical path around the nose against which the Goldman nasal mask fitted and the contour around the glottis when examining anatomical specimens of the glottis.

The first prototype was constructed from the cuff of a Goldman nasal mask for dental anesthesia stretched over a diagonally cut size 10 mm tracheal tube and fixed

Table 1.1 Key historical points

Event	*Year*
LMA conceived and designed	1981 (June)
First use in human patient	1981 (August)
First meeting Robert Gaines-Cooper	1983 (February)
First publication (*British Journal of Anaesthesia*)	1983 (August)
First clinical series published (*Anaesthesia*)	1985 (April)
LMA first constructed from latex	1986 (July)
New silicone prototype shown to John Nunn	1986 (December)
First production models available for testing	1987 (December)
Full production	1988 (February)
First purchase – Royal East Sussex Hospital	1988 (April)
First publication of production model (*Anaesthesia*)	1988
First independent assessment of LMA (*Anaesthesia*)	1989
All UK hospitals with operating rooms purchased LMA	1990 (Autumn)
Approval for use in USA	1991 (August)
Queen's award for industry	1993
Included in ASA algorithm for difficult airway	1993
Available in 80 countries	1995
Used in 30 million patients	1996
Expanded role in ASA algorithm (Benumof)	1996

into position with acrylic glue (Figure 1.1). The intention was that the cuff portion would sit in the pharyngeal sack where it would form a circumferential low pressure seal around the glottis. This prototype was first used on a human patient undergoing a routine hernia repair at the William Harvey Hospital, Ashford, Kent, in the summer of 1981. The new device was inserted blindly under halothane anesthesia; a clear airway was immediately obtained and positive pressure ventilation (PPV) was possible. As a result of this experience three more prototypes were assembled and a pilot study of 23 patients followed at the London Hospital. The results were published in the *British Journal of Anaesthesia* in August 1983[27]. The study included 16 patients undergoing gynecological laparoscopy who were successfully ventilated (a procedure for which use of the LMA is currently controversial – see Chapter 13, *Gynecological laparoscopy*). The results of the study and the ease with which he found he could insert the device into his own pharynx convinced Brain that considerable further research was justified, but it aroused neither commercial nor academic interest. It became clear that any further development would have to be carried out by the inventor and, after obtaining local ethical committee approval, ongoing trials were commenced in which the fundamental design was explored, refined and then tested on the inventor's patients at a rate of approximately 1000 per year.

The first clinical series was reported in *Anaesthesia* in 1985 and described the successful use of Goldman cuff based prototypes in over 500 patients undergoing a wide variety of surgical procedures[28]. By late 1985 it was clear, however, that no further progress could be made with the Goldman cuff. The Dunlop Rubber Company provided Brain with a silicone elliptical torus surrounding a flat silicone membrane. By piercing this membrane with slots and deforming the flat surface into a shallow bowl, the inventor was able to construct a prototype with significant advantages over its predecessors. The mask aperture bars so formed prevented epiglottic entrapment and the uniform shape of the cuff allowed it to be fully deflated, creating a thin leading edge for improved placement. The Dunlop cuff was clearly superior to previous prototypes, but was too small for use in adults, and in July 1986 Brain purchased a supply of liquid

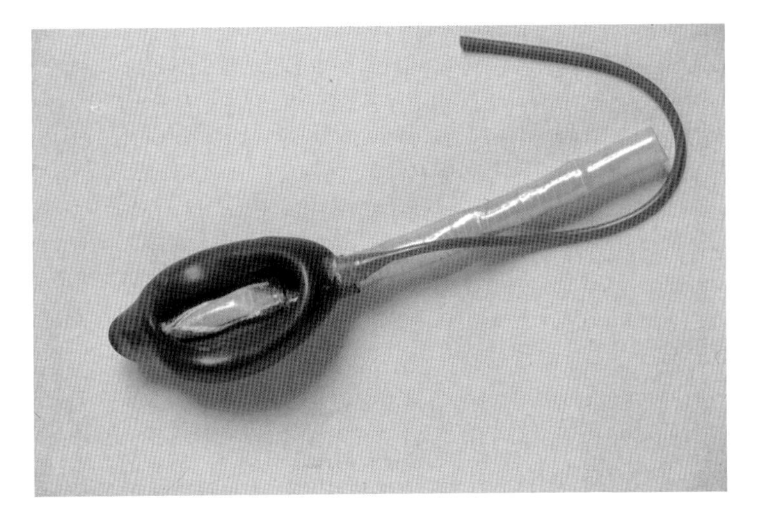

Figure 1.1 Early prototype LMA.

latex and began to make plaster of Paris casts to test a wide range of design ideas. Over 60 different designs of latex LMA were constructed and tested clinically (Figure 1.2).

In searching for the optimal characteristics for a laryngeal mask one of the criteria was to achieve a high pressure seal. It was found possible to do this by increasing the expandable volume of the cuff, but this caused cyanosis of the tongue. Another approach was to increase the surface contact of the mask with the larynx, and a number of anatomically accurate models were built including solid rubber and foam versions which were designed to completely cover the posterior-facing surface of the larynx (Figure 1.3); however this wedging effect was found to be too stimulating to be acceptable clinically, presumably because the posterior aspect of the larynx is richly innervated[29]. Interestingly, this latter approach has been revisited recently in an American design[30]. Finally it was realized that a high pressure seal could be achieved by addition of a posterior cuff, but the inventor was wary of producing this without some form of vent to prevent possible damming back of vomited material with the resulting danger of esophageal rupture, a situation which has been known to occur when vomiting occurs in the presence of cricoid pressure[31].

By September 1986 extensive testing of latex and silicone variants had shown that: (1) reliability of insertion and airway maintenance were best achieved by keeping the cross-sectional area of the cuff torus as near constant as possible at all points, so that inflation resulted in equal expansion in all areas; (2) the Dunlop cuff was too small for effective sealing in adults, but offered the best characteristics for smooth insertion; (3) seal pressures higher than 30 cm H_2O could not be safely achieved without injecting such large volumes into special laterally unfolding cuffs that tongue cyanosis

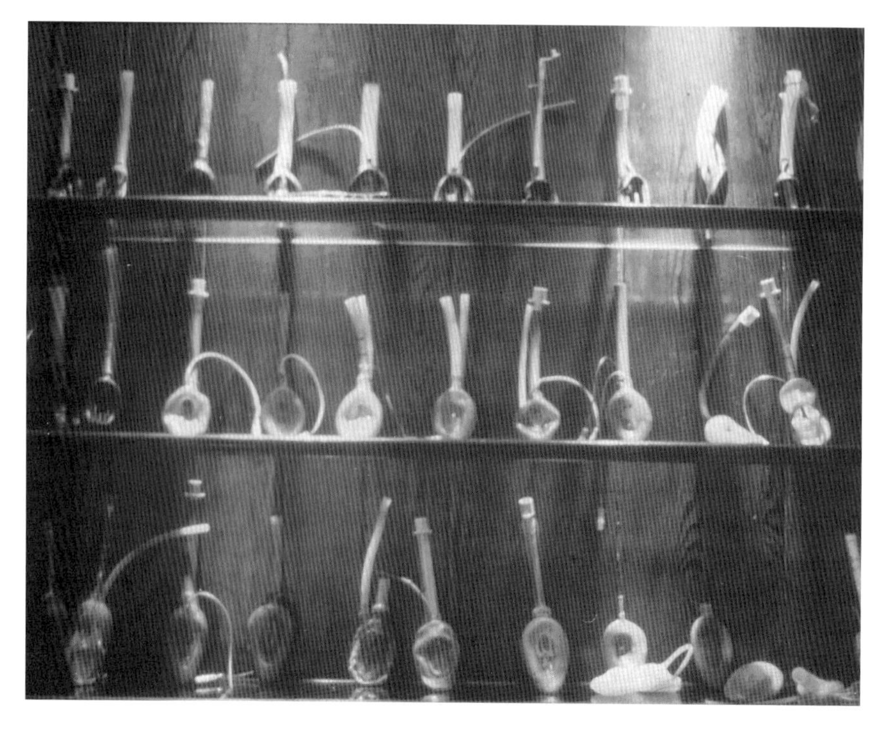

Figure 1.2 Early prototypes – over 60 different latex prototypes were produced before 1988.

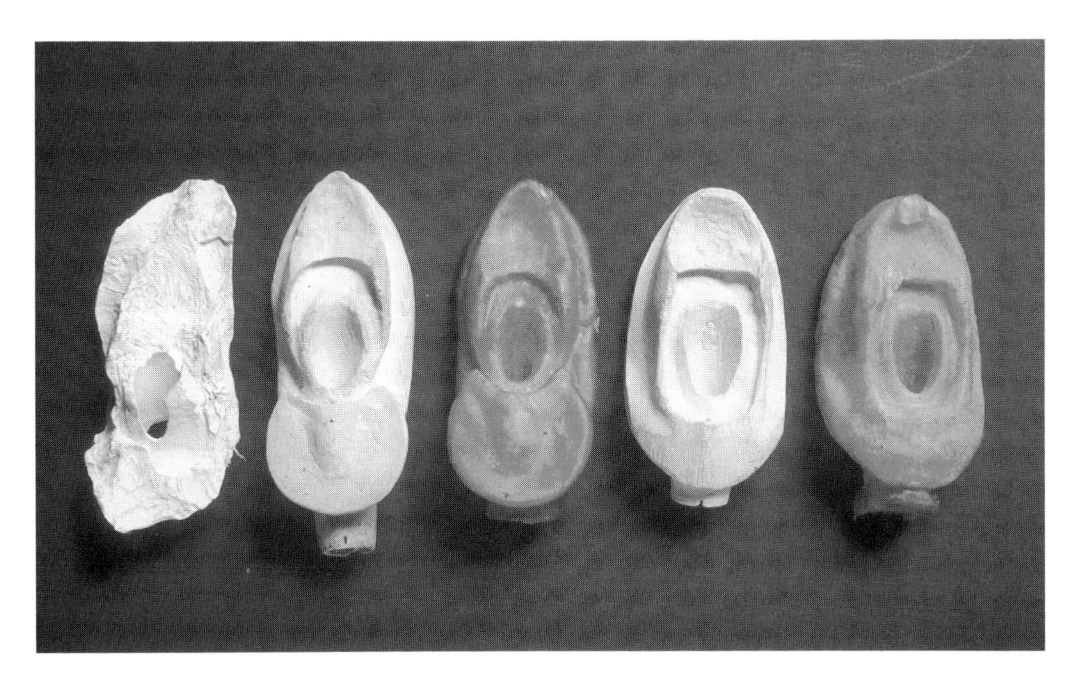

Figure 1.3 Prototype laryngeal wedge-type airways. From the left, cast of posterior aspect of larynx, dipping mandrel and corresponding latex mask (long), dipping mandrel and corresponding latex mask (short).

developed. The search for high seal pressures was proving difficult and in late 1986 a larger version of the Dunlop cuff was produced which provided a clinically acceptable seal of approximately 20 cm H_2O. This prototype was demonstrated to an eminent UK anesthesiologist, Professor John Nunn, on 4 December 1986, following which the search for higher seal pressures was abandoned.

The final design was a compromise between ease of insertion and the quality of the seal with the glottis, since to a certain extent these two goals were mutually exclusive in design terms[32]. By December 1987 the first all-factory made LMA was ready for trial and the initial results exceeded expectations since the new silicone cuff was softer and larger than the Dunlop cuff, making a more extensive contact with the laryngeal perimeter. The LMA went into production in the UK in early 1988 following extensive clinical trials. By the time it became commercially available it had been used in over 7000 patients. Interestingly, a British anesthesiologist, Dr S Buchan, made his own versions of Brain's original prototype and was using it in clinical practice from 1985 onwards.

The Royal East Sussex Hospital, UK, was the first to purchase the LMA and, in 1988, anesthesiologists working there published a favorable preliminary report about its use in 150 patients[33]. Soon the new device had tapped into a vast unrecognized market for a noninvasive airway which avoided the hazards of intubation, yet provided 'hands free' anesthesia. Within 12 months over 500 other hospitals were using the LMA and, by Autumn 1990, all UK hospitals with operating rooms had purchased them[26]. By 1991 it had been used in over 2 million patients in the UK[32]. Much of the success of the LMA has been attributed to the widespread availability of propofol and the development of the silicone cuff[34]. A handful of individuals also played a critical role in its success. The LMA would probably never have become a commercial reality without the vision and energy of entrepreneur Robert Gaines-Cooper. He recognized the potential of the device, and not only provided the venture capital to take it from prototype to finished product, but went on to build up a worldwide distribution network, establishing manufacturing bases around the world. Professor John Nunn (UK) was the first influential anesthesiologist to investigate the LMA and recognize its potential. Professor Andranic Ovassapian (USA) was one of the first to appreciate its potential in failed intubation, and Professor Jonathan Benumof (USA) also helped establish the LMA as a tool for difficult airway management by including it in the American Society of Anesthesiologists' algorithm[35,36]. Professor Paul White (USA) and his team have provided useful data supporting its value as an airway tool in routine anesthesia[34,37–41].

In 1989, the first independent assessment of the LMA was made by Brodrick et al who obtained a clear and unobstructed airway in 98/100 patients[42]. They described the LMA as the 'missing link' between the face mask and tracheal tube, and confirmed that the device had three outstanding features: excellent airway patency; no manual support of jaw required; good for transfer to the post anesthesia care unit. In the same year, Tate described the LMA as 'possibly the greatest advance in airway maintenance since Magill introduced the tracheal tube'[43].

Not all early publications were favorable. Using a fiberoptic scope, Payne noted that the esophagus was visible on 6% of occasions (now recognized as a malposition – see Chapter 6: *Malposition*), confirming that the LMA did not isolate the gastrointestinal tract from the respiratory tract[44]. In a cluster of letters entitled 'The laryngeal mask: cautionary tales', Wilkinson reported a case of stridor; Cyna and MacLeod reported eight cases of regurgitation out of 546 'fasted' patients including two cases of aspiration; and Campbell, Criswell and John also reported cases of aspiration[45]. Brain was quick to emphasize that problems could be avoided if patients were appropriately selected and the recommended insertion techniques adhered to[46]. Practitioners were also reminded that the LMA was best thought of as a new technique of administering anesthesia rather than simply as a new device; use of the LMA is an art that must be acquired before it can be directly amenable to criticism.

News of the LMA rapidly spread outside the UK. British trainee anesthesiologists working overseas and visitors to the UK helped to disseminate 'hands on' information about the LMA prior to its formal release in other countries. Between 1989 and 1990, preliminary reports about the LMA appeared in journals from Malaysia[47], Singapore[48], Scandinavia[49], France[50], Japan[51,52], Norway[53] and Canada[54] as did the first studies reporting its successful use in children[55]. The first Australian[56], German[57] Dutch[58] and Brazilian[59] papers were published in 1991, the first Spanish[60] and Korean papers in 1992[61], the first Italian papers in 1995[62], and the first Russian papers in 1996[63,64]. The LMA was approved for use in the USA in August 1991. Since then the three major US anesthetic journals (*Anesthesiology*, *Anesthesia and Analgesia*, and *Journal of Clinical Anesthesia*) have published 217 articles on the LMA.

Current status

Over the last 8 years, the LMA has gained widespread acceptance in the UK as a general purpose airway for routine anesthesia where usage rates are in the range of

30–60% of all anesthesias given[65–67]. The Conquest Hospital in the UK where the device was first sold report usage rates of 75%[68]. Day surgery units in the USA have recently reported LMA usage rates of 28%, with the tracheal tube 52% and the face mask 20%[69]. Several advanced uses have emerged, aided by the development of the flexible LMA (Table 1.2). It has been the subject of numerous reviews[26,34,36,70–107] and editorials[32,108–123]. Published data from large studies and reports (>1000 patients) have confirmed the safety and efficacy of the device for spontaneous and controlled ventilation during routine use[66,72,124–134] (Table 1.3). Prospective randomized studies

Table 1.2 Advanced uses of the LMA

Patients and clinical situations	*Techniques*	*Surgery*
Infants[137]	Endoscopy[138]	Ear and nose surgery[89]
Obesity[129]	Prolonged procedures[139]	Oral/dental surgery[79]
Respiratory disease[140]	Non-supine positions[141]	Adenotonsillectomy[142]
Oropharyngeal pathology[143]	Awake insertion[144]	Laser surgery[145]
Laryngotracheal pathology[146]	Drug dispersal[147,148]	Major head/neck surgery[149]
Non-fasted[150]	Airway exchange[151]	Carotid endarterectomy[152]
Burns[153]		Tracheostomy[154]
Difficult airway[87]		Microlaryngeal surgery[26]
Intensive care[80]		Tracheal/carinal surgery[155]
		Thyroid/parathyroid/thymic surgery[156]
		Ophthalmic surgery[133]
		Remote and repeat anesthesia[127]
		Gynecological laparoscopy[157]
		Lower abdominal surgery[66,158]
		Upper abdominal surgery[159]
		Cardiothoracic surgery[160]
		Minimally invasive neurosurgery[161]
		Major neurosurgery[151]
		Electroencephalographic mapping[162]
		Bronchoscopy[144]

Table 1.3 Large-scale data

Authors	*Year*	*Patients*
Leach and Alexander[72]	1991	7000
Brain[124,125]	1991	8500
Haden et al[126]	1993	5655
Moylan and Luce[127]	1993	2500
Langer et al[128]	1993	1925
Verghese et al[129]	1993	2359
Van Damme[130]	1994	5000
Braun and Fritz[131]	1994	3000
Wainwright[133]	1995	1879
Brimacombe[132]	1995	1500
Verghese and Brimacombe[66]	1995	11 910
Lopez-Gil et al[134]	1996	1400

from peer review journals (n = 52) have demonstrated that the LMA is superior to the tracheal tube and face mask in some areas of airway management, although outcome studies are currently lacking[135]. It also has a role in the management of difficult intubation, both as a substitute airway and as an aid to intubation[87]. It has been included in the American Society of Anesthesiologists' algorithm for management of the difficult airway[35,36]. To date, the LMA has been the subject of over 1000 publications and been used in more than 30 million anesthetized patients (manufacturers estimate) in at least 80 countries[110]. No fatalities have been reported to the manufacturer resulting from its use for more than 6 years[68]. It has been estimated that there are approximately 600 deaths a year from use of the tracheal tube[136].

Literature statistics and limitations

The volume of literature on the LMA has grown rapidly and currently represents a significant proportion of clinical anesthesia research worldwide. Most issues of most anesthesia journals over the last 4 years have published work or commentary on the LMA. Two journals (*European Journal of Anaesthesiology* and *Minerva Anestesiologia*) have devoted entire supplements to the LMA. At the 11th World Congress of Anaesthesiology in Sydney in 1996, 1.2% (24/2000) of all papers concerned the LMA[163]. By the end of 1995 there were 1072 publications comprising: 202 papers, 168 abstracts, 51 mini-papers (letters containing study data), 80 full case reports, 118 case reports as letters to the editor, 335 other letters, 38 reviews, 15 editorials and 65 other publications, including coincidental use of the LMA in other studies, articles and manuals (Table 1.4). Of the 202 LMA papers, over 75% have been published in peer review journals. In the first half of 1996 there were over 140 LMA publications.

Several criticisms have been levelled at the LMA literature[34,88,120]. Firstly, it has been suggested that the literature is dominated by anecdotal case reports and letters to the editor. Secondly, that there are insufficient large-scale studies demonstrating safety and efficacy. Thirdly, that there is a lack of randomized prospective trials in peer review journals demonstrating any advantages over the face mask or tracheal tube. Finally, it is clear that the scientific appraisal of the LMA is complicated by the existence of a

Table 1.4 Analysis of LMA literature

	1983	*1984*	*1985*	*1986*	*1987*	*1988*	*1989*	*1990*	*1991*	*1992*	*1993*	*1994*	*1995*	*Total*
Papers	1	0	1	0	0	0	5	11	24	38	37	43	42	202
Abstracts	0	0	0	0	0	1	2	3	12	36	43	35	36	168
Mini-papers (letters)	0	0	0	0	0	1	0	5	8	13	10	3	11	51
Case reports	0	1	1	0	0	1	3	5	14	14	16	6	19	80
Case reports (letters)	0	0	0	0	0	0	4	13	14	26	25	23	13	118
Other letters	0	1	0	1	0	1	15	16	33	41	78	101	48	335
Reviews	0	0	0	0	0	0	0	0	1	6	13	3	15	38
Editorials	0	0	0	0	0	0	0	0	0	2	7	5	1	15
Others	0	0	0	1	1	0	2	2	3	4	19	4	29	65
Total	1	2	2	2	1	4	31	55	109	180	248	223	214	1072

learning curve extending well beyond the experience level of many of those taking part in controlled trials designed to evaluate the device[46,132].

References

1 Drummond GB. Influence of thiopentone on upper airway muscles. *Br J Anaesth* 1989;**63**:12–21.

2 Fouke JM, Strohl KP. Effect of position and lung volume on upper airway geometry. *J Appl Physiol* 1987;**63**:375–380.

3 Marsh AM, Nunn JF, Taylor SJ, Charlesworth CH. Airway obstruction associated with the use of the Guedel airway. *Br J Anaesth* 1991;**67**:517–523.

4 Joh SJ, Matsura H, Kotani Y, et al. Change in tracheal blood flow during endotracheal intubation. *Acta Anaesthesiol Scand* 1987;**31**:300–304.

5 Seegobin RD, van Hasselt GL. Endotracheal cuff pressure and tracheal mucosal blood flow: endoscopic study of effects of four large volume cuffs. *Br Med J* 1984;**288**:965–968.

6 Harmer M. Complications of tracheal intubation. In: Latto IP, Rosen M, eds. *Difficulties in tracheal intubation.* London: Baillière Tindall, 1987;36–48.

7 Rose DK, Cohen MM. The airway: problems and predictions in 18,500 patients. *Can J Anaesth* 1994;**41**:372–383.

8 Caplan RA, Posner KL, Ward RJ, Cheney FW. Adverse respiratory events in anesthesia: a closed claims analysis. *Anesthesiology* 1990;**72**:828–833.

9 Northrup WP. Apparatus for prolonged artificial forcible respiration. *Br Med J* 1894;697.

10 Hewitt F. Clinical observations upon respiration during anaesthesia. *Proc Roy Med Chirurg Soc* 1891;**3**:31–38.

11 Guedel AE. A nontraumatic pharyngeal airway. *J Am Med Assoc* 1933;**100**:1862.

12 Shipway F. Airway for intranasal operations. *Br Med J* 1935;767.

13 Leech BC. The pharyngeal bulb gasway: a new aid in cyclopropane anesthesia. *Anesth Analg* 1937;**16**:22–25.

14 Fink BR. Roentgen ray studies of airway problems. I. The oropharyngeal airway. *Anesthesiology* 1957;**18**:162–163.

15 Baskett PJF. The laryngeal mask in resuscitation. *11th World Congress of Anesthesiology, Sydney, 14–20 April 1996, Abstract Handbook* p.530 (Abstract).

16 Mehta S. A supraglottic oropharyngeal airway. *Anaesthesia* 1990;**45**:893–894.

17 Greenberg RS, Toung T. The cuffed oro-pharyngeal airway – a pilot study. *Anesthesiology* 1992;**77**:A558 (Abstract).

18 Greenberg RS, Kay NH. Evaluation of the cuffed oropharngeal airway (COPA) in outpatients. *11th World Congress of Anesthesiology, Sydney, 14–20 April 1996, Abstract Handbook* p.477 (Abstract).

19 Greenberg RS, Chapolini RJ. Radiologic evaluation of the cuffed oropharyngeal airway (COPA) in adult cadavers. *11th World Congress of Anesthesiology, Sydney, 14–20 April 1996, Abstract Handbook* p.617 (Abstract).

20 Greenberg RS, Kay NH. Propofol dose required for placement of the cuffed oropharyngeal airway (COPA) in outpatients. *11th World Congress of Anesthesiology, Sydney, 14–20 April 1996, Abstract Handbook* p.617 (Abstract).

21 Greenberg RS, Kay NH. Indicators of 'best fit' cuffed oropharyngeal airway (COPA) size in adults. *11th World Congress of Anesthesiology, Sydney, 14–20 April 1996, Abstract Handbook* p.618 (Abstract).

22 Berry A, Brimacombe J. An evaluation of the cuffed oropharyngeal airway (COPA). *Combined Scientific Meeting ANZCA and ASA, Perth, 26–30 October,* p.104 (Abstract).

★ 23 McIntyre JWR. History of anaesthesia: oropharyngeal and nasopharyngeal airways: I (1880–1995). *Can J Anaesth* 1996;**43**:629–635.
Historical review showing that the multiple objectives of the LMA had not been described collectively at the time of Hewitt's presentation on the oropharyngeal airway in 1908 and were largely neglected until the present time. Suggests that for supraglottic airway management four types of airway should be available: a Guedel airway, a nasopharyngeal airway, a laryngeal mask airway and an airway specifically to facilitate blind tracheal intubation.

24 Burwell DR, Jones JG. The airways and anaesthesia I. Anatomy, physiology and fluid mechanics. *Anaesthesia* 1996;**51**:849–857.

25 Burwell DR, Jones JG. The airways and anaesthesia II. Pathophysiology. *Anaesthesia* 1996;**51**:943–954.

★ 26 Brain AIJ. The development of the laryngeal mask – a brief history of the invention, early clinical studies and experimental work from which the laryngeal mask evolved. *Eur J Anaesthesiol* 1991;**4**:5–17.
The most comprehensive account of the history and development of the LMA from conception to commercial release and beyond. It includes the results of an unpublished trial in which the LMA was used with the new induction agent propofol and describes the evolution of the insertion technique.

★ 27 Brain AIJ. The laryngeal mask – a new concept in airway management. *Br J Anaesth* 1983;**55**:801–805.
The first and most frequently cited paper on the laryngeal mask airway. Brain describes the successful use of a

prototype made from a Goldman dental nasal mask attached to a tracheal tube with acrylic glue. The prototype was used in 23 patients, 16 of whom underwent gynecological laparoscopy.

★ **28** Brain AI, McGhee TD, McAteer EJ, Thomas A, Abu Saad MA, Bushman JA. The laryngeal mask airway. Development and preliminary trials of a new type of airway. *Anaesthesia* 1985;**40**:356–361.
The second paper describing the further development of the LMA and 18 months of clinical experience. The LMA was used successfully in 118 patients, 17 of whom underwent controlled ventilation. It was used in place of a face mask for routine anesthesia, and was of particular value in ophthalmic, dental, ENT and where difficulties with the airway were expected. The incidence of sore throat was low. This paper also describes the use of an introducer tool that was subsequently abandoned.

29 Sant'Ambrogio G, Mathew OP, Fisher JT, Sant'Ambrogio FB. Laryngeal receptors responding to transmural pressure, airflow and local muscle activity. *Resp Physiol* 1983;**54**:317–330.

30 Benumof JL. The laryngeal mask airway and the ASA algorithm. *Anesthesiol News* 1996;4–56.

31 Ralph SJ, Wareham CA. Rupture of the oesophagus during cricoid pressure. *Anaesthesia* 1991;**46**:40–41.

32 White DC. The laryngeal mask – a non-invasive airway. *Eur J Anaesthesiol* 1991;**4**:1–4.

33 Alexander CA, Leach AB, Thompson AR, Lister JB. Use your Brain! *Anaesthesia* 1988;**43**:893–894.

34 Pennant JH, White PF. The laryngeal mask airway. Its uses in anesthesiology. *Anesthesiology* 1993;**79**:144–163.

35 Practice Guidelines for Management of the Difficult Airway – a Report by the American Society of Anesthesiologists Task Force on Management of the Difficult Airway. *Anesthesiology* 1993;**78**:597–602.

36 Benumof J. The laryngeal mask airway and the ASA difficult airway algorithm. *Anesthesiology* 1996;**84**:686–699.

37 Watcha MF, White PF, Tychsen L, Steven JL. Comparative effects of laryngeal mask airway and endotracheal tube insertion on intraocular pressure in children. *Anesth Analg* 1992;**75**:355–360.

38 Smith I, White PF. Use of the laryngeal mask airway as an alternative to a face mask during outpatient arthroscopy. *Anesthesiology* 1992;**77**:850–855.

39 Watcha MF, Garner FT, White PF, Lusk R. Laryngeal mask airway vs face mask and Guedel airway during pediatric myringotomy. *Arch Otolaryngol Head Neck Surg* 1994;**120**:877–880.

40 Pace NA, Gajraj NM, Pennant JH, Victory RA, Johnson ER, White PF. Use of the laryngeal mask airway after oesophageal intubation. *Br J Anaesth* 1994;**73**:688–689.

41 Joshi GP, Morrison SG, Okonkwo NA, White PF. Continuous hypopharyngeal pH measurements in spontaneously breathing anesthetised outpatients: laryngeal mask airway versus tracheal intubation. *Anesth Analg* 1996;**82**:254–257.

★ **42** Brodrick PM, Webster NR, Nunn JF. The laryngeal mask airway. A study of 100 patients during spontaneous breathing. *Anaesthesia* 1989;**44**:238–241.
The first independent paper in which the LMA was used in 100 patients by 18 anesthesiologists with no previous experience in its use. A clear and unobstructed airway was obtained in 98% without the need for jaw support, thus leaving the anesthesiologist's hands entirely free. The seal was adequate for controlled ventilation with a leak pressure of 17 kPa. Three major advantages were noted: excellent airway patency, no manual support of jaw and good for transfer to recovery. The LMA was described as the 'missing link' between the face mask and tracheal tube.

43 Tate N. Laryngeal mask airway. *Today's Anaesthetist* 1989;**4**:63–64.

44 Payne J. The use of the fibreoptic laryngoscope to confirm the position of the laryngeal mask. *Anaesthesia* 1989;**44**:465.

45 Wilkinson PA, Cyna AM, MacLeod DM, Campbell JR, Criswell J, John R. The laryngeal mask: cautionary tales. *Anaesthesia* 1990;**45**:167–168.

46 Brain AIJ. Studies on the laryngeal mask: first, learn the art. *Anaesthesia* 1991;**46**:417–427.

47 Miranda AF, Reddy SVG. Controlled ventilation with Brain laryngeal mask. *Med J Malaysia* 1991;**45**:65–69.

48 Reddy SVG, Win N. Brain laryngeal mask – study in 50 spontaneously breathing patients. *Sing Med J* 1990;**31**:338–340.

49 Sarma VJ. The use of a laryngeal mask airway in spontaneously breathing patients. *Acta Anaesthesiol Scand* 1990;**34**:669–672.

50 Poltronieri J. [The laryngeal mask]. *Ann Fr Anesth Reanim* 1990;**9**:362–366.

51 Yasuda I, Amaha K, Irimada M, Hirano T, Sasaki I. [Clinical application of laryngeal mask airway]. *Jpn J Anaesth* 1989;**38**:1641–1646.

52 Amaha K, Yasuda I, Makita K, Toyooka H. Laryngeal mask – a newly designed oral airway. *Jpn J Anaesth* 1989;**38**:1383–1386.

53 Brattebo G, Wisborg T, Rodt SA. [The laryngeal mask: a new tool for creating a free airway]. *Nord Med* 1991;**106**:109–111.

54 Maltby JR, Loken RG, Watson NC. The laryngeal mask airway: clinical appraisal in 250 patients. *Can J Anaesth* 1990;**37**:509–513.

55 Mason DG, Bingham RM. The laryngeal mask airway in children. *Anaesthesia* 1990;**45**:760–763.

56 McCrirrick A, Ramage DT, Pracilio JA, Hickman JA. Experience with the laryngeal mask airway in two hundred patients. *Anaesth Intens Care* 1991;**19**:256–260.

57 Hensel M, Stober HD. Erfahrungen mit der Kehlkopfmaske. *Anasthesiol Intensivmed* 1991;**12**:339–342.

58 Slappendel R, Harbers JBM, ten Have FTM, Moll JE. Eerste ervaringen met het larynxmasker. *Nederlands Tijdschrift Anaesth* 1991;**May**:16–20.

59 Oliveira, I, Poterio GMB, Schiavuzzo JM, Valejo MA. Mascara laringea: nova opcao em anestesia inhalatoria? *Rev Brasil Anestesiol* 1991;**41**:CBA 5

60 Vaca JM, Cabal JV, Camarero EJ, Vega A. La masca laringea. *Rev Esp Anestesiol Reanim* 1992;**39**:28–33.

61 Jae-Hun Jeong, Hong-Seuk Yang, Hyung-Sang Cho. Clinical investigation of the laryngeal mask airway. *J Kor Soc Anesthesiol* 1992;**25**:708–718.

62 Cristalli A, Rezzani S. La maschera laringea in chirurgia generale. *Minerva Anestesiol* 1995;**61**:23–27.

63 Smirnova V, Lickvantsev V, Sitnikov V, Vinogradov V. Low flow anaesthesia with laryngeal mask. *11th World Congress of Anesthesiology, Sydney, 14–20 April 1996, Abstract Handbook* p.406 (Abstract).

64 Mizikov V, Variuschina T, Esakov I. The laryngeal mask in paediatric anaesthesia: the first experience in Russia. *11th World Congress of Anesthesiology, Sydney, 14–20 April 1996, Abstract Handbook* p.465 (Abstract).

65 Alexander CA, Leach AB. The laryngeal mask – experience of its use in a District General Hospital. *Today's Anaesthetist* 1989;**4**:200–205.

66 Verghese C, Brimacombe J. Survey of laryngeal mask usage in 11 910 patients – safety and efficacy for conventional and nonconventional usage. *Anesth Analg* 1996;**82**:129–133.

67 Dingley J, Asai T. Insertion methods of the laryngeal mask airway. A survey of current practice in Wales. *Anaesthesia* 1996;**51**:596–599.

68 Brain AIJ. Use of the laryngeal mask airway (LMA) in general anaesthesia. *Minerva Anestesiol* 1996;**61**:9–11.

69 Wat LI, Templin PA, Lynch ME, Hammamura RK, White PF. Use of the laryngeal mask airway for ambulatory anesthesia: utilization, longevity and cost. *American Society of Anesthesiologists' Annual General Meeting, New Orleans, October 1996* (Abstract).

70 McEwan AI, Mason DG. The laryngeal mask airway. *J Clin Anesth* 1992;**4**:252–257.

71 Haynes SR, Morton NS. The laryngeal mask airway: a review of its use in paediatric anaesthesia. *Paediatr Anaesth* 1993;**3**:65–73.

72 Leach AB, Alexander CA. The laryngeal mask – an overview. *Eur J Anaesthesiol* 1991;**4**:19–31.

73 Brimacombe J, Shorney N. The laryngeal mask airway. *Br J Hosp Med* 1992;**47**:252–256.

74 Brimacombe J, Shorney N. The laryngeal mask airway – a review and update. In: Kaufman L, ed. *Anaesthesia review 10*. London: Churchill Livingstone, 1993;183–202.

75 Brimacombe J. AANA Journal Course: Update for nurse anesthetist – part IV. The laryngeal mask airway: a review for the nurse anesthetist. *Am Assoc Nurse Anesthet J* 1992;**60**:490–499.

76 Brimacombe J. The laryngeal mask airway: tool for airway management. *J Post Anaesth Nurs* 1993;**8**:88–95.

77 Janssens M, Lamy M. Laryngeal mask. *Intens Care World* 1993;**10**:99–102.

78 Wedekind LV, Krier C. Kehlkopfmaske – Eine Ubersicht 1983–1993. *Anaesthesiol Intensivmed Notfalmed Schmerzther* 1993;**28**:137–147.

79 Brimacombe J, Berry A. The laryngeal mask airway for dental surgery – a review. *Aust Dent J* 1995;**40**:10–14.

80 Brimacombe J, Berry A, Verghese C. The laryngeal mask airway in critical care medicine. *Intens Care Med* 1995;**21**:361–364.

81 Yasumoto K. Laryngeal mask airway: A new method of airway management. *J Clin Exp Med* 1992;**12**:865–868.

82 Doyle DJ. Clinical applications of the laryngeal mask airway. *Contemporary Anaesth* 1993;**4**:8–15.

83 McGoldrick KE. The laryngeal mask airway. *Day Surg Patient* 1993;**2**:1–5.

84 Smith I, Joshi G. The laryngeal mask airway for outpatient anesthesia. *J Clin Anesth* 1993;**5**:22S–28S.

85 Brimacombe J. The laryngeal mask airway for neonatal resuscitation. *Neonatal Intens Care* 1994;**7**:14–17.

86 Brimacombe J, Berry A. The laryngeal mask airway for obstetric anaesthesia and neonatal resuscitation. *Int J Obstet Anesth* 1994;**3**:211–218.

87 Brimacombe J, Berry A, Brain A. The laryngeal mask airway. In: Sandler AN, Doyle DJ, eds. *The difficult airway I*. Philadelphia: WB Saunders, 1995;411–437.

88 Asai T, Morris S. The laryngeal mask airway: its features, effects and role. *Can J Anaesth* 1994;**41**:930–960.

89 Brimacombe J, Berry A. Use of the laryngeal mask airway in otolaryngology. *J Otolaryngol* 1995;**24**:125–133.

90 Brimacombe J. Emergency airway management in rural practice: use of the laryngeal mask airway. *Aust J Rural Hlth* 1995;**3**:10–19.

91 Brimacombe J, Berry A. The laryngeal mask airway – anatomical and physiological implications. *Acta Anaesthesiol Scand* 1996;**40**:201–209.

92 Springer DK, Jahr JS. The laryngeal mask airway – safety, efficacy and current use. *Am J Anesthesiol* 1995;**2**:65–69.

93 Brimacombe J, Brain AIJ. The laryngeal mask airway. *Curr Opin Anaesthesiol* 1995;**8**:478–484.

94 Brimacombe J, Berry A, Daves S. The laryngeal mask airway. In: Hanowell L, Waldron R, eds. *Principles of airway management*. Philadelphia: Lippincott – Raven, 1996;195–212.

95 Raphael JH, Langton JA. Uses and abuses of the laryngeal mask airway. *Curr Anaesth Crit Care* 1995;**6**:250–254.

96 Lorenzini C. Mascara laringea. *Anestesia em Revista – Soc Brazil Anestesiol* 1995;**44**:17–18.

97 Lorenzini C. Mascara laringea – uno novo conceito na manutencao da via aerea. *Atual Anestesiol* 1994;**3**:9–12.
98 Brain AIJ. The laryngeal mask airway. *Aether* 1995;**1**:7–10.
99 Cortes J, Franco A, Bouzada M, Cortinas J, Pedraza I, Alvarez J. La mascarilla laringea. *Actual Anesthesiol Reanim* 1995;**5**:21–28.
100 Brimacombe J, Berry A, Brain AIJ, Verghese C. The laryngeal mask airway. *Anaesth Rev 13* (in press).
101 Brimacombe J, Gandini D. The laryngeal mask airway – potential applications in perinatal medicine. *J Obstet Gynecol Neonatal Nurs* (in press).
102 McGoldrick KE. The laryngeal mask airway: an overview. *Surv Anesthesiol* 1995;**39**:203–207.
103 Ruby RRF, Webster AC, Morley-Forster PK, Dain S. Laryngeal mask airway in paediatric otolaryngologic surgery. *J Otolaryngol* 1996;**24**:288–291.
104 Longo S. Mascara Laringea. *Rev Argentina Anesth* 1996;**54**:91–93.
105 Brimacombe J, Costa e Silva L. The laryngeal mask airway – a review. *Portugese J Anaesth* (in press).
106 Brimacombe J, Costa e Silva L. The laryngeal mask airway – practical considerations for anaesthesia. *Rev Brasil Anestesiol* 1997;**47**:48–60.
107 Brimacombe J, Loudianov M, Campbell RCH. The laryngeal mask airway – a new concept in airway management. *Russ J Anaesth* (in press).
108 Laryngeal mask airway. *Lancet* 1991;**338**:1046–1047.
109 Fisher JA, Ananthanarayan C, Edelist G. Role of the laryngeal mask in airway management. *Can J Anaesth* 1992;**39**:1–3.
110 Brimacombe J, Berry A. The laryngeal mask airway – the first ten years. *Anaesth Intens Care* 1993;**21**:225–226.
111 O'Meara ME, Jones JG. The laryngeal mask – useful for spontaneous breathing, controlled ventilation, and difficult intubations. *Br Med J* 1993;**306**:224–225.
112 Benumof JL. Laryngeal mask airway – indications and contraindications. *Anesthesiology* 1992;**77**:843–846.
113 Wilson IG. The laryngeal mask airway in paediatric practice. *Br J Anaesth* 1993;**70**:124–125.
114 Ward ME. A new look at the breath of life. *Br J Anaesth* 1993;**69**:339–340.
115 Brain AIJ. Einsatz der Kehlkopfmaske in England. *Anaesthesiol Intensivmed Notfalmed Schmerzther* 1993;**28**:135–136.
116 Schulte am Esch J. Die Kehlkopfmaske – Ein weiteres Konzept zur Atemwegssicherung. *Anaesthesiol Intensivmed Notfalmed Schmerzther* 1993;**28**:133–134.
117 Asai T, Vaughan RS. Misuse of the laryngeal mask airway. *Anaesthesia* 1994;**49**:467–469.
118 Robotham JL. Neonatal resuscitation using the laryngeal mask airway. *Anesthesiology* 1994;**80**:27A
119 Krier C, Hempel V. Kehlkopfmaske. *Anaesthesiol Intensivmed Notfalmed Schmerzther* 1994;**29**:282–283.
120 Maltby JR. The laryngeal mask airway in anaesthesia. *Can J Anaesth* 1994;**41**:888–893.
121 Schulte am Esch J. New challenges require adaptation of anaesthetic management. *Curr Opinion Anaesthesiol* 1995;**8**:475–477.
122 Curry P. The laryngeal mask in pre-hospital care. *J Br Assoc Immediate Care* 1994;**17**:55–57.
123 Nair I, Bailey PM. Review of uses of the laryngeal mask in ENT anaesthesia. *Anaesthesia* 1995;**50**:898–900.
124 Brain AIJ. The laryngeal mask and the oesophagus. *Anaesthesia* 1991;**46**:701–702.
125 Lee JJ, Brain AIJ. Laryngeal mask and trauma to uvula. *Anaesthesia* 1989;**44**:1014–1015.
126 Haden RM, Pinnock CA, Campbell RL. The laryngeal mask for intraocular surgery. *Br J Anaesth* 1993;**71**:772
127 Moylan SL, Luce MA. The reinforced laryngeal mask airway in paediatric radiotherapy. *Br J Anaesth* 1993;**71**:172
128 Langer A, Hempel V, Ahlhelm T, Heipertz W. Die Kehlkopfmaske bei > 1900 Allgemeinanasthesien – Erfahrungsbericht. *Anaesthesiol Intensivmed Notfalmed Schmerzther* 1993;**28**:156–160.
129 Verghese C, Smith TGC, Young E. Prospective survey of the use of the laryngeal mask airway in 2359 patients. *Anaesthesia* 1993;**48**:58–60.
130 Van Damme E. Die Kehlopfmaske in der ambulanten Anasthesie – Eine Auswertung von 5000 ambulanten Narkosen. *Anaesthesiol Intensivmed Notfalmed Schmerzther* 1994;**29**:284–286.
131 Braun U, Fritz U. Die Kehlopfmaske in der Kinderanasthesie. *Anaesthesiol Intensivmed Notfalmed Schmerzther* 1994;**29**:286–288.
132 Brimacombe J. Analysis of 1500 laryngeal mask uses by one anaesthetist in adults undergoing routine anaesthesia. *Anaesthesia* 1996;**51**:76–80.
133 Wainwright AC. Positive pressure ventilation and the laryngeal mask airway in ophthalmic anaesthesia. *Br J Anaesth* 1995;**75**:249–250.
134 Lopez-Gil M, Brimacombe J, Alvarez M. Safety and efficacy of the laryngeal mask airway – a prospective survey of 1400 paediatric patients. *Anaesthesia* 1996;**51**:969–972.
135 Brimacombe J. The advantages of the LMA over the tracheal tube or facemask: a meta-analysis. *Can J Anaesth* 1995;**42**:1017–1023.
136 Bellhouse CP, Dore C. Criteria for estimating likelihood of difficulty of endotracheal intubation with the Macintosh laryngoscope. *Anaesth Intens Care* 1988;**16**:329–337.

137 Mizushima A, Wardall GJ, Simpson DL. The laryngeal mask airway in infants. *Anaesthesia* 1992;**47**:849–851.

138 Brimacombe J. The laryngeal mask airway for access to the upper gastrointestinal tract. *Anesthesiology* 1996;**84**:1009–1010.

139 Brimacombe J, Archdeacon J. The laryngeal mask airway for unplanned prolonged procedures. *Can J Anaesth* 1995;**42**:1176

140 Ferrari LR, Goudsouzian NG. The use of the laryngeal mask airway in children with bronchopulmonary dysplasia. *Anesth Analg* 1995;**81**:310–313.

141 Chen CH, Lin CC, Tan PP. [Clinical experience of laryngeal mask airway in lateral position during anesthesia]. *Acta Anaesthesiol Sin* 1995;**33**:31–34.

142 Williams PJ, Bailey PM. Comparison of the reinforced laryngeal mask airway and tracheal intubation for adenotonsillectomy. *Br J Anaesth* 1993;**70**:30–33.

143 Brimacombe J, Berry A, van Duren P. Use of a size 2 laryngeal mask airway to relieve life threatening hypoxia in an adult with quinsy. *Anaesth Intens Care* 1993;**21**:475–476.

144 Brimacombe J, Tucker P, Simons S. The laryngeal mask airway for awake diagnostic bronchoscopy – a study of 200 consecutive patients. *Eur J Anaesthesiol* 1995;**12**:357–361.

145 Sher M, Brimacombe J, Laing D. Anaesthesia for laser pharyngoplasty – a comparison of the tracheal tube versus reinforced laryngeal mask airway. *Anaesth Intens Care* 1995;**23**:149–154.

146 Smith TGC, Whittet H, Heyworth T. Laryngomalacia – a specific indication for the laryngeal mask. *Anaesthesia* 1992;**47**:910.

147 Spain BT, Riley RH. Salbutamol via the laryngeal mask airway for relief of bronchospasm. *Anaesthesia* 1992;**47**:1107.

148 Albertsen P, Eschen C, Verder H. Laryngeal mask used as a guideway for brief access to the intratracheal space in premature infants. *8th International Workshop on Surfactant Replacement, Oslo, 20–22 May 1993* (Abstract).

149 Kalapac S, Donald S, Brimacombe J. Laryngeal mask biopsy! *Anaesth Intens Care* 1996;**24**:283.

150 Asai T. Use of the laryngeal mask for tracheal intubation in patients at increased risk of aspiration of gastric contents. *Anesthesiology* 1992;**77**:1029–1030.

151 Costa e Silva L, Brimacombe J. Tracheal tube/laryngeal mask exchange for emergence. *Anesthesiology* 1996;**85**:218.

152 Costa e Silva L, Brimacombe J. The laryngeal mask for carotid endarterectomy. *J Cardiothoracic and Vascular Anesth* 1996;**10**:972–973.

153 Russell R, Judkins KC. The laryngeal mask airway and facial burns. *Anaesthesia* 1990;**45**:894.

154 Thomson KD. Laryngeal mask airway for elective tracheostomy. *Anaesthesia* 1992;**47**:76.

155 Slinger P, Robinson R, Shennib H, Benumof JL, Eisenkraft JB. Alternative technique for laser resection of a carinal obstruction. *J Cardiothoracic Anesth* 1992;**6**:749–755.

156 Hobbiger HE, Allen JG, Greatorex RG, Denny NM. The laryngeal mask airway for thyroid and parathyroid surgery. *Anaesthesia* 1996;**51**:972–974.

157 Brimacombe J, Berry A. Airway management during gynaecological laparoscopy – is it safe to use the laryngeal mask airway? *Ambulatory Surg* 1995;**3**:65–70.

158 Brimacombe J. The laryngeal mask airway for abdominal surgery. *J Clin Exp Med* 1994;**171**:949–951.

159 Brimacombe J. Airway protection with the new laryngeal mask prototype. *Anaesthesia* 1996;**51**:602–603.

160 Llagunes J, Rodriguez-Hesles C, Aguar F. Laryngeal mask airway in cardiac surgery. *Can J Anaesth* 1994;**41**:1016.

161 Costa e Silva L, Brimacombe J. The laryngeal mask airway for stereotactic implantation of fetal hypophysis. *Anesth Analg* 1996;**82**:430–431.

162 Ammar T, Towey RM. The laryngeal mask airway. *Anaesthesia* 1990;**45**:75.

163 *Abstract Book. 11th World Congress of Anaesthesiologists, 14–20 April 1996, Sydney, Australia.*

2 Anatomical implications

Anatomy

Anatomical structures relevant to LMA placement include the mouth, oropharynx, laryngopharynx and hypopharynx.

Mouth

The roof of the mouth is formed by the vaulted palate comprising the bony hard palate (anterior 2/3) and the soft palate (posterior 1/3). The general shape of the hard palate is such that a food bolus is directed into the oropharyngeal inlet with the stiffened soft palate shielding the nasopharynx. The precise shape of the hard palate is highly variable and this may account for some difficulty in passing the LMA into the oropharynx, particularly if the angle of approach between the hard palate and posterior oropharyngeal wall is less than 90 degrees[1]. The general size and shape of the tongue has little bearing on LMA placement since the tongue is an anterior structure and LMA placement follows a posterior path[2]. Mouth opening is essential for LMA placement. The average distance between the upper and lower incisor teeth in adult patients with normal temporomandibular joint function is 47 mm with a range of 31–55 mm[3]. It is possible to insert the LMA with an incisal opening of 12 mm[4].

Oropharynx

To enter the laryngopharynx the LMA passes through the oropharynx. This is bounded anteriorly by the palatoglossal arch and the tongue. Immediately posterior to the tongue is the epiglottis, a leaf-shaped plate of elastic cartilage covered with mucous membrane. The median glosso-epiglottic fold runs between the front of the epiglottis and the back of the tongue and on each side are lateral depressions, the epiglottic valleculae. The palatine tonsils lie in the lateral walls of the oropharynx and if grossly enlarged may impede passage of the LMA[5,6]. The posterior part of the oropharynx is bounded by the anterior aspect of the cervical vertebrae covered in muscle and mucosa.

Laryngopharynx and hypopharynx

The posterior and lateral walls of the laryngopharynx are bounded by the inferior and middle constrictor muscles which taper rapidly towards the esophagus. The anterior wall is formed by the inlet of the larynx superiorly and the pyriform fossae, the inter-arytenoid muscles, the posterior cricopharyngeus muscles and the attachments of the longitudinal muscles of the esophagus. The hypopharynx is the space behind the arytenoid and cricoid cartilages. It is approximately 3.5 cm in length. The superior 1.5 cm lies behind the arytenoid cartilages and the inferior 2 cm lies behind the cricoid cartilage[7].

Neurovascular considerations

Several nerves and blood vessels within the tissues of the oropharynx may theoretically be compressed by a malpositioned and/or overinflated laryngeal mask. Examples are the lingual artery as it enters the base of the tongue; the glossopharyngeal nerve as it passes between the superior and middle constrictor muscles; the recurrent laryngeal nerve as it enters the larynx by passing deep to the lower border of the inferior constrictor; and the lingual nerve as it enters the mouth below the inferior border of the superior constrictor and continues against the periosteum of the mandible posterior to the third molar (see Chapter 9, *Pharyngolaryngeal morbidity: Major morbidity* and *Vocal cord function*).

Position of the LMA

When fully and correctly inserted, the LMA tip occupies the entire hypopharynx and rests against the upper esophageal sphincter behind the cricoid cartilage at the approximate level of the 6–7th cervical vertebrae[8,9]. The sides of the LMA face the pyriform fossae with the upper surface behind the base of the tongue, below the level of the tonsils[10,11] (Figure 2.1). The epiglottis rests either within the bowl of the mask or under the proximal cuff at an angle probably determined by the extent to which passage of the mask has deflected it downwards (Figure 2.2a). The effect of the LMA on the surrounding pharyngeal and laryngeal muscle groups and their action on the LMA itself as it alters pharyngeal geometry is unknown. It is certainly possible that the posterior cricoarytenoid and cricothyroid muscles may be affected and that the presence of the LMA has a direct mechanical effect on laryngeal resistance to gas flow.

Although ideally the correctly placed tip forms a plug over the upper esophageal sphincter, rather like a ball valve, this position may frequently not be achieved. It is presently unknown whether there is a relationship between incomplete occlusion of the upper sphincter and the incidence of aspiration. Figure 2.2b shows an incompletely

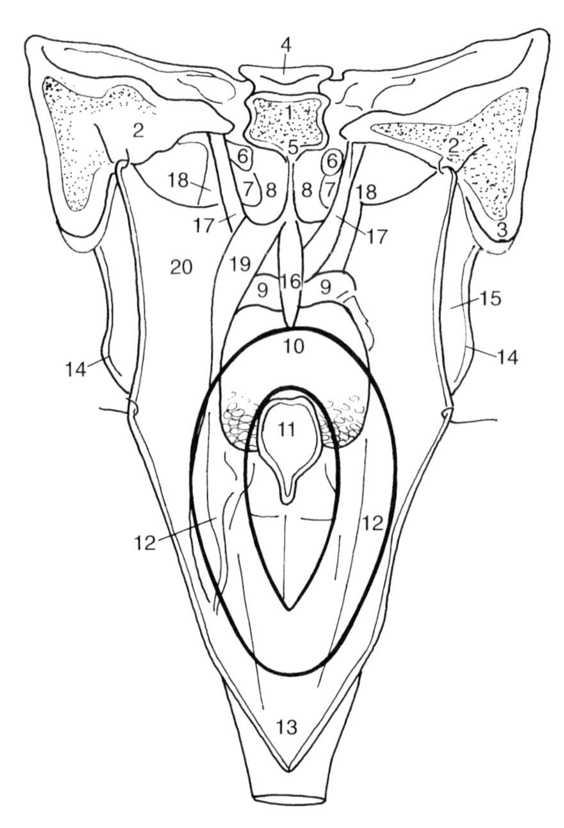

Figure 2.1 Schematic representation of position of LMA in hypopharynx. 1, basilar process of occipital bone; 2, petrous part of temporal bone; 3, mastoid processes; 4, part of splenoid bone; 5, vomer; 6, extremities of Eustachean tubes; 7, extremities of spongy bones of nose; 8, posterior openings of nose; 9, fauces; 10, upper surface of tongue; 11, epiglottis; 12, lateral borders of thyroid cartilage; 13, tube of oesophagus; 14, angle of the mandible; 15, internal pterygoid muscle; 16, azygos uvulae muscle; 17, elevators of soft palate; 18, tensors of soft palate; 19, palatopharyngeus; 20, superior constrictor (everted).

inserted mask with the pyriform fossa clearly visible on the left in spite of an excellent clinical seal. It has been suggested that the LMA preferentially directs regurgitated fluid into the trachea[12]. The counterarguments are that since the LMA obliterates the pharyngeal reservoir, there is less fluid available to be aspirated at any one moment, and that regurgitated fluid will follow the low pressure pathway up the LMA tube on expiration[13].

Exact positioning is not crucial for a clinically acceptable/patent airway. Asai points out that if the mask is judged to be correctly placed when only the glottis or the glottis and posterior surface of the epiglottis is seen through the fiberoptic scope the incidence of anatomical misplacement is 20–35%[14]. Fiberoptic[15–24], radiological[22,25], computerized tomography (CT)[26] and magnetic resonance[27] studies have revealed that the actual position of the LMA is not always ideal, yet function remains satisfactory (Figure 2.3). In fact, there are reports in which X-rays revealed the mask in the oral cavity or bending completely backwards, neither of which had been detected clinically[25,28,29]. In 13–60% of adults the epiglottis may become downfolded over the vocal cords; this is more likely if insertion techniques other than the currently recommended one are

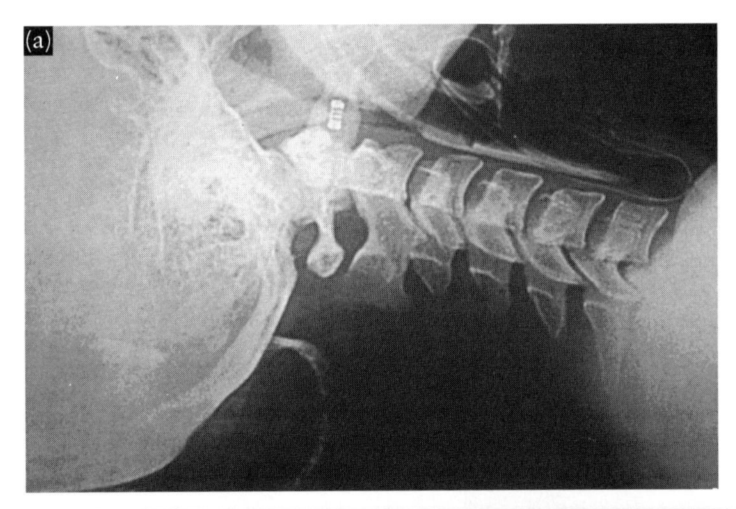

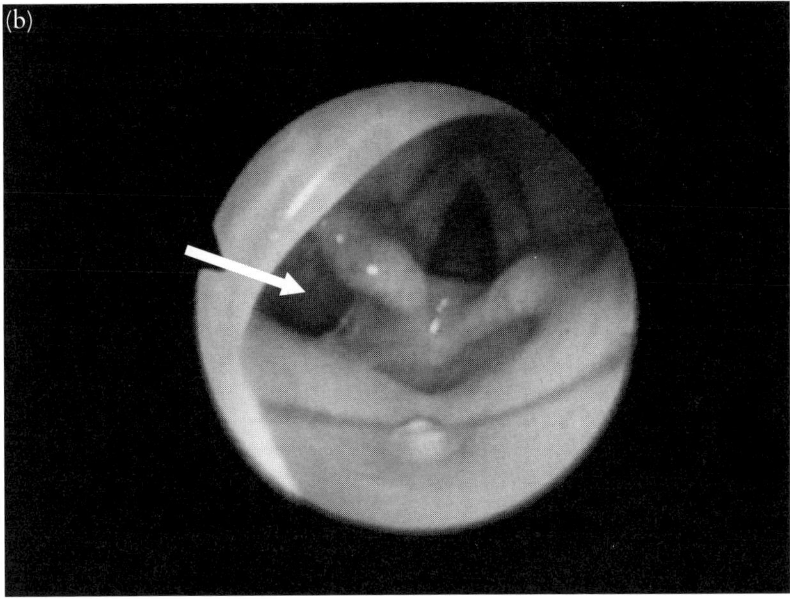

Figure 2.2 (a) Correctly inserted LMA, lateral X-ray. Note the position of the hyoid bone near the proximal mask. The mask tip lies in contact with the upper esophageal sphincter (b) Fiberoptic view of LMA with tip incompletely wedged behind the cricoid cartilage. In this position the pyriform fossa is clearly seen (arrowed) on the left hand side and is not blocked by the mask, providing a route for regurgitated fluid to enter the glottis.

employed or where user skill is limited[15,30]. Fiberoptic studies generally demonstrate a lower figure for epiglottic downfolding due to the inability of the fiberscope to detect any epiglottic downfolding occurring above the mask aperture bars[31]. The esophageal inlet is visible in the bowl of the mask in 0–10%[15–17,32–34] and is considered to be a malposition. This may be related to poor insertion technique, inappropriate size selection, or to overpressure (>25 cm H_2O) applied during PPV which may displace the LMA tip from the hypopharynx and thus expose the esophagus[35]. One study showed that the aryepiglottic folds were infolded towards the vocal cords in 40% of patients, although it is likely that this high figure was related to malposition[30].

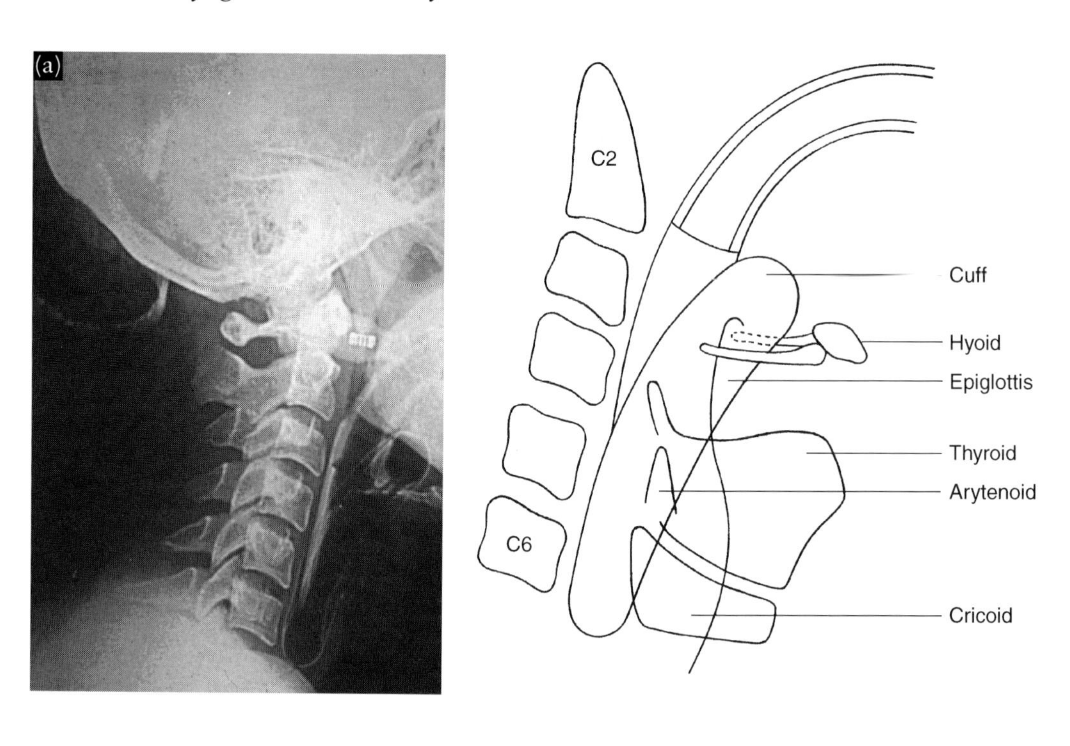

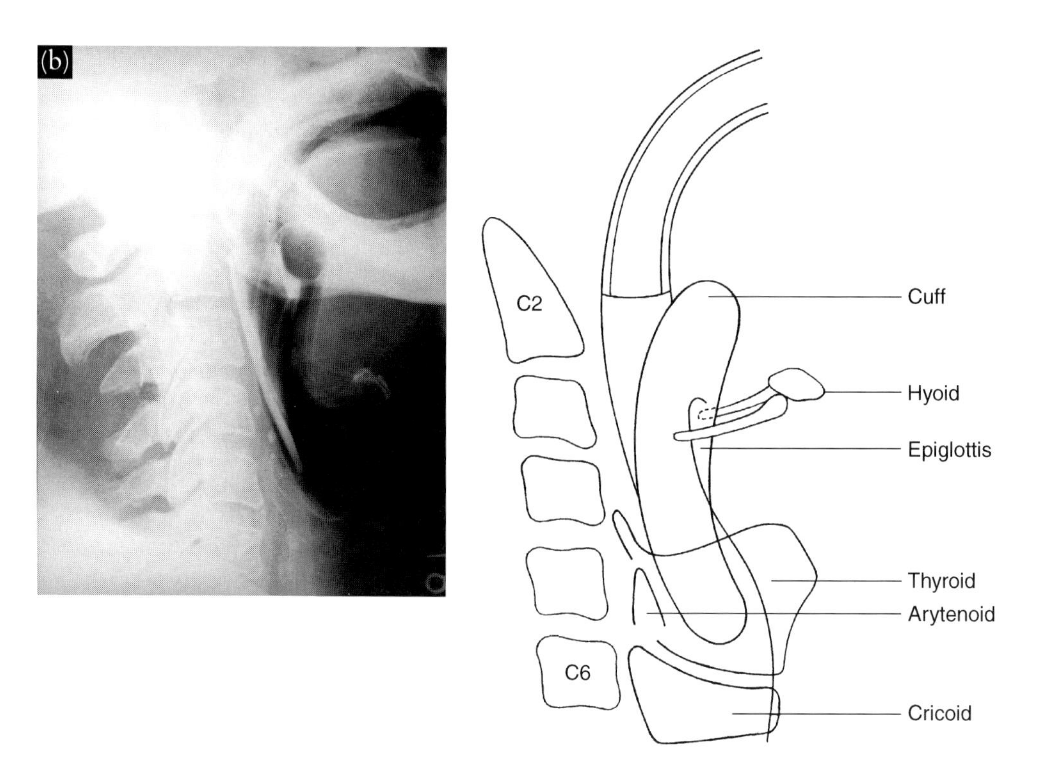

Figure 2.3 X-ray scan of LMA in (a) correct and (b) incorrect position. X-ray (b), from Reference 25, with permission from Blackwell Scientific Publications.

Dye and radiological studies have demonstrated that the LMA cuff forms an effective seal across the pharynx, preventing contamination of the glottis and trachea by oropharyngeal secretions, blood and other debris[32–34,36,37].

Implications for the laryngopharynx

When the cuff is inflated, the thyroid, arytenoid and cricoid cartilages are pressed anteriorly and the tissues overlying the larynx bulge slightly. Inflation of the cuff usually causes slight upward movement of the whole device as the expanding mask tip is partly squeezed out of the triangular-shaped base of the hypopharynx. The resulting position brings the glottic and the LMA apertures in line with each other. The efficacy of the seal depends on the fit between the oval-shaped cuff of the LMA and the oval-shaped groove surrounding the glottic inlet.

Reaction to insertion may take several forms, varying from complete rejection to slight swallowing movements, depending on anesthetic depth and user proficiency. The common occurrence of swallowing following insertion and preceding removal during emergence from anesthesia is accounted for by the anatomical situation of the mask. Swallowing is initiated by stimulation of the numerous receptors in the mucous membrane of the pharynx and larynx, especially on the laryngeal aspect of the epiglottis, aryepiglottic folds, ventricular bands and interarytenoid area, mediated via the cranial ninth and tenth nerves as an involuntary reflex[38]. At the same time there is reflex closure of the glottic sphincter (transient glottic closure), caused by stimulation of the internal branch of the superior laryngeal nerve. The latter reflex explains why premature insertion of the LMA is often associated with inability to inflate the lungs until the glottic sphincter relaxes, usually about 20 s later. This phenomenon needs to be recognized, because it is otherwise easily mistaken for misplacement of the LMA or laryngeal spasm. Misplacement may indeed occur but becomes progressively less as experience is gained, provided the recommended insertion technique is carefully followed[39].

The fact that the LMA occupies a different position to the tracheal tube has some important consequences. The large bulk of the LMA normally prevents it passing through either the glottic or the upper esophageal sphincters, making it both less invasive and less uncertain with respect to position than the tracheal tube. Avoidance of tracheal intubation means there is no danger of accidental bronchial occlusion. The fact that the vocal cords are not normally encroached on avoids the problems of laryngeal spasm associated with insertion or removal of the tracheal tube[40]. Because the vocal cords are free to move normally during respiration, inspiratory dilatation and expiratory constriction of the glottis can still occur. Inspiratory dilatation reduces the work of breathing while expiratory constriction may be important in intrapulmonary gas mixing and possibly in maintaining the functional residual capacity. Both mechanisms are neutralized by tracheal intubation.

When positive pressure ventilation is used, paralysis is reversed before removal of the tracheal tube, allowing the vocal cords to 'bite-down' onto the tube, which is then forcibly withdrawn through them. Reversal of paralysis using the LMA allows the vocal cords to recover their function undisturbed. The patient is able to generate an effective cough even when the LMA is still in place. This may be important in patients whose survival depends on frequent coughing, as in chronic obstructive airways disease. The tracheal tube exerts a powerful stimulus, so that a smooth anesthetic technique usually dictates its removal at a plane of anesthesia at which reflex responses are obtunded. The LMA, if undisturbed, provokes very little stimulus and consequently can be left in place until protective reflexes have recovered to the point at which the patient can maintain the airway unassisted.

Two clear dangers derive from the position of the LMA. As it does not penetrate sphincters, it cannot prevent the effects of their inappropriate opening or closing. Hence the patient with gastric contents may still regurgitate through the upper esophageal sphincter and soiling of the pulmonary tree may occur because the mask does not prevent passage of material into the larynx via the pyriform fossae. Also, the glottic sphincter may close or laryngeal spasm may occur as a response to surgical stimulation at inadequate levels of anesthesia, a common problem encountered by the inexperienced.

The second danger derives from the fact that the LMA needs to be correctly oriented if the glottic and LMA apertures are to remain facing each other. Unlike the tracheal tube, rotation of the LMA may cause complete obstruction. The black line on the tube should always face the upper lip of the patient. Other malpositions of the LMA can sometimes occur following insertion even in experienced hands. It is important to recognize this and to learn to make the distinction between malposition and inadequate anesthetic depth when the airway is clinically obstructed, so that appropriate action may be taken.

Cricoid pressure

Cricoid pressure (CP) was reintroduced into medicine by Sellick as a mechanical means of protecting patients at risk of aspiration of gastric contents[41] and preventing gastric insufflation during mask ventilation[42]. It has been described as the 'linchpin of the rapid sequence induction'[43] and over the last 35 years has become widely accepted as a standard of practice during anesthesia[43–45] and to a lesser extent resuscitation[46–48]. However, although a superficially simple and anatomically appropriate maneuver, there have been increasing concerns about its safety and efficacy[49–53]. Not only are there fewer than 40 studies investigating its use and none confirming its clinical benefits, but there is reliable evidence that it is often ineffective (even when applied by experienced personnel)[54–56], tentative evidence that it is detrimental to overall patient safety[52,57,58], and recent evidence that it reduces lower esophageal sphincter tone[59]. The most important limitation clinically with CP is that it may interfere with tracheal intubation and face mask ventilation. This is of major significance since failure to manage the airway is a more frequent cause of morbidity/mortality than aspiration[60]. LMA usage may also be impeded by CP. The hypopharynx extends to the lower border of the cricoid cartilage where it becomes the esophagus and the correctly placed LMA tip lies at a variable depth behind the cricoid cartilage (Figure 2.4). In theory, the LMA cannot be placed correctly in the entire length of the hypopharynx with applied CP. This may therefore reduce the ease of insertion of the LMA, reduce the efficacy of CP, and may also make the LMA less effective as an aid to intubation.

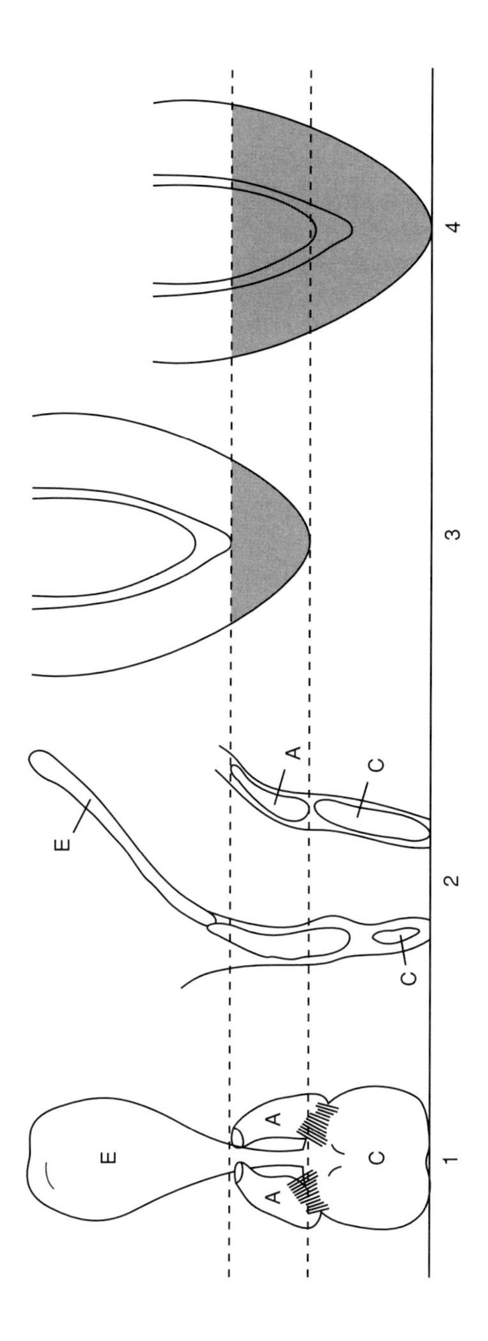

Figure 2.4 Schematic view of the anatomical position of the LMA tip with cricoid pressure[76]. The hatched area indicates the distal part of the mask that occupies the hypopharynx. 1 = Lateral view of the pharynx; 2 = posterior view of the pharynx; 3 = position of the tip of the mask when cricoid pressure is applied before placement, the mask, in theory, might be wedged in the hypopharynx, but it can occupy only the space behind the arytenoid cartilages. The mask is positioned at least 2 cm more proximal than usual. The arytenoid cartilages can then be pushed anteriorly, and thus the mask is more likely to become dislodged. 4 = Position of the tip of the mask when no cricoid pressure is applied. When the mask is placed correctly the distal part of the mask should occupy fully the hypopharynx, the pharyngeal space behind both the arytenoid and cricoid cartilages. *Key*: E = epiglottis; A = arytenoid cartilages; C = cricoid cartilages. Reproduced with permission, *British Journal of Anaesthesia*.

Effect of cricoid pressure on ease of insertion

Although case reports have suggested that LMA placement is generally unimpeded by cricoid pressure[61–71] this has not been confirmed by prospective studies and current opinion is polarized on the effect of CP on LMA insertion[72–76]. Composite data from all trials, while limited by different methodologies, suggest that LMA insertion is more likely to be successful without CP (92% versus 66%)[16,77–82] (Table 2.1). It is possible that the differing findings are related to:

1. The mode of application of CP: the cricoid yoke or double handed CP appears to make LMA insertion more difficult than single handed CP[73,74]. This may be related to incomplete compression of the retrolaryngeal tissues by single handed CP[83];
2. Head and neck extension, which may make insertion more difficult[75,76];
3. The degree of force applied to the cricoid cartilage compared with that used to place the LMA[84,85];
4. Inexperience or poor technique in LMA insertion[82];
5. Failure to deflate the mask tip correctly prior to insertion[82].

Asai has suggested that the LMA cannot occupy the entire hypopharynx if CP is correctly applied and has demonstrated that placement was successful in only 3/22 patients when a standardized cricoid force was applied[81]. Gabbott and Sasada demonstrated that placement was possible in 29/40 within two 10 s attempts using cricoid pressure with manual in-line neck stabilization[82]. The clinical implications of the CP/LMA interaction for failed intubation are discussed in Chapter 14: *Unpredicted difficult airway*.

Table 2.1 Studies investigating the interaction between the LMA and cricoid pressure in vivo

Researchers	*CP*	*Control (no CP)*	*Cricoid mode*
Heath and Allagain[78]	50/50		SH
Brimacombe[16]	34/40	37/40	SH
Ansermino and Blogg[79]	3/20	19/22	Yoke
Brimacombe et al[77]	45/50*	49/50	SH
Asai et al[80]	10/20	19/20	DH‡
Asai et al[81]	3/22	22/22	Yoke
Gabbott and Sasada[82]	14/40 (29/40)†	33/40	SH + MIT
Total	159/242 (66%)	179/194 (92%)	

* Simulated failed intubation; † improved at second attempt; ‡ with pillow.

Key: SH = single handed; DH = double handed; yoke = cricoid yoke; SH + MIT = single handed plus manual in-line traction.

Efficacy of cricoid pressure

Strang demonstrated in 10 cadavers[86], using a cricoid force of 43 N and esophageal pressures of 7.8 kPa, that the presence of the LMA itself does not compromise CP[86]. Asai et al have confirmed this in anesthetized humans[87]. They studied 50 patients and demonstrated that the incidence of gastric insufflation is significantly reduced at peak airway pressures of 30 cm H_2O when CP is applied at 30 N with the LMA in situ. The authors also showed that the correctly placed LMA is not dislodged by CP, but that it may impede ventilation, particularly if the neck is unsupported.

Anatomical consequences

It is well known that CP makes laryngoscopy and tracheal intubation more difficult by distorting laryngeal architecture, particularly if it is incorrectly applied. There is a consensus that the application of CP produces a deterioration in the fiberoptic view ranging from slight[16,77] to gross[80–82] distortion. The effect of application of CP after placement of the LMA on success rate for fiberoptic intubation is not known although Asai has suggested it does not become difficult[88]. It has been suggested that the laryngeal inlet can be tipped anteriorly by the inflated LMA cuff when CP is applied[16]. This may explain why intubation via the LMA is more difficult with CP applied since the angle of approach is less favorable[78]. The degree of tilt has been postulated to increase with increasing penetration of the tip into the space behind the arytenoids and the hypopharynx. It is possible that by tilting the cricoid cartilage cranially during the application of cricoid pressure, this effect may be partially counteracted[89]. Difficulty may also rarely be related to CP causing mechanical closure of the cords[90]. This may be due to internal rotation of the arytenoids as they are compressed against the LMA cuff. In theory, the application of cricoid pressure may make dislodgment more likely, but this has not been documented in clinical trials[16] and is probably uncommon[88].

References

1 Ishimura H, Minami K, Sata T, Shigematsu A, Kadoya T. Impossible insertion of the laryngeal mask airway and oropharyngeal axes. *Anesthesiology* 1995;**83**:867–869.
2 Brimacombe J, Berry A. Mallampati grade and laryngeal mask placement. *Anesth Analg* 1996;**82**:1112–1113.
3 Sheppard IM, Sheppard FM. Maximal incisal opening: a diagnostic index. *J Dent Med* 1965;**20**:13–15.
4 Maltby JR, Loken RG, Beriault MT, Archer DP. Laryngeal mask airway with mouth opening less than 20 mm. *Can J Anaesth* 1995;**42**:1140–1142.
5 Mason DG, Bingham RM. The laryngeal mask airway in children. *Anaesthesia* 1990;**45**:760–763.
6 van Heerden PV, Kirrage D. Large tonsils and the laryngeal mask airway. *Anaesthesia* 1989;**44**:703.
7 Romanes GJ. *Cunningham's manual of practical anatomy. Head and neck and brain.* Oxford: Oxford University Press, 1978;117–118.
8 Brain AIJ. Laryngeal mask misplacement – causes, consequences and solutions. *Anaesthesia* 1992;**47**:531–532.
9 Brain AIJ. Studies on the laryngeal mask: first, learn the art. *Anaesthesia* 1991;**46**:417–427.
10 Williams PJ, Bailey PM. Comparison of the reinforced laryngeal mask airway and tracheal intubation for adenotonsillectomy. *Br J Anaesth* 1993;**70**:30–33.
11 Webster AC, Morley-Forster PK, Dain S, et al. Anaesthesia for adenotonsillectomy: a comparison between tracheal intubation and the armoured laryngeal mask airway. *Can J Anaesth* 1993;**40**:1171–1177.
12 Koehli N. Aspiration and the laryngeal mask airway. *Anaesthesia* 1991;**46**:419.
13 Brain AIJ. The laryngeal mask and the oesophagus. *Anaesthesia* 1991;**46**:701–702.
14 Asai T, Morris S. The laryngeal mask airway: its features, effects and role. *Can J Anaesth* 1994;**41**:930–960.
15 Brimacombe J, Berry A. Insertion of the laryngeal mask airway – a prospective study of four techniques. *Anaesth Intens Care* 1993;**21**:89–92.
16 Brimacombe J. Cricoid pressure and the laryngeal mask airway. *Anaesthesia* 1991;**46**:986–987.
17 Du Plessis MC, Marshall Barr A, Verghese C, Lyall JRW. Fibreoptic bronchoscopy under general anaesthesia using the laryngeal mask airway. *Eur J Anaesthesiol* 1993;**10**:363–365.
18 Rowbottom SJ, Simpson DL, Grubb D. The laryngeal mask airway in children. A fibreoptic assessment of positioning. *Anaesthesia* 1991;**46**:489–491.

19 Mizushima A, Wardall GJ, Simpson DL. The laryngeal mask airway in infants. *Anaesthesia* 1992;**47**:849–851.

20 Wilson IG. The laryngeal mask airway in paediatric practice. *Br J Anaesth* 1993;**70**:124–125.

21 Dubreuil M, Laffon M, Plaud B, Penon C, Ecoffey C. Complications and fiberoptic assessment of size 1 laryngeal mask airway. *Anesth Analg* 1993;**76**:527–529.

22 Aoyama K, Takenaka I, Sata T, Shigematsu A. The triple airway manoeuvre for insertion of the laryngeal mask airway in paralysed patients. *Can J Anaesth* 1996;**42**:1010–1016.

23 Elwood T, Cox RG. Laryngeal mask insertion with a laryngoscope in paediatric patients. *Can J Anaesth* 1996;**43**:435–437.

24 Gurpinar A, Yavascaoglu B, Korfali G, Dogruyol H. Fibreoptic assessment of positioning of the laryngeal mask airway in children. *European Society of Anaesthesiologists Annual Congress, London, 1–5 June 1996,* A306 (Abstract).

★ 25 Nandi PR, Nunn JF, Charlesworth CH, Taylor SJ. Radiological study of the laryngeal mask. *Eur J Anaesthesiol* 1991;**4**:33–39.
The first radiological study of the LMA. Twenty-four elderly males had lateral neck X-rays with the LMA in situ. Showed that the epiglottis was within the bowl in 16/24 patients and that the device could function well despite poor positioning.

★ 26 Goudsouzian NG, Denman W, Cleveland R, Shorten G. Radiologic localisation of the laryngeal mask airway in children. *Anesthesiology* 1992;**77**:1085–1089.
The first CT and NMR study of the position of the LMA in children. Fifty children were investigated and there was little correlation between position and function. In 46/50 patients the cuff was in the pharynx and covered the laryngeal opening.

27 Shorten GD, Opie NJ, Graziotti P, Morris I, Khangure M. Assessment of upper airway anatomy in awake, sedated and anaesthetised patients using magnetic resonance imaging. *Anaesth Intens Care* 1994;**22**:165–169.

28 Molloy AR. Unexpected position of the laryngeal mask airway. *Anaesthesia* 1991;**46**:592.

29 Ball AJ. Laryngeal mask misplacement – a nonproblem. *Anesth Analg* 1995;**81**:204.

30 Payne J. The use of the fibreoptic laryngoscope to confirm the position of the laryngeal mask. *Anaesthesia* 1989;**44**:465.

31 Asai T. Difficulty in assessing the correct position of the laryngeal mask airway. *Br J Anaesth* 1994;**72**:366.

★ 32 John RE, Hill S, Hughes TJ. Airway protection by the laryngeal mask – a barrier to dye placed in the pharynx. *Anaesthesia* 1991;**46**:366–367.
The first study investigating the efficacy of the LMA as a throat pack. Methylene blue dye was placed in the pharynx of 64 patients with the LMA in situ and no leak of dye was detected on the larynx using a fiberoptic scope.

33 Samarkandi AH, Ali MS, Elgammal M, Bakhamees HS. Airway protection by the laryngeal mask airway in children. *Middle East J Anesthesiol* 1995;**13**:107–113.

34 Cork RC, Depa RM, Standen JR. Prospective comparison of use of the laryngeal mask and endotracheal tube for ambulatory surgery. *Anesth Analg* 1994;**79**:719–727.

35 Fullekrug B, Pothmann W, Werner C, am Esch JS. The laryngeal mask airway: anesthetic gas leakage and fiberoptic control of positioning. *J Clin Anesth* 1993;**5**:357–363.

36 Cork RC, Kaul B, Frink EJ, Jr, Standen JR, Depa R. Comparison of laryneal mask with endotracheal tube for airway control. *Anesthesiology* 1992;**75**:A1112 (Abstract).

37 Fujii T, Watanabe S, Taguchi N, Takeshima R. Airway protection by the laryngeal mask during various neck positions and during protracted surgeries: sealing to dye placed in the pharynx. *Anesth Analg* 1996;**82**:S118 (Abstract).

38 Sant'Ambrogio G, Mathew OP, Fisher JT, Sant'Ambrogio FB. Laryngeal receptors responding to transmural pressure, airflow and local muscle activity. *Resp Physiol* 1983;**54**:317–330.

39 Lopez-Gil M, Brimacombe J, Cebrian J, Arranz J. The laryngeal mask airway in pediatric practice – a prospective study of skill acquisition by resident anesthesiologists. *Anesthesiology* 1996;**84**:807–811.

40 Harmer M. Complications of tracheal intubation. In: Latto IP, Rosen M, eds. *Difficulties in tracheal intubation.* London: Baillière Tindall, 1987;36–48.

41 Sellick BA. Cricoid pressure to prevent regurgitation of stomach contents during induction of anaesthesia. *Lancet* 1961;**ii**:404–406.

42 Salem MR, Wong AY, Mani M, Sellick BA. Efficacy of cricoid pressure in preventing gastric inflation during bag-mask ventilation in pediatric patients. *Anesthesiology* 1974;**40**:96–98.

43 Rosen M. Editorial. *Anaesthesia* 1981;**36**:142.

44 Davies JM, Weets S, Crone LA, Paulin E. Difficult intubation in the parturient. *Can J Anaesth* 1989;**36**:668–674.

45 Tunstall ME. Failed intubation in the parturient. *Can J Anaesth* 1989;**36**:611–613.

46 Standards and guidelines for cardiopulmonary resuscitation and emergency cardiac care. *J Am Mec Assoc* 1985;**255**:2905–2984.

47 Bircher NG. Wolf Creek III: a time to look forward, a time to look back. *Crit Care Med* 1985;**13**:950.

48 Melker RJ. Recommendations for ventilation during cardiopulmonary resuscitation: time for change? *Crit Care Med* 1986;**13**:882.

49 Gwinnutt CL. Cricoid pressure and advanced life support. *Anaesthesia* 1995;**50**:912.

50 Smurthwaite GJ. Cricoid pressure and advanced life support. *Anaesthesia* 1995;**50**:912.

51 Elcock DH. Cricoid pressure and advanced life support. *Anaesthesia* 1995;**50**:912–913.

52 Kron SS. Questionable effectiveness of cricoid pressure in preventing aspiration. *Anesthesiology* 1995;**83**:431.

53 Schwartz DE, Cohen NH. Questionable effectiveness of cricoid pressure in preventing aspiration. *Anesthesiology* 1995;**83**:432.

54 Howells TH, Chamney AR, Wraight WJ, Simons RS. The application of cricoid pressure. An assessment and a survey of its practice. *Anaesthesia* 1983;**38**:457–460.

55 Lawes EG. Cricoid pressure with or without the 'cricoid yoke'. *Br J Anaesth* 1986;**58**:1376–1379.

56 Vanner RG, O'Dwyer JP, Pryle BJ, Reynolds F. Upper oesophageal sphincter pressure and the effect of cricoid pressure. *Anaesthesia* 1992;**47**:95–100.

57 Schwartz DE, Mathhay MA, Cohen NH. Death and other complications of emergency airway management in critically ill adults. *Anesthesiology* 1995;**82**:367–376.

58 Vanner RG. Mechanisms of regurgitation and its prevention with cricoid pressure. *Int J Obstet Anesth* 1993;**3**:207–215.

59 Tournadre JP, Chassard D, Berrada K, Bouletreau P. Lower oesophageal sphincter pressure during application of cricoid pressure in conscious volunteers. *Br J Anaesth* 1996;**76**:A50.

60 Caplan RA, Posner KL, Ward RJ, Cheney FW. Adverse respiratory events in anesthesia: a closed claims analysis. *Anesthesiology* 1990;**72**:828–833.

61 McClune S, Regan M, Moore J. Laryngeal mask airway for caesarean section. *Anaesthesia* 1990;**45**:227–228.

62 Storey J. The laryngeal mask for failed intubation at caesarean section. *Anaesth Intens Care* 1992;**20**:118–119.

63 Chadwick LS, Vohra A. Anaesthesia for emergency caesarean section using the Brain laryngeal mask airway. *Anaesthesia* 1989;**44**:261–262.

64 Lim W, Wareham C, de Mello WF, Kocan M. The laryngeal mask in failed intubation. *Anaesthesia* 1990;**41**:689–690.

65 Hasham FM, Andrews PJD, Juneja MM, Ackermann III WE. The laryngeal mask airway facilitates intubation at cesarean section. A case report of difficult intubation. *Int J Obstet Anesth* 1993;**2**:181–182.

66 McFarlane C. Failed intubation in an obese obstetric patient and the laryngeal mask. *Int J Obstet Anesth* 1993;**2**:183–184.

67 Brimacombe J. Emergency airway management in rural practice: use of the laryngeal mask airway. *Aust J Rural Hlth* 1995;**3**:10–19.

68 Swayne P, Greenslade GL. Emergency intubation through the laryngeal mask airway. The effective application of cricoid pressure. *Anaesthesia* 1994;**49**:696–697.

69 Kokkinis K. The use of the laryngeal mask airway in CPR. *Resuscitation* 1994;**27**:9–12.

70 Myles PS, Venema HR, Lindholm DE. Trauma patient managed with the laryngeal mask airway and percutaneous tracheostomy after failed intubation. *Med J Aust* 1994;**161**:640.

71 Dalmeida RE, Mayhew J, Gallagher T, Herring LE. The laryngeal mask airway: a must in the obstetric suite. *J Clin Anesth* (in press).

72 Brimacombe J, Berry A, Heath ML, Allagain J, Blogg CE, Ansermino JM. Cricoid pressure and the laryngeal mask airway. *Br J Anaesth* 1993;**70**:596.

73 Brimacombe J, Berry A, White A. Single- compared to double-handed cricoid pressure for LMA insertion. *Br J Anaesth* 1994;**72**:732–734.

74 Asai T, Barclay K, Power I, Vaughan RS. Single- compared to double-handed cricoid pressure for insertion of an LMA. *Br J Anaesth* 1994;**72**:733–734.

75 Brimacombe J, Berry A. Cricoid pressure and the LMA: efficacy and interpretation. *Br J Anaesth* 1994;**49**:862–863.

76 Asai T, Barclay K, Power I, Vaughan RS. Cricoid pressure and the LMA: efficacy and interpretation. *Br J Anaesth* 1994;**49**:863–865.

★ **77** Brimacombe J, White A, Berry A. Effect of cricoid pressure on ease of insertion of the laryngeal mask airway. *Br J Anaesth* 1993;**71**:800–802.
Randomized prospective trial comparing LMA insertion with and without cricoid pressure following a simulated failed intubation with thiopentone and suxamethonium. Showed that LMA insertion was 90% successful with single-handed cricoid pressure applied.

78 Heath ML, Allagain J. Intubation through the laryngeal mask – a technique for unexpected difficult intubation. *Anaesthesia* 1991;**46**:545–548.

79 Ansermino JM, Blogg CE. Cricoid pressure may prevent insertion of the laryngeal mask airway. *Br J Anaesth* 1992;**69**:465–467.

★ **80** Asai T, Barkley K, Power I, Vaughan RS. Cricoid pressure impedes placement of the laryngeal mask airway and subsequent tracheal intubation. *Br J Anaesth* 1994;**72**:47–51.
Randomized prospective trial of 40 patients comparing LMA insertion with and without cricoid pressure. Showed that LMA insertion was successful in 50% with double-handed cricoid pressure applied.

81 Asai T, Barclay K, Power I, Vaughan RS. Cricoid pressure impedes placement of the laryngeal mask airway. *Br J Anaesth* 1995;**74**:521–525.

82 Gabbott DA, Sasada MP. Laryngeal mask airway insertion using cricoid pressure and manual in-line neck stabilisation. *Anaesthesia* 1995;**50**:674–676.

83 Vanner RG, Pryle BJ. Nasogastric tubes and cricoid pressure. *Anaesthesia* 1993;**48**:1112–1113.

84 Asai T, Barkley K, Power I, Vaughan RS. The role of the laryngeal mask in obstetric anaesthesia. *Int J Obstet Anesth* 1995;**4**:190–191.

85 Brimacombe J, Berry A. The role of the laryngeal mask in obstetric anaesthesia. *Int J Obstet Anesth* 1995;**4**:192–194.

★ **86** Strang TI. Does the laryngeal mask airway compromise cricoid pressure? *Anaesthesia* 1992;**47**:829–831.
Prize-winning paper in which cricoid pressure was shown to be effective with the LMA in situ in 10 cadavers. When cricoid pressure was released, barium dye placed in the esophagus was found in the lungs of 6/10.

87 Asai T, Barclay K, McBeth C, Vaughan RS. Cricoid pressure applied after placement of the laryngeal mask prevents gastric insufflation but inhibits ventilation. *Br J Anaesth* 1996;**76**:772–776.

88 Asai T. Use of the laryngeal mask for tracheal intubation in patients at increased risk of aspiration of gastric contents. *Anesthesiology* 1992;77:1029–1030.

89 Salem MR, Heyman JH, Livschultz V, Mahdi M. Cephalad displacement of the larynx facilitates tracheal intubation. *Anesthesiology* 1987;**67**:3A (Abstract).

90 Brimacombe J, Berry A. Mechanical airway obstruction following cricoid pressure with the laryngeal mask airway. *Anesth Analg* 1994;78:604–605.

3 Physiological implications

Gastrointestinal system

The swallowing reflex

The normal practice of anesthesia is to manipulate the upper airway with head position and/or laryngoscopy to produce a direct view of the vocal cords. Most blind techniques are difficult maneuvers because, without a laryngoscope, it is not possible to produce this straightening out of the upper airway curve. LMA insertion is highly successful as a blind technique (up to 98% successful insertion within 20 s)[1] as it utilizes a normal existing physiological mechanism – that of swallowing – to follow the natural curve and direction of the upper airway, the inserting finger imitating the tongue's action in swallowing food. However, the swallowing reflex itself must be suppressed for the insertion and then tolerance of the LMA cuff in the pharynx. Clinical experience with the LMA in awake and sedated patients suggests that the swallowing reflex remains intact under topical anesthesia[2] or light general anesthesia[3].

Receptors which specifically trigger swallowing have not been identified histologically. Fluid and slowly adapting pressure receptors are distributed over the pharyngeal and laryngeal regions and swallowing may be triggered by fluid and light touch, with different fluids appearing to have a variable influence over swallowing[4]. It is possible to postulate that a flavored LMA could be beneficial for LMA insertion in awake/sedated patients if this were to promote the swallowing reflex. During emergence from LMA anesthesia, swallowing activity is commonly used to indicate that the patient is emerging close to the point at which the LMA may be safely removed without triggering laryngeal spasm[5].

Insertion of the LMA in the nonanesthetized patient triggers a variety of protective and digestive reflexes including coughing, gagging, retching, swallowing and hypersalivation[2]. With increasing anesthetic depth, either local or general, these reflexes are suppressed to a varying degree. If LMA insertion occurs at inadequate anesthetic depth a single incomplete swallow may occur and the glottis, instead of transiently closing as in the normal swallow, remains closed for a period of 20–30 s, leading to a misdiagnosis of laryngeal spasm or malposition, a frequent clinical error made by inexperienced LMA users[6]. Coughing is more likely to occur if the LMA tip impacts with the glottic inlet, but may also occur if pharyngeal secretions are driven into the glottis by the mask as it is inserted.

The ability to utilize the swallowing pathway for insertion, which does not normally require a person to assume a different head position, makes possible the successful use of the LMA in patients in whom movement of the cervical spine is impossible or contraindicated due to pathology stiffening the bony architecture or endangering the spinal cord[7,8].

The esophagus

The presence of the mask in the pharynx and the stimulation provoked by insertion inevitably involve the upper gastrointestinal tract reflexes. It has been known for nearly 40 years that sustained distension of the pharynx induces prolonged relaxation of the lower esophageal sphincter (LOS)[9]. The pharynx contains mechano- and chemo-receptors which play a part in triggering the primary peristaltic wave of deglutition[10]. However, inappropriate stimulation or bypassing of these trigger zones may produce a less coordinated response including secondary peristalsis which lacks both the speed of completion and the coordination of primary peristalsis and can result in relaxation of the LOS without subsequent immediate restoration of tone. There is some evidence from one dye study[11], one study using a pressure probe pull-through technique[12], and two studies using an esophageal pH probe[13,14] that LOS tone may be reduced with the LMA when compared with the face mask[11,12,14] or tracheal tube[13]. However, this theory remains controversial[15–18]; repeat dye and pH studies in both ventilated and spontaneously breathing patients[19–24] have failed to confirm these findings. The variable figures found in the differing studies may relate to differing mean cuff pressures or may simply reflect the sensitivities of the detection techniques or the skill of the LMA users. A confounding factor in the interpretation of pH studies comparing the LMA and face mask is that the presence of the mask blocks passage of alkaline secretions from the upper pharynx from reaching the lower esophagus[14]. One factor preventing aspiration may be the persistent function of the upper esophageal sphincter (UOS)[25]. Using Dent Sleeve manometry, Vanner et al showed that during spontaneous ventilation anesthesia UOS pressure does not fall significantly with an LMA in situ, suggesting that the pharyngo-upper esophageal sphincter contractile reflex may be intact[26]. Furthermore, the UOS is known to constrict in response to the presence of acidic fluids in the lower esophagus[27].

Pharyngeal mucosa

The precise mechanical effects of the LMA on the pharyngeal tissues are unknown. In theory, the inflated LMA cuff could generate sufficient compression and shearing forces to cause a reduction in pharyngeal mucosal blood flow and direct tissue trauma, as can occur during tracheal intubation[28,29]. It has also been suggested that parts of the pharynx compressed against rigid tissues such as the hyoid bone or cervical vertebrae may be more susceptible to damage[30]. The pharynx, however, is a highly distensible structure which is normally subject to large transient pressure changes and distortion under many physiological conditions. Marjot has shown that calculated transmitted mucosal pressures potentially exceed the capillary perfusion pressure of the adjacent pharyngeal mucosa[31], but there is no evidence that this is harmful even over prolonged periods[3,32,33]. Hamakawa has directly measured the pressure on the middle part of the outside of the LMA in 40 patients and shown that extracuff pressure is approximately 25 mm Hg and does not increase during O_2/N_2O anesthesia despite increases in intracuff pressure[34]. Although there are obvious limitations to measuring pressure at one arbitrary point, this study may help to explain why pharyngeal morbidity is uncommon. It also confirms that the relationship between intracuff and pharyngeal mucosal pressure is nonlinear, making guidelines based on intracuff pressures alone less useful. No major pharyngeal trauma has been reported in several million LMA anesthetics and minor morbidity, such as sore throat, which occurs in approximately 10% of patients, is usually mild and is less than for the tracheal tube and similar to the face mask[35]. This might be partly explained by progressive accommodation of the pharyngeal muscles to the mask[31,33], but to avoid pharyngeal mucosal damage it has been postulated that either the pressure on the pharyngeal mucosa must be lower than calculated values, or the pharyngeal mucosa must be resistant to ischemic damage, or adaptation of the pharyngeal blood vessels must occur, either due to the uneven distribution of pressure exerted by the LMA or to a redistribution of blood flow[33]. A further possible consequence of pharyngeal mucosal trauma is transient bacteremia, but, in contrast to tracheal intubation[36,37], this does not appear to occur during LMA insertion[38,39]. Factors affecting LMA cuff pressure are given in Table 3.1.

Respiratory system

Pulmonary defenses

The upper airway has a major role in the defense of the lung. Afferent neural pathways respond to invading noxious stimuli by reflex cough and/or bronchoconstriction and, in the semi-anesthetized patient, laryngeal spasm. At cellular level, cilia are responsible for clearance of mucous, and phagocytes and other cells of the immune series are responsible for protection against invasion by foreign particles and organisms.

Little is known about the specific pharyngolaryngeal receptors except that some react mainly to changes in pressure and to a much lesser extent to air flow[40]. The effect of the LMA on pharyngolaryngeal receptors[40] and the possible physiological implications for the tracheobronchial tree are unknown. In theory, the LMA should cause

Table 3.1 Factors affecting LMA cuff pressure in vivo

Gas inside the LMA cuff
- volume
- temperature of gas
- gas partial pressures

Gas outside the LMA cuff
- partial pressure in tissues touching cuff (affected by tissue perfusion)
- partial pressure of inspiratory gases in tube and bowl of the LMA

Properties of the LMA
- permeability of cuff and pilot balloon to various gases
- may change with age of LMA and volume
- thickness of cuff wall (varies with size)

Mechanical pressures
- pharyngeal anatomy
- pharyngeal muscle tone – anesthetic depth/respiratory effort
- position of the LMA
- head and neck movement
- pressure on neck
- bending LMA tube
- swallowing, retching or coughing

minimal triggering of[41,42], or interference with[43], lung defenses because they are distal to the device. Support for this idea comes from clinical data which suggest that laryngeal spasm[42], bronchospasm[44–47] and coughing[41] occur less frequently than with the tracheal tube. Tracheal intubation is known to interfere with mucociliary clearance[48] and the LMA probably does not impede this mechanically although anesthesia itself may interfere with ciliary function[49]. It is thus possible that the LMA may be of benefit in maintaining the tracheobronchial climate and this may have implications for patients with pulmonary pathology[50]. Postoperative laryngeal competence is not impaired by the LMA and may be similar to that with the tracheal tube[51]. Gal found that tracheal intubation in conscious volunteers markedly reduced flow-volume curves, raising residual volume and causing gas trapping[52]. Whether the LMA would lessen this effect, so reducing the risk of postoperative atelectasis, and also enable the cough reflex to return at an earlier stage is still under speculation. There is clinical evidence that it may offer benefits in patients with respiratory disease[53–55]. For instance it has been suggested that pediatric patients with mild upper respiratory tract infections may have improved postoperative oxygen saturation with the LMA compared with the tracheal tube[53].

Pulmonary mechanics

Surface and tissue forces within the alveoli primarily affect lung compliance whilst smooth muscle contraction primarily affects lung resistance[56]. The larynx normally contributes up to 25% of total airways resistance. During normal respiration this is adjusted by flow or pressure sensors in the larger airways which alter local airway diameter, increasing resistance during expiration and decreasing it during inspiration[57]. The effects of cricothyroid (CT) and posterior cricoarytenoid (PCA) muscle activity on the vocal cords and on pressure–flow relationships of the larynx have been studied in awake normal subjects[57–62]. This interaction is complex and is thought to be critical in determining the effective compliance and patency of the upper airway[57,58]. The activity of the PCA and probably also the CT precedes inspiration by abduction of the vocal cords and directly increases the laryngeal diameter[62].

The LMA bypasses the narrowed laryngopharyngeal space, providing an unobstructed, low resistance airway. Dead space is approximately 50% less than with the face mask[47], but more than when the trachea is intubated[63]. Work of breathing is similar between the LMA and tracheal tube. It appears that the larger bore of the LMA tube offsets the laryngeal resistance factor[64–69]. Reignier et al have shown that in children aged 6–24 months anesthetized with halothane there is less paradoxic inspiratory movement breathing through the LMA than tracheal tube[70]. Work of breathing with the flexible LMA (FLMA) will be higher since the tube is narrower and longer. It has also been shown that the LMA can accommodate a larger fiberoptic scope (FOS) than either the FLMA or tracheal tube while permitting an acceptable ventilatory flow[71].

Cardiovascular system

The larynx has the greatest afferent nerve supply of all the airways, being largely supplied by fibers from the internal branch of the superior laryngeal nerve[40]. The response to laryngeal pressure and flow receptor stimulation is an increase in upper airway muscle activity. Reflex responses to a number of mechanical and chemical stimuli are also mediated by the superior laryngeal nerve and lead to sympathetic stimulation and rises in blood pressure and tachycardia. Laryngoscopy and subsequent tracheal intubation are associated with a 25–50% rise in blood pressure and a similar increase in heart rate[72]. Slogoff and Keats have shown that tachycardia is the primary cause of myocardial ischemia occurring under anesthesia with hypertension and hypotension as the next most important causes[73]. There is a direct correlation between tachycardia and hypertension and postoperative myocardial infarction[74].

Insertion of the LMA is associated with only a 0–20% rise in blood pressure and heart rate in both adults[75–82] and children[83–85] (Figure 3.1). This is comparable to the face mask and Guedel airway and can be related to the avoidance of sensitive anterior structures on insertion and the lack of instrumentation of the larynx[77]. LMA insertion produces less hemodynamic stress response than fiberoptic guided orotracheal intubation[80]. Plasma concentrations of adrenaline and noradrenaline are higher following tracheal intubation than LMA insertion[86]. Kayashima and Fukutome have shown that the RR wave intervals on the EKG, as measured by the fast Fourier transformation method, and heart rate variability may be good predictors of the hemodynamic response during LMA placement[87]. Fiberoptic guided intubation through the LMA in normal children produces few significant hemodynamic changes[88]. Patients with an LMA require significantly less anesthetic agent to maintain depth of anesthesia than those who are intubated[89–91] and have less hypertension during emergence[86,92,93]. This benefit may extend into the postoperative period with a reduced

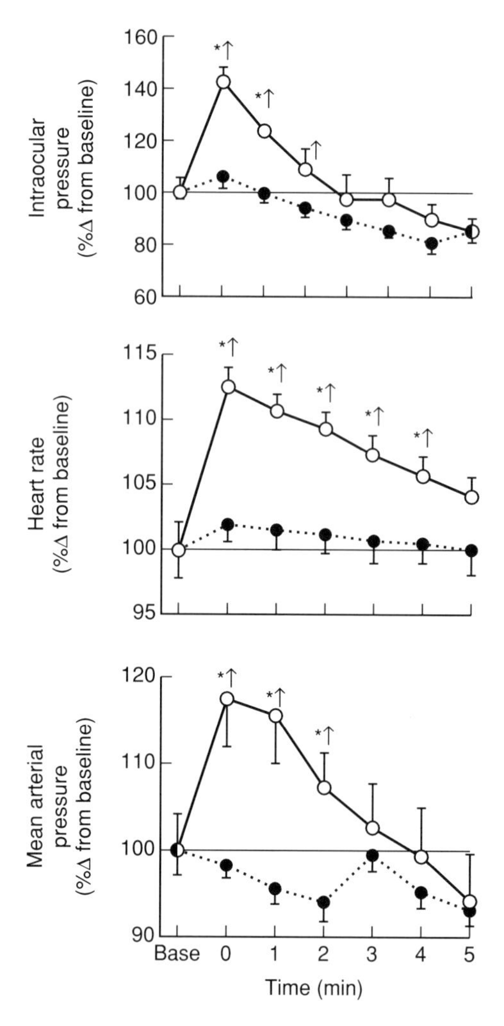

Figure 3.1 Hemodynamic stress response to LMA insertion. Comparison of the percentage change (%Δ) in intraocular pressure, heart rate and mean arterial blood pressure over baseline (Base) values (100%) after the insertion of a laryngeal mask airway (●) or tracheal tube (○). Time zero is the time of insertion of the airway device. Error bars are ± SEM. *$P < 0.05$ versus baseline values. _ $p < 0.05$ versus laryngeal mask group. Reproduced with kind permission of the International Anesthesia Research Society[83].

requirement for postoperative analgesia during recovery[94]. The cardiovascular effects of general anesthetic agents will by inference also be reduced when the LMA is used since lower concentrations will be required. The LMA may offer advantages over the tracheal tube in the anesthetic management of patients with cardiovascular disease such as hypertension[95], ischemic heart disease[96] and acute cerebrovascular disease[97]. The benefits for patients with normal cardiovascular systems are less clear.

Intraocular pressure

The effect of LMA insertion compared with tracheal intubation on intraocular pressure is influenced by the induction agent and whether the eye is normal or not. Sympathetic responses to laryngoscopy and intubation cause a 25% rise in intraocular pressure (IOP) compared with only 5–10% for the LMA when anesthesia is induced with thiopentone[86], etomidate[98] or halothane[83]. When propofol is used neither the tracheal tube nor LMA produce a rise in intraocular pressure in patients with normal eyes[99]. Propofol decreases intraocular pressure compared with thiopentone and following tracheal intubation[100,101]. In patients with glaucoma given propofol, however, there is a rise in intraocular pressure following tracheal intubation, but not following LMA insertion[102]. On recovery from anesthesia, intraocular pressures remain lower with the LMA[86,103]. Intubated patients are also more likely to cough and so increase their IOP more dramatically: one study reported a 30-fold reduction in coughing compared with the tracheal tube on emergence from anesthesia[41].

Intracranial pressure

There are no studies investigating the effect of LMA placement on intracranial pressure (ICP), but Ferson et al have reported use of the LMA as an aid to tracheal intubation in a patient undergoing neurosurgery for a cerebellar tumor with intracranial pressure monitoring in situ (D. Ferson, personal communication, 1996). They found no significant increases in ICP during LMA insertion and only a modest increase (4 mm Hg) during intubation via the LMA.

Monitoring

The supraglottic location of the LMA cuff implies that it is uniquely positioned to detect laryngopharyngeal activity and it has been suggested that it could be used as an indicator of depth of anesthesia in nonparalyzed patients[104]. Vocal cord activity is a commonly used clinical sign of inadequate anesthetic depth in nonintubated patients. Sudden cord closure can be precipitated by intense surgical stimulation[105], but it is possible that milder noxious stimuli may be associated with lesser degrees of cord closure. Subtle glottic movement can be readily observed, and perhaps quantified, during LMA anesthesia without muscle relaxation. An increase in glottic movement can be detected through direct observation of the cords[6], alterations in airways resistance, or by auscultation of abnormal breath sounds by placing a stethoscope over the side of the neck, as described by Brain[106]. If there is a reduction in anesthetic depth, vocal cord activity will increase. If a flow-volume monitor is used, changes in the flow-volume loops may show the alteration in the laryngeal resistor component of the airway. Preliminary work suggests that glottic movement occurs at deeper planes of anesthesia than gross motor response for a fixed noxious stimulus[104].

Pharyngeal muscle movement may be detected by linking the LMA cuff to a pressure transducer. Cuff pressures will tend to increase as anesthesia lightens and muscle activity increases. Sudden rises of over 50 mm Hg have been noted during straining and coughing. However, other factors such as nitrous oxide diffusion into the cuff, warming of cuff gases[33] and changes in head position need also be taken into account.

Capnography and analysis of other airway gases can be readily conducted with the LMA and these correlate well with arterial blood gas values, particularly if the sample is taken from the distal tube[107-112]. Kobayashi et al showed that the discrepancy between end-tidal CO_2 and arterial CO_2 was significantly greater during LMA anesthesia than preoperatively (5.8 versus 10 mm Hg)[113]. There was a positive correlation with $Pa\text{CO}_2$, respiratory rate and volatile concentration and a negative correlation with tidal volume. Chibber et al have shown that, in infants and children weighing >10 kg who are mechanically ventilated via the LMA, end-tidal CO_2 is as accurate an indicator of $Pa\text{CO}_2$ as when patients are ventilated via a tracheal tube[112]. Estimation of $Pa\text{CO}_2$ is more reliable with the LMA than with the face mask, particularly at small tidal volumes[111].

References

1 Brimacombe J, Berry A. Insertion of the laryngeal mask airway – a prospective study of four techniques. *Anaesth Intens Care* 1993;**21**:89–92.

2 Brimacombe J, Newell S, Swainston R, Thompson J. A potential new technique for awake fibreoptic bronchoscopy – use of the laryngeal mask airway. *Med J Aust* 1992;**156**:876–877.

3 Brimacombe J. Laryngeal mask anaesthesia and recurrent swallowing. *Anaesth Intens Care* 1991;**19**:275–276.

4 Nishino T. Swallowing as a protective reflex for the upper respiratory tract. *Anesthesiology* 1993;**79**:588–601.

5 Brain AIJ. *The Intavent laryngeal mask – instruction manual.* London: Intavent, 1991;1–58.

6 Brimacombe J. Laryngoscopy through the LMA – a useful skill to acquire. *Anaesth Intens Care* 1992;**20**:535.

7 Brimacombe J, Berry A. Laryngeal mask airway insertion. A comparison of the standard versus neutral position in normal patients with a view to its use in cervical spine instability. *Anaesthesia* 1993;**48**:670–671.

8 Pennant JH, Pace NA, Gajraj NM. Role of the laryngeal mask airway in the immobile cervical spine. *J Clin Anesth* 1993;**5**:226–230.

9 Ingelfinger FJ. Esophageal motility. *Physiol Rev* 1958;**38**:533–584.

10 Brain AIJ. Modification of laryngeal mask insertion technique in children. *Anesth Analg* 1995;**81**:212.

11 Barker P, Langton JA, Murphy PJ, Rowbotham DJ. Regurgitation of gastric contents during general anaesthesia using the laryngeal mask airway. *Br J Anaesth* 1992;**69**:314–315.

12 Rabey PG, Murphy PJ, Langton JA, Barker P, Rowbotham DJ. Effect of the laryngeal mask airway on lower oesophageal sphincter pressure in patients during general anaesthesia. *Br J Anaesth* 1992;**69**:346–348.

13 Valentine J, Stakes AF, Bellamy MC. Reflux during positive pressure ventilation through the laryngeal mask. *Br J Anaesth* 1994;**74**:543–545.

★ 14 Owens TM, Robertson P, Twomey C, Doyle M, McDonald N, McShane AJ. The incidence of gastroesophageal reflux with the laryngeal mask: a comparison with the facemask using esophageal lumen pH electrodes. *Anesth Analg* 1995;**80**:980–984.

Study of 55 patients using esophageal pH monitoring during LMA compared with face mask anesthesia. Showed that pharyngeal pH similar, but there was a higher incidence of reflux in the mid to lower esophagus with the LMA. This study was subsequently criticized[17,18].

15 Vanner RG. Regurgitation and the laryngeal mask airway. *Br J Anaesth* 1993;**70**:380.

16 Brimacombe J, Berry A. Aspiration pneumonitis and the laryngeal mask airway. *Anesth Analg* 1994;**78**:816.

17 Brimacombe J. Gastroesophageal reflux with the laryngeal mask. *Anesth Analg* 1996;**82**:215.

18 Owens TM, McShane AJ. Gastroesophageal reflux with the laryngeal mask. *Anesth Analg* 1996;**82**:215.

19 Akhtar TM, Street MK. Risk of aspiration with the laryngeal mask. *Br J Anaesth* 1994;**72**:447–450.

20 El Mikatti N, Luthra AD, Healy TEJ, Mortimer AJ. Gastric regurgitation during general anaesthesia in the supine position with the laryngeal and face mask airways. *Br J Anaesth* 1992;**68**:529P–530P (Abstract).

21 Lefort P, Visseaux H, Gabriel R, Palot M, Pire JC. Utilisation du masque larynge pour la coelioscopie. *Ann Fr Anesth Reanim* 1993;**12**:R231 (Abstract).

22 Hogu H, Barlas S, Dogu D, Gelis M, Ozay K, Arikan Z. Regurgitation with laryngeal mask airway (LMA) and endotracheal tube (ETT). *Br J Anaesth* 1995;**74**:14 (Abstract).

★ 23 Joshi GP, Morrison SG, Okonkwo NA, White PF. Continuous hypopharyngeal pH measurements in spontaneously breathing anesthetised outpatients: laryngeal mask airway versus tracheal intubation. *Anesth Analg* 1996;**82**:254–257.

Study of 60 patients in which hypopharyngeal pH was measured during spontaneously breathing anesthesia with the LMA or tracheal tube. There were no episodes of hypopharyngeal regurgitation (pH < 4) in either group.

24 El Mikatti N, Luthra AD, Healy TEJ, Mortimer AJ. Gastric regurgitation during general anaesthesia in different positions with the laryngeal mask airway. *Anaesthesia* 1995;**50**:1053–1055.

25 Lund WS. Deglutition. In: Wright DA, ed. *Scott-Brown otolaryngology basic sciences*. London: Butterworth, 1987;284–295.

★ 26 Vanner RG, Pryle BJ, O'Dwyer JP, Reynolds F. Upper oesophageal sphincter pressure during inhalational anaesthesia. *Anaesthesia* 1992;**47**:950–954.
Study investigating the effect of various maneuvers on upper esophageal sphincter tone. Showed that tone was unaffected by LMA insertion in seven unparalyzed patients. Maintained upper esophageal sphincter tone may account in part for the low incidence of aspiration with the LMA.

27 Cohen S. The pathogenesis of gastroesophageal reflux disease: a challenge in clinical physiology. *Ann Intern Med* 1992;**117**:1051–1052.

28 Joh SJ, Matsura H, Kotani Y, et al. Change in tracheal blood flow during endotracheal intubation. *Acta Anaesthesiol Scand* 1987;**31**:300–304.

29 Seegobin RD, van Hasselt GL. Endotracheal cuff pressure and tracheal mucosal blood flow: endoscopic study of effects of four large volume cuffs. *Br Med J* 1984;**288**:965–968.

30 Lumb AB, Wrigley MW. The effect of nitrous oxide on laryngeal mask cuff pressure. In vitro and in vivo studies. *Anaesthesia* 1992;**47**:320–323.

31 Marjot R. Pressure exerted by the laryngeal mask airway cuff upon the pharyngeal mucosa. *Br J Anaesth* 1993;**70**:25–29.

32 Brimacombe J, Shorney N. The laryngeal mask airway and prolonged balanced anaesthesia. *Can J Anaesth* 1993;**40**:360–364.

33 Brimacombe J, Berry A. Laryngeal mask airway cuff pressure and position during anaesthesia lasting 1–2 hours. *Can J Anaesth* 1994;**41**:589–593.

★ 34 Hamakawa T, Nakamura S, Kawasaki Y. Intracuff pressure of the LM and pressure on the pharynx. *J Clin Anesth (Rinsho-Masui)* 1993;**17**:1165–1167.
Study of 40 patients in which extracuff pressure was measured on the middle part of the outside of the LMA during O_2/N_2O *anesthesia using a PSL-200GA sensor. Shows that extracuff pressure is approximately 25 mm Hg and does not increase despite increases in intracuff pressure. This may explain in part why pharyngeal trauma is uncommon with the LMA despite high intracuff pressures.*

35 Alexander CA, Leach AB. Incidence of sore throats with the laryngeal mask. *Anaesthesia* 1989;**44**:791.

36 Gerber MA, Gastanaduy AS, Buckley JJ, Kaplan EL. Risk of bacteraemia after endotracheal intubation for general anaesthesia. *Southern Med J* 1980;**73**:1478–1480.

37 Cannon LA, Gardner W, Treen L, Litlan GI, Dougherty J. The incidence of bacteraemia associated with emergency intubation – relevance to prophylaxis against endocarditis. *Ohio Medicine* 1990;**86**:596–599.

38 Brimacombe J, Shorney N, Swainston R, Bapty G. The incidence of bacteraemia following laryngeal mask insertion. *Anaesth Intens Care* 1992;**20**:484–486.

39 Stone JM, Karalliedde LD, Carter ML, Cumerland NS. Bacteraemia and insertion of laryngeal mask airways. *Anaesthesia* 1992;**47**:77

40 Sant'Ambrogio G, Mathew OP, Fisher JT, Sant'Ambrogio FB. Laryngeal receptors responding to transmural pressure, airflow and local muscle activity. *Resp Physiol* 1983;**54**:317–330.

41 Thomson KD. The effect of the laryngeal mask airway on coughing after eye surgery under general anaesthetic. *Ophthalmic Surg* 1992;**23**:630–631.

42 Haden RM, Pinnock CA, Campbell RL. The laryngeal mask for intraocular surgery. *Br J Anaesth* 1993;**71**:772

43 White DC. The laryngeal mask – a non-invasive airway. *Eur J Anaesthesiol* 1991;**4**:1–4.

44 Langer A, Hempel V, Ahlhelm T, Heipertz W. Die Kehlkopfmaske bei > 1900 Allgemeinanasthesien – Erfahrungsbericht. *Anaesthesiol Intensivmed Notfalmed Schmerzther* 1993;**28**:156–160.

45 Shnider SM, Papper EM. Anesthesia for the asthmatic patient. *Anesthesiology* 1961;**22**:886.

46 Lew JKL, Spence AA, Elton RA. Cross-sectional study of complications of inhalational anaesthesia in 16995 patients. *Anaesthesia* 1991;**46**:810–815.

47 Langenstein H, Moller F, Krause R, Kluge R, Vogelsang H. Die handhabung der Larynxmaske bei Augenoperationen. *Congress on Anaesthesia in Eye Surgery, Congress-Centrum Stadtpark, Hannover, 10–11 May 1996* (Abstract).

48 Klainer AS, Turndorf H, Wu W, Maewal H, Allender P. Surface alterations due to endotracheal intubation. *Am J Med* 1975;**58**:674–683.

49 Phadhana S, Anger C, von Bommel T, Deitmer T. Die Reaktionen des Flimmerepithels des Respirationstraktes auf eine Intubationsnarkose. *Laryngorhinootologie* 1989;**68**:319–322.

★ 50 Ferrari LR, Goudsouzian NG. The use of the laryngeal mask airway in children with bronchopulmonary dysplasia. *Anesth Analg* 1995;**81**:310–313.
Study of 27 former premature infants with bronchopulmonary dysplasia undergoing general anesthesia for open eye vitrectomy with either the tracheal tube or the LMA. The incidence of postoperative complications was lower in the

LMA group and patients were discharged earlier. Shows the value of the LMA in patients with mild chronic respiratory disease.

51 Stanley GD, Bastianpillai BA, Mulcahy K, Langton JA. Postoperative laryngeal competence. The laryngeal mask airway and tracheal tube compared. *Anaesthesia* 1995;**50**:985–986.

52 Gal TJ. Pulmonary mechanics in normal subjects following endotracheal intubation. *Anesthesiology* 1980;**52**:27–35.

53 Cros AM, Boudey C, Esteben D, Milacic M, Dardel E. Intubation versus masque larynge – incidence des spasmes et des desaturations en per et postoperatoire. *Ann Fr Anesth Reanim* 1994;**12**:R87 (Abstract).

54 Webster AC, Reid WD, Siebert LF, Taylor MD. Laryngeal mask airway for anaesthesia for cryopexy in low birth weight infants. *Can J Anaesth* 1995;**42**:361–362.

55 Lonnqvist PA. Successful use of laryngeal mask airway in low-weight expremature infants with bronchopulmonary dysplasia undergoing cryotherapy for retinopathy of the premature. *Anesthesiology* 1995;**83**:422–424.

56 Mitzner W, Blosser S, Yager D, Wagner E. Effect of bronchial smooth muscle contraction on lung compliance. *J Appl Physiol* 1992;**72**:158–167.

57 Tully A, Brantiscano T, Loring SH, Engel LA. Influence of posterior cricoarytenoid muscle activity on pressure-flow relationship of the larynx. *J Appl Physiol* 1991;**70**:2252–2258.

58 Wheatley JR, Kelly WT, Tully A, Engel LA. Pressure-diameter relationships of the upper airway in awake supine subjects. *J Appl Physiol* 1991;**70**:2242–2251.

59 Brantiscano T, Collett PW, Engel LA. Respiratory movements of the vocal cords. *J Appl Physiol* 1983;**54**:1269–1276.

60 Wheatley JR, Brantiscano T, Engel LA. Cricothyroid muscle responses to increased chemical drive in awake normal humans. *J Appl Physiol* 1991;**70**:2233–2241.

61 Wheatley JR, Brantiscano T, Engel LA. Respiratory-related activity of cricothyroid muscle in awake normal humans. *J Appl Physiol* 1991;**70**:2226–2232.

62 Brantiscano T, Dodd DS, Engel LA. Respiratory activity of posterior cricoarytenoid muscle and vocal cords in humans. *J Appl Physiol* 1984;**57**:1143–1149.

63 Asai T, Morris S. The laryngeal mask airway: its features, effects and role. *Can J Anaesth* 1994;**41**:930–960.

64 Bhatt SB, Kendall AP, Lin ES, Oh TE. Resistance and additional inspiratory work imposed by the laryngeal mask airway. A comparison with tracheal tubes. *Anaesthesia* 1992;**47**:343–347.

65 Al-Hasani A. Resistance to constant air flow imposed by the standard laryngeal mask, the reinforced laryngeal mask airway and RAE tubes. *Br J Anaesth* 1993;**71**:594–596.

66 Ooi R, Soni N. The work of ventilation imposed by the laryngeal mask airway. *Anesthesiology* 1993;**79**:A499 (Abstract).

67 Berry A, Verghese C. Changes in pulmonary mechanics during IPPV with the laryngeal mask airway compared to the tracheal tube. *Anesth Analg* 1994;**78**:S38 (Abstract).

★ 68 Boisson-Bertrand D, Hannhart B, Rousselot JM, Duvivier C, Quilici N, Peslin R. Comparative effects of laryngeal mask and tracheal tube on total respiratory resistance in anaesthetised patients. *Anaesthesia* 1994;**49**:846–849.
Study comparing work of breathing of the LMA with that of the tracheal tube in 10 patients. Found that work of breathing was similar despite the fact that glottic resistance (which accounts for 25% of airway resistance) is not bypassed by the LMA.

69 Pothmann W, Reissmann H. Upper airway resistance with laryngeal mask airway and endotracheal tube. *Anesthesiology* 1995;**83**:A493 (Abstract).

70 Reignier J, Ameur MB, Ecoffey C. Spontaneous ventilation with halothane in children. A comparison between endotracheal tube and laryngeal mask airway. *Anesthesiology* 1995;**83**:674–678.

71 Brimacombe J, Dunbar-Reid K. The effect of introducing fibreoptic bronchoscopes on gas flow in laryngeal masks and tracheal tubes. *Anaesthesia* 1996;**51**:923–928.

72 Ng WS. Pathophysiological effects of tracheal intubation. In: Latto IP, Rosen M, eds. *Difficulties in tracheal intubation.* London: Baillière Tindall, 1984;12–35.

73 Slogoff S, Keats AS. Does perioperative myocardial ischemia lead to postoperative myocardial infarction? *Anesthesiology* 1985;**62**:107–114.

74 Slogoff S, Keats AS. Further observations on perioperative myocardial ischemia. *Anesthesiology* 1986;**65**:539–542.

75 Braude N, Clements EA, Hodges UM, Andrews BP. The pressor response and laryngeal mask insertion. A comparison with tracheal intubation. *Anaesthesia* 1989;**44**:551–554.

76 Wilson IG, Fell D, Robinson SL, Smith G. Cardiovascular responses to insertion of the laryngeal mask. *Anaesthesia* 1992;**47**:300–302.

77 Hickey S, Cameron AE, Asbury AJ. Cardiovascular response to insertion of Brain's laryngeal mask. *Anaesthesia* 1990;**45**:629–633.

78 Wood MLB, Forrest ETS. Haemodynamic response to insertion of laryngeal mask. *Anaesthesia* 1989;**44**:1001.

79 Smigovec E, Sakic K, Tripkovic B. [The laryngeal mask – news in orthopedic anesthesia]. *Lijec Vjesn* 1993;**115**:166–169.

80 Imai M, Matsumura C, Hanaoka Y, Kemmotsu O. Comparison of cardiovascular responses to airway management: using a new adaptor, laryngeal mask insertion, or conventional laryngoscopic intubation. *J Clin Anesth* 1995;7:14–18.

81 Teles ASS, Gerez MC, Fortuna A. Alteracoes cardiovasculares na colocacao da mascara laringea (ML): inducao com etomidato e alfentanyl. *Rev Brasil Anestesiol* 1992;**42**:CBA 011.

82 Jeong J, Yang H, Cho H. Clinical investigation of laryngeal mask airway. *J Kor Soc Anesthesiol* 1993;**25**:708–718.

★ **83** Watcha MF, White PF, Tychsen L, Steven JL. Comparative effects of laryngeal mask airway and endotracheal tube insertion on intraocular pressure in children. *Anesth Analg* 1992;**75**:355–360.
Study comparing the cardiovascular and intraocular pressure responses to LMA insertion versus tracheal intubation in 41 children. Showed the LMA to be superior.

84 Fujii Y, Tanaka H, Toyooka H. [Effects of laryngeal mask airway on circulation and on incidence of postoperative sore throat and hoarseness]. *Masui* 1993;**42**:1559–1562.

85 Jung K, Cho C, Yang H. Clinical investigation of the laryngeal mask airway in children. *J Kor Soc Anesthesiol* 1993;**26**:763–769.

86 Lamb K, James MFM, Janicki PK. The laryngeal mask airway for intraocular surgery: effects on intraocular pressure and stress responses. *Br J Anaesth* 1992;**69**:143–147.

87 Kayashima K, Fututome T. Heart rate variability and hemodynamic response during placement of the laryngeal mask airway. *11th World Congress of Anesthesiology, Sydney, 14–20 April 1996, Abstract Handbook* p.181 (Abstract).

88 Heard CMB, Caldicott LD, Fletcher JE, Selsby DS. Fiberoptic guided endotracheal intubation via the laryngeal mask airway in paediatric patients. A report of a series of cases. *Anesth Analg* 1996;**82**:1287–1289.

89 Taguchi M, Watanabe S, Asakura N, Inomata S. End-tidal sevoflurane concentrations for laryngeal mask airway insertion and for tracheal intubation in children. *Anesthesiology* 1994;**81**:628–631.

90 Fiani N, Scandella C, Giolitto N, Prudhomme G, Leon A. Comparison of reinforced laryngeal mask vs endotracheal tube in tonsillectomy. *Anesthesiology* 1994;**81**:A491 (Abstract).

91 Wilkins CJ, Cramp PG, Staples J, Stevens WC. Comparison of the anesthetic requirement for tolerance of laryngeal mask airway and endotracheal tube. *Anesth Analg* 1992;**75**:794–797.

92 Webster AC, Morley-Forster PK, Dain S, et al. Anaesthesia for adenotonsillectomy: a comparison between tracheal intubation and the armoured laryngeal mask airway. *Can J Anaesth* 1993;**40**:1171–1177.

93 Joshi GP, Morrison SG, Gajraj NM, Okonkwo N, White PF. Hemodynamic changes during emergence from anesthesia: use of the laryngeal mask airway vs endotracheal tube. *Anesth Analg* 1994;**78**:S185 (Abstract).

94 Cork RC, Depa RM, Standen JR. Prospective comparison of use of the laryngeal mask and endotracheal tube for ambulatory surgery. *Anesth Analg* 1994;**79**:719–727.

95 Fujii Y, Tanaka H, Toyooka H. Circulatory responses to laryngeal mask airway insertion or tracheal intubation in normotensive and hypertensive patients. *Can J Anaesth* 1995;**42**:32–36.

96 Llagunes J, Rodriguez-Hesles C, Aguar F. Laryngeal mask airway in cardiac surgery. *Can J Anaesth* 1994;**41**:1016.

97 Ito N, Aikawa N, Hori S, et al. Laryngeal mask airway in acute cerebrovascular disease. *Lancet* 1992;**339**:69.

98 Holden R, Morsman CD, Butler J, Clark GS, Hughes DS, Bacon PJ. Intra-ocular pressure changes using the laryngeal mask airway and tracheal tube. *Anaesthesia* 1991;**46**:922–924.

99 Akhtar TM, McMurray P, Kerr WJ, Kenny GNC. A comparison of laryngeal mask airway with tracheal tube for intra-ocular ophthalmic surgery. *Anaesthesia* 1992;**47**:668–671.

100 Mirakhur RK, Shepherd WFI. Intraocular pressure changes with propofol ('Diprivan'): comparison with thiopentone. *Postgrad Med J* 1985;**61**:41–44.

101 Mirakhur RK, Elliot P, Shepherd WFI, Archer DB. Intraocular pressure changes during induction of anaesthesia and tracheal intubation. A comparison of thiopentone and propofol followed by vecuronium. *Anaesthesia* 1988;**43**:54–57.

102 Barclay K, Wall T, Wareham K, Asai T. Intra-ocular pressure changes in patients with glaucoma – comparison between the laryngeal mask airway and tracheal tube. *Anaesthesia* 1994;**49**:159–162.

103 Myint Y, Singh AK, Peacock JE, Padfield A. Changes in intra-ocular pressure during general anaesthesia. A comparison of spontaneous breathing through a laryngeal mask with positive pressure ventilation through a tracheal tube. *Anaesthesia* 1995;**50**:126–129.

104 Brimacombe J, Berry A. Monitoring anesthetic depth during laryngeal mask anesthesia. *J Clin Anesth* 1994;**6**:525–526.

105 Brewer N, Luckhardt AB, Lees WM, Bryant DS. Reflex closure of glottis by stimulation of visceral afferent nerves. *Anesth Analg* 1934;**13**:257–259.

106 Brain AIJ. Studies on the laryngeal mask: first, learn the art. *Anaesthesia* 1991;**46**:417–427.

107 Ivens D, Verborgh C. Is correlation of arterial and end-tidal carbon dioxide pressure during inhalational anaesthesia better with laryngeal mask as compared to face mask? *Br J Anaesth* 1993;**70**:9S (Abstract).

108 Hicks IR, Soni NC, Shephard JN. Comparison of end-tidal and arterial carbon dioxide measurements during anaesthesia with the laryngeal mask airway. *Br J Anaesth* 1993;**71**:734–735.

109 Spahr-Schopfer IA, Bissonnette B, Hartley EJ. Capnometry and the paediatric laryngeal mask airway. *Can J Anaesth* 1993;**40**:1038–1043.

110 Newell S, Brimacombe J. A modified tracheal tube mount for sampling gases from the distal shaft of the laryngeal mask airway. *J Clin Anesth* 1995;444–445.

111 Ivens D, Verborgh C, Phan Thi H, Camu F. The quality of breathing and capnography during laryngeal mask and facemask ventilation. *Anaesthesia* 1995;**50**:858–862.

112 Chibber AK, Kolano JW, Roberts WA. Relationship between end-tidal and arterial carbon dioxide with laryngeal mask airways and endotracheal tubes in children. *Anesth Analg* 1996;**82**:247–250.

113 Kobayashi Y, Iwasaki H, Namiki A. Discrepancy between end-tidal and arterial carbon dioxide pressures during sevoflurane anesthesia with the laryngeal mask airway. *11th World Congress of Anesthesiology, Sydney, 14–20 April 1996, Abstract Handbook* p.622 (Abstract).

4 Device details

The standard laryngeal mask airway

The currently available LMA is composed of medical-grade silicone rubber and is reuseable, being sterilized by steam autoclaving (Figure 4.1). It consists of a curved tube opening at the distal end into the lumen of a small elliptical mask that has an inflatable outer rim. Two vertical elastic bars, mask aperture bars, are present across the opening to prevent obstruction of the tube by the epiglottis. The flexibility of the mask aperture bars does not limit the diameter of instrumentation passed through the LMA tube. Proximally the tube is joined to a standard polysulfone connector. The tube is attached

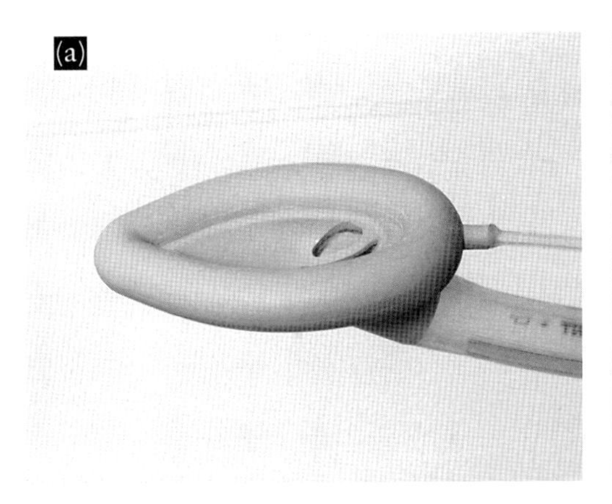
(a)

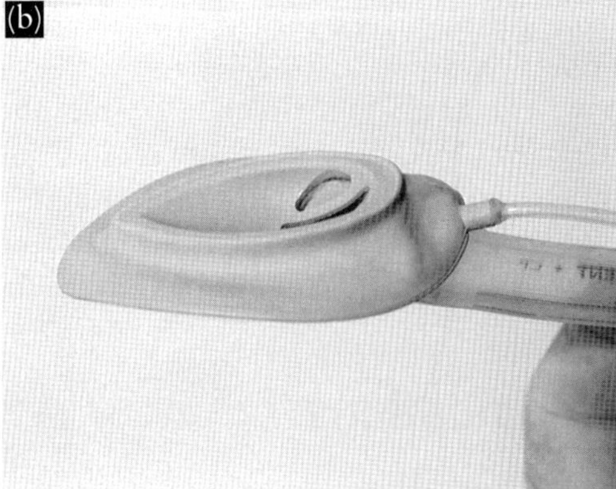
(b)

Figure 4.1 The adult LMA with cuff (a) inflated and (b) deflated.

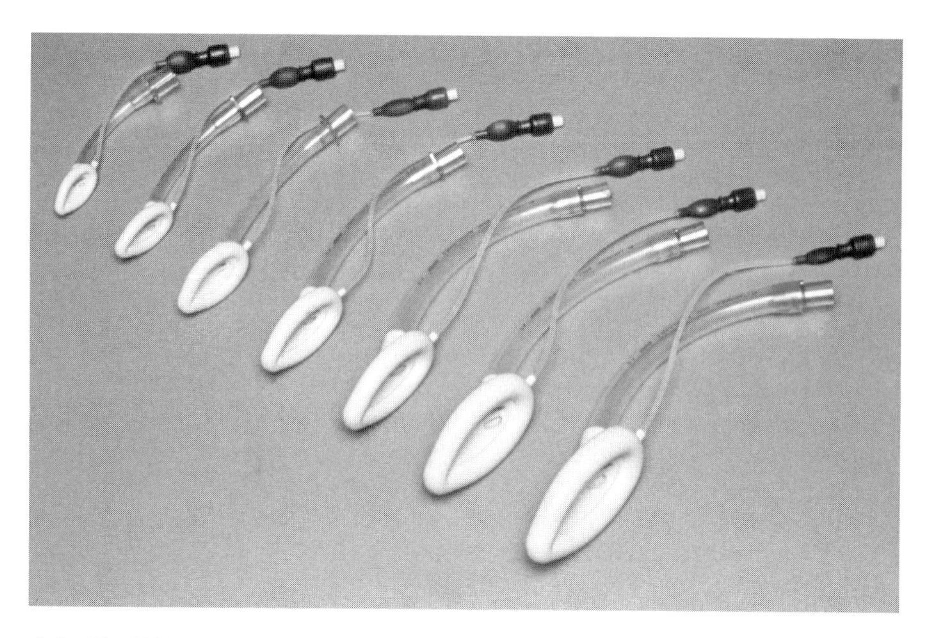

Figure 4.2 The LMA is currently available in seven sizes, from neonates to large adults.

to the back of the mask at an angle of 30 degrees. This angle was chosen because it was found to be the optimal angle for tracheal intubation via the LMA[1]. A black line runs longitudinally along the posterior curvature of the shaft to aid in orienting the tube in situ. A pilot tube and self-sealing pilot balloon are attached to the surface of the inflatable rim. The valve is made from polypropylene and has a metallic spring (not metallic in the magnetic resonance imaging version). There is no latex in any part of the LMA. The LMA is currently available in seven different sizes for use in patients from neonates to large adults (Figure 4.2).

The flexible laryngeal mask airway

The flexible laryngeal mask airway (FLMA) (called 'reinforced LMA' in UK) was specifically designed for use in ear, nose and throat (ENT), head and neck, and dental surgery, and was first described by Alexander in 1990[2]. It consists of a normal LMA bowl connected to a floppy, flexometallic tube which has a narrower bore than the standard LMA and is relatively crush-proof[2,3] (Figure 4.3). As it is of narrow gauge and can be moved easily within the mouth, it provides better surgical access than the standard LMA during head and neck surgery. It became commercially available in 1992 and is available in all sizes except size 1 and 1.5.

Modifications

Two other modifications have been developed by the UK manufacturer which extend the range of use of the LMA: a short tube LMA (2 cm shorter than the standard device)

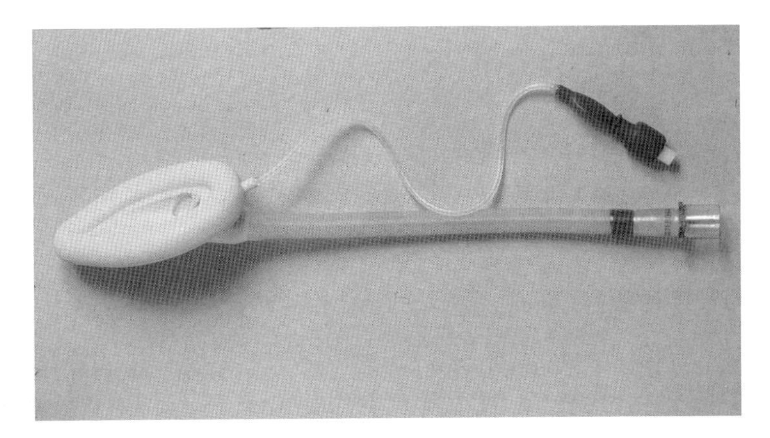

Figure 4.3 The flexible laryngeal mask airway.

to facilitate tracheal intubation (UK only) and color coded LMAs with nonmetallic valves for magnetic resonance imaging (MRI)[4]. A dedicated intubating LMA (ILM) with a wide bore tube and guiding handle should become commercially avalable in 1997 (see Chapter 17, *Future modifications*).

Accessory equipment

A wide variety of accessory equipment has been described to facilitate use of the LMA to aid cuff deflation[5], placement[6–15], removal[16–20], fixation[21–26], monitoring[27–29], prevention of kinking[30] or biting[21,31–36], or to facilitate intubation via the LMA[37–46] or function as a throat pack[26,47]. There have been several suggestions for providing supplementary oxygen during recovery including a modified Bain's circuit[48], a T-piece[49,50], a Portex Thermovent T[51] and a pediatric breathing circuit[52,53] (Table 4.1).

Diffusion of gases

The silicone cuff of the LMA is permeable to a variety of gases, depending on their solubility in silicone and their partial pressure[56]. Carbon dioxide and nitrous oxide readily diffuse through the membrane whereas oxygen and nitrogen diffuse more slowly (Figure 4.4). There have been no studies directly measuring the permeability to different volatile agents, but it is likely that they will also diffuse rapidly. When the LMA cuff is filled with air in vitro it gradually deflates[57] (Figure 4.5). Similarly the fully evacuated LMA cuff will spontaneously re-inflate over several hours, reinforcing the fact that the cuff must be fully deflated prior to autoclaving[58] (Figure 4.6). During oxygen/nitrous oxide (O_2/N_2O) anesthesia, nitrous oxide rapidly diffuses into the air-filled cuff causing a rise in cuff pressure[56,57,59–69] (Figure 4.7). It has been suggested that cuff pressure can be controlled during O_2/N_2O anesthesia by inflating the cuff with a similar O_2/N_2O mixture[70]. This technique works well for the tracheal tube[71], but there are too many variable factors for a given concentration of nitrous oxide to stabilize

Table 4.1 Accessory equipment

Bite block
- bite guard[34]
- silicone rubber cylinders[36]
- translucent PVC tubing[32,33]
- tracheal tube holder[21]
- U-shaped aluminum rod[35]

Deflation tool[5]

Fixation
- circle anesthetic breathing system[24]
- dormett bandage[23]
- fixation knot[22]
- short flexible silicone hose[25]
- tracheal tube holder[21]
- modified 'V-pack' (Dentmed Ltd, Bristol, UK)[26]

Insertion aids
- Dingley's insertion tool[10] (Portex, UK)
- J-forceps[12]
- laryngoscope[6]
- modified Magill's forceps (FLMA)[13]
- modified stylet (FLMA)
- skid[7]
- stylet (FLMA)[8,9]
- sugar spoon[11]
- tracheal tube (FLMA)[14]

Intubation aids
- bougie[44]
- exchange catheter[39,40]
- rectal tube[37]
- hollow bougie[38]
- extender[54]
- guide tube[43]
- PVC tube[41]
- two membrane-covered elbow connectors[45]
- guide wire[44,46]

Kinking prevention
- armored tube[30]

Monitoring
- butterfly needle tubing (distal capnography)[28]
- esophageal detector device[27]
- self-inflating bulb[29]

Throat pack
- suction catheter between stem and cuff[47]
- foam 'V-pack'[26]

Recovery – oxygenation
- modified Bain's circuit[48]
- T-piece[49,50]
- Portex Thermovent T[51]
- Pediatric breathing circuit[52]

Removal aids (following tracheal intubation)
- extenders[17–20]
- Magill's forceps[55]
- Bulldog forceps[20]

LMA cuff pressure[59] (Figure 4.8). There is evidence that minimizing cuff pressure reduces the incidence of sore throat[66,69]. Epstein et al have determined the elastance of the LMA both in vitro and in vivo[65] (Table 4.2). The authors considered that the diffusion of N_2O into the cuff was not a cause for clinical concern. The inventor's advice is to keep intracuff pressures in the region of 60 cm H_2O for all sizes[72].

Table 4.2 LMA elastance in vitro and in vivo

LMA size	*In vitro volume range (ml)*	*In vitro elastance (mm Hg ml^{-1})*	*In vivo elastance (mm ml^{-1})*
1	4–8	45.4 ± 1.3	Not done
2	8–15	22.4 ± 0.6	21.9 ± 3.1
2.5	12–20	19.0 ± 0.1	17.6 ± 2.2
3	21–33	11.8 ± 0.1	Not done
4	30–60	6.00 ± 0.0	Not done

Reproduced with permission from the *Journal of Clinical Anesthesia*[65].

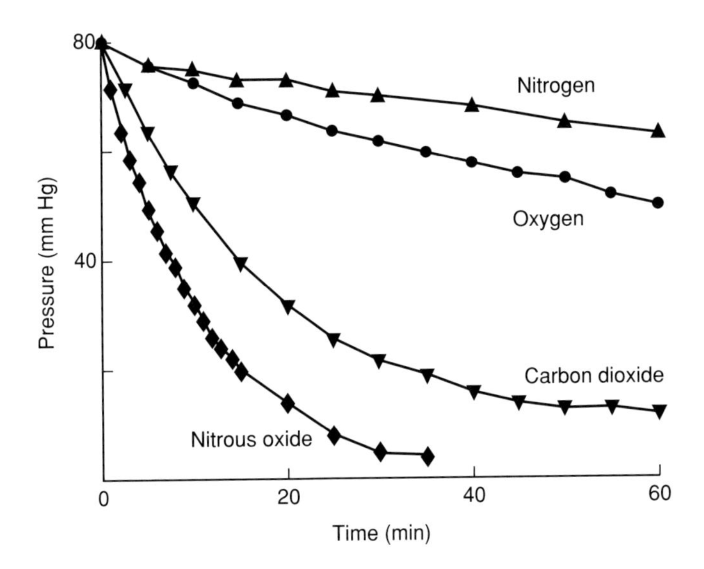

Figure 4.4 Pressure changes with the same gas both inside and outside the LMA cuff, reflecting ability of gases to diffuse across the LMA cuff wall down a pressure gradient of 80 mm Hg. Reproduced with permission from *Anaesthesia*[56].

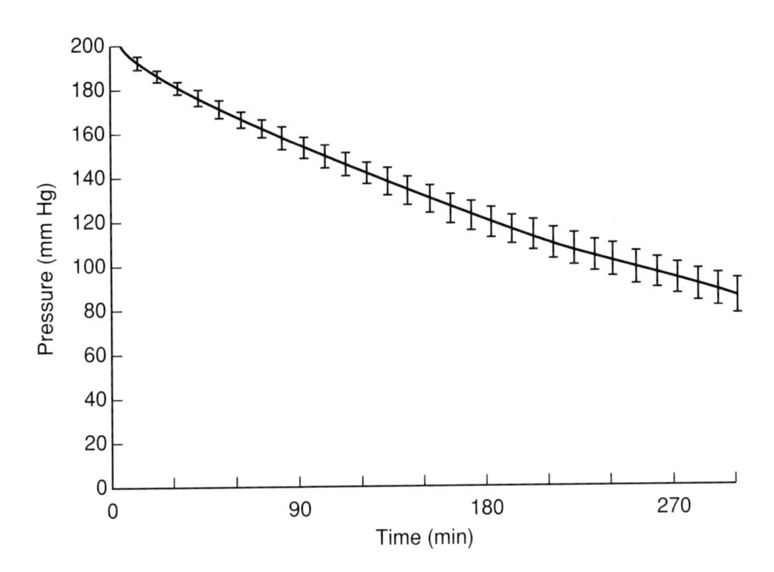

Figure 4.5 Spontaneous deflation characteristics. Reproduced with permission from the Canadian Society of Anaesthetists.[57]

Magnetic resonance imaging

Magnetic resonance imaging presents particular problems for the anesthesiologist in that monitoring and airway maintenance must be done from a remote location[73]. Laryngoscopes are magnetically attracted to the scanner and may be difficult to use.

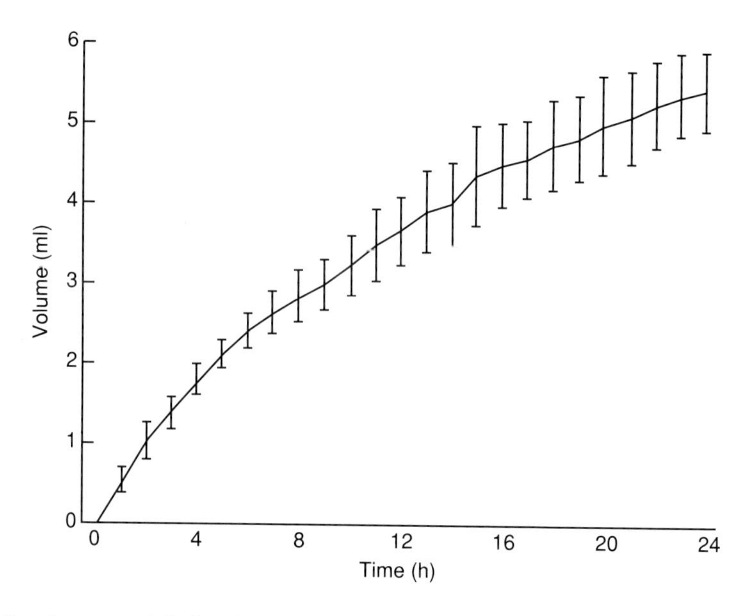

Figure 4.6 Spontaneous re-inflation characteristics. Reproduced with permission from the Canadian Society of Anaesthetists.[58]

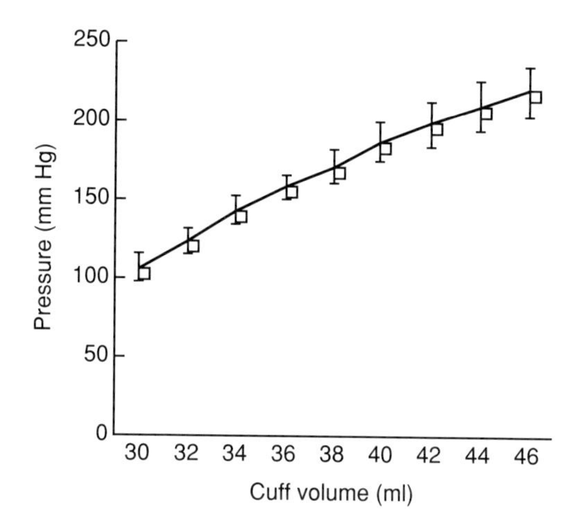

Figure 4.7 Cuff pressure increases as nitrous oxide concentration in the cuff increases during anesthesia. Reproduced with permission from the Canadian Society of Anaesthetists.[57]

The LMA contains no ferromagnetic components although there is a tiny metallic spring in the valve which can interfere with scanning[74]. A color coded version of the LMA is available in the UK with a nonmetallic valve[4]. The LMA is unsuitable if magnetic resonance spectroscopy is performed since the resonance of some silicone-containing materials is identical to that of human tissue[75]. The flexible LMA produces a distorted image along the tube and some tissue distortion further out and is unsuitable for MRI scanning[76].

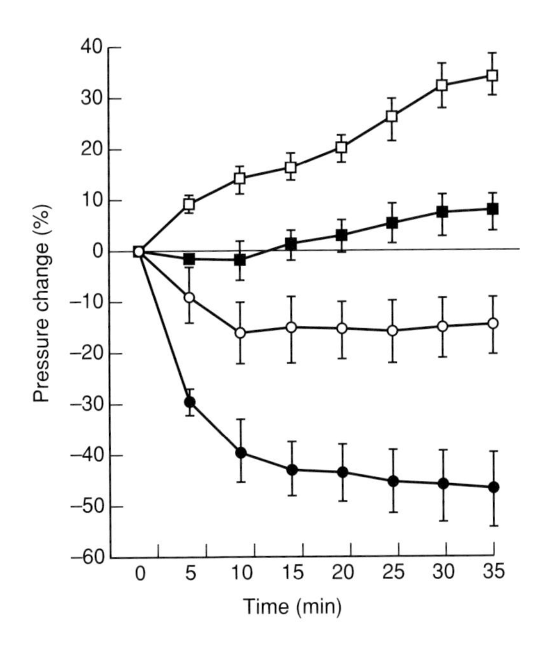

Figure 4.8 Influence of adding various concentrations of nitrous oxide on cuff pressure during N_2O/O_2 anaesthesia. Reproduced with permission from the American Society of Anesthesiologists.[59]
Key: □ = air; ■ =33% N_2O; ○ = 50% N_2O; ● = 66% N_2O.

Laser

The LMA and FLMA are constructed from silicone rubber, which contains silica fillers that provide high temperature resistance and some flame retardation. The 'ash' produced at the impact site is the silica reinforcing filler remaining after the polymer has burnt away. Silicone rubber has some fire retardant properties and has been used to manufacture laser resistant tracheal tubes[77]. Published data about the incendiary characteristics of the LMA/FLMA are limited. Early reports suggested that the LMA tube is resistant to CO_2 lasers at power densities below $1.2–2.25 \times 10^3$ W cm^{-2} [78,79], but that 1.2×10^4 W cm^{-2} produces immediate ignition[78] (Figure 4.9). McCulloch et al showed that the LMA could not be ignited or penetrated with the flash-pumped dye laser at an energy density of 7 J cm^{-2} used for port wine stains[80].

At power densities of less than 4.7×10^3 W cm^{-2}, the LMA/FLMA are noticeably more resistant to the CO_2 laser than are PVC tubes. At 2.25×10^3 W cm^{-2}, the power density used for laser pharyngoplasty[81], the LMA and FLMA tubing could not be ignited. Interestingly, the Laser Shield tracheal tube (Xomed, Inc., Laser Shield, USA), which is made from silicone rubber, ignites after 2–6 s at a power density of 2.6×10^3 W cm^{-2} [77], suggesting that the LMA/FLMA is more resistant to laser attack. This may be related to the increased thickness of the LMA/FLMA tubing. By comparison, tracheal tubes wrapped in stainless steel and foil are unaffected by power densities of up to 1.9×10^4 W cm^{-2} after 1 min of continuous laser exposure[82]. The weakest point of the LMA is the cuff, which is penetrated at 3–5 s at 2.25×10^3 W cm^{-2}. Further studies are required to confirm these data and assess the resistance of the LMA to Nd-YAG and other lasers.

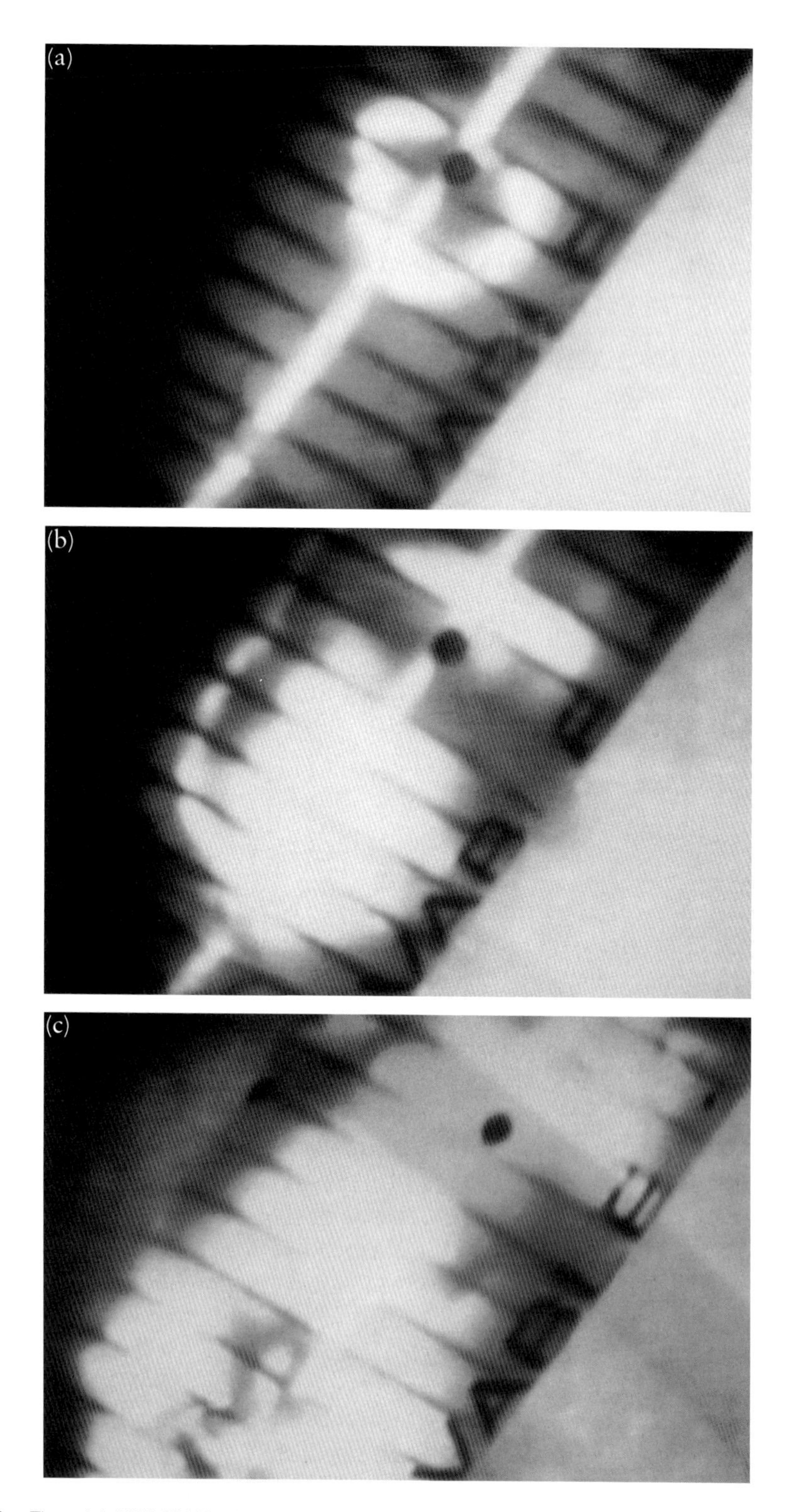

Figure 4.9 The adult LMA/FLMA tube is resistant to CO_2 laser strike at power densities below $1.2–2.25 \times 10^3$ W cm^{-2}. At 1.2×10^4 W cm^{-2} there is immediate ignition. Progressive blowtorch fire (a–c).

Life expectancy/cost-effectiveness

The LMA may be re-used within the manufacturer's warranty (UK only) up to 40 times, but many authors report its use when recycled 200–250 times[83,84]. Wat et al studied the longevity of 20 LMAs and found the average number of uses per device to be 92[85]. Four of the devices were lost or discarded. The lifespan of the LMA is prolonged by careful use, strict adherence to cleaning and sterilization procedures, and by avoiding forceful removal of the device through partially clenched teeth. As with any re-usable device, careful performance of the recommended pre-use checks is the only reliable means of ensuring that it is safe to use, irrespective of the number of re-uses. It may be a problem to keep track of how many usage cycles an individual LMA has undergone. Verification of the number of uses is possible by documenting the serial number of each LMA, which is printed near the connector end, and noting each time the LMA is autoclaved. The UK company commissioned an independent study on the LMA by the Rubber and Plastics Research Association (Rapra) (UK) which showed that tear strength of the airway tube dropped from 3.46 N mm^{-1} at 10 uses to 1.09 N mm^{-1} at 40 uses and that the curing effect of repeat autoclaving progressively hardens the silicon cuff, the modulus increasing from 1.16 MPa to 1.67 MPa after 40 uses (personal communication, Rapra). Silicone has an indefinite shelf life. In practice mechanical, chemical and thermal stresses are the factors responsible for deterioration. Maroof has suggested using a stylet to increase the life expectancy of the aging LMA by stiffening the LMA tube[86]. This is not recommended since, even if the stylet aids placement, a defective LMA will be left in situ which is more likely to kink and may compromise patient care[87,88]. McLure has reported damage to the LMA cuff by a sharp metal post protruding from an extensively decayed tooth[89].

There can be few countries where the cost of medical care is not becoming increasingly difficult to reconcile with perceived acceptable standards. In intensive care and anesthesiology considerable advances in sophisticated monitoring equipment have played no small part in the acceleration of costs in this field which has been accepted almost without question even where the benefits are unproven[90,91]. It may be too early to make a meaningful cost–benefit analysis of the LMA, but several groups have attempted to quantify its cost-effectiveness. It has been suggested that if the LMA is only re-used 30 times it will prove to be financially and environmentally beneficial compared with disposable face masks and tracheal tubes[70]. Further aspects to cost-saving are avoidance of drugs which would have been used to achieve intubation[92], low or minimal flow anesthesia[93], reduced intraoperative anesthetic requirements, reduced emergence times compared with the tracheal tube[94], a potential increase in patient turnover[95], a reduced incidence of postoperative morbidity (sore throat, suxamethonium pains) and reduced postoperative analgesic requirements[96]. Langenstein et al showed that the time spent in the postanesthesia care unit (PACU) was reduced in children undergoing eye surgery with the LMA compared with the tracheal tube[97]. Joshi et al showed the LMA equally cost-effective to the tracheal tube if it is used > 10 times as an alternative to a vecuronium technique[98]. Use of suxamethonium greatly reduces the cost of tracheal tube anesthesia, and the LMA only becomes cost equal after 150 uses[98], but this does not take into account the cost to the patient of suxamethonium pains. Macario et al performed an in-depth cost analysis of the LMA for elective surgery in adult outpatients taking into account many of the above factors[99]. They found that if the LMA was used 40 times for more than 40 min it was a cost-efficient airway in this setting. This finding does not change if the cost of neuromuscular blockade or the incidence of airway-related complications is varied over a clinically relevant range. Wat et al showed that the LMA was cost-effective compared with use of a tracheal tube and nondepolarizing agent after only 10 uses per device[85]. However, when compared with a tracheal tube with a depolarizing muscle relaxant, 40 uses are required per LMA device. The cost-effectiveness of making the LMA available on all resuscitation carts has been questioned by Mansfield and Miller[100]. It has been suggested that pretreating patients with midazolam may facilitate induction with thiopentone and thus reduce costs by avoiding propofol[101]. A cheaper disposable LMA may be more appropriate in the context of emergency medicine and prototypes are currently undergoing trials in the UK.

References

1 Brain AIJ. The development of the laryngeal mask – a brief history of the invention, early clinical studies and experimental work from which the laryngeal mask evolved. *Eur J Anaesthesiol* 1991;**4**:5–17.

★ 2 Alexander CA. A modified Intavent laryngeal mask for ENT and dental anaesthesia. *Anaesthesia* 1990;**45**:892–893.
First description of the flexible LMA. Reports its use in 20 patients undergoing molar extraction or tonsillectomy.

3 Brain AIJ. *The role of the reinforced tube laryngeal mask.* London: Intavent, 1992.

4 Asai T, Morris S. The laryngeal mask airway: its features, effects and role. *Can J Anaesth* 1994;**41**:930–960.

5 Brimacombe J, Brain AIJ, Branagan H, Spry M, Schofield J. Optimal shape of the laryngeal mask cuff: the influence of three deflation techniques. *Anaesthesia* 1996;**51**:673–676.

6 Chow BF, Lewis M, Jones SE. Laryngeal mask airway in children: insertion technique. *Anaesthesia* 1991;**46**:590–591.

7 Harding JB. A 'skid' for easier insertion of the laryngeal mask airway. *Anaesthesia* 1993;**48**:80.

8 Williams PJ, Bailey PM. Insertion technique for reinforced laryngeal mask airway and its use in recovery. *Anaesthesia* 1993;**48**:733–734.

9 Asai T, Stacey M, Barclay K. Stylet for reinforced laryngeal mask airway. *Anaesthesia* 1993;**48**:636.

10 Dingley J, Whitehead MJ. A comparative study of sore throat with the laryngeal mask airway. *Anaesthesia* 1994;**49**:251–254.

11 Rabenstein K. Alternative techniques for laryngeal mask insertion. *Anaesthesia* 1994;**49**:80–81.

12 Omi A, Fukuhara T, Isshiki A, Arakawa K, Goto H. Effectiveness of the J-shaped LMA-holding forceps (J-forceps) for LMA insertion. *Anesthesiology* 1994;**81**:A627 (Abstract).

13 Welsh BE. Use of a modified Magill's forceps to place a flexible laryngeal mask. *Anaesthesia* 1995;**50**:1002–1003.

14 Palmer JHM. Introducing the re-inforced laryngeal mask airway. *Anaesthesia* 1994;**49**:1098.

15 Welsh BE. A modified placement stilette. *Today's Anaesthetist* 1995;129.

16 Chadd GD, Crane DL, Phillips RM, Tunell WP. Extubation and reintubation guided by the laryngeal mask airway in a child with the Pierre Robin syndrome. *Anesthesiology* 1992;**76**:640–641.

17 Chadd GD, Walford AJ, Crane DL. The 3.5/4.5 modification for fiberscope-guided tracheal intubation using the laryngeal mask airway. *Anesth Analg* 1992;**75**:307–308.

18 Reynolds PI, O'Kelly SW. Fiberoptic intubation and the laryngeal mask airway. *Anesthesiology* 1993;**79**:1144.

19 Zagnoev M, McCloskey J, Martin T. Fiberoptic intubation via the laryngeal mask airway. *Anesth Analg* 1994;**78**:813–814.

20 Breen PH. Simple technique to remove laryngeal mask airway 'guide' after endotracheal intubation. *Anesth Analg* 1996;**82**:1302.

21 Worsley MH, Howie CC. Fixation of the laryngeal mask airway. *Anaesthesia* 1990;**45**:1001.

22 Nott MR. A tie for the laryngeal mask airway. *Anaesthesia* 1993;**48**:1013.

23 Conacher ID. A method of fixing of laryngeal mask airways. *Anaesthesia* 1993;**48**:638.

24 Bignell S, Brimacombe J. LMA stability and fixation. *Anaesth Intens Care* 1994;**22**:745.

25 Baum J, Sachs G. The laryngeal mask airway – fixation, gags and stability. *Anaesthesiol Intensivmed Notfalmed Schmerzther* 1995;**30**:130.

26 Christie IW. A means of stabilising laryngeal mask airways during dental procedures. *Anaesthesia* 1996;**51**:604.

27 Ainsworth QP, Calder I. The oesophageal detector device and the laryngeal mask. *Anaesthesia* 1990;**45**:794.

28 Newell S, Brimacombe J. A modified tracheal tube mount for sampling gases from the distal shaft of the laryngeal mask airway. *J Clin Anesth* 1995;**7**:444–445.

29 Wafai Y, Salem MR, Tartaglione A, Joseph NJ. Facilitation of positioning of the laryngeal mask airway by the self-inflating bulb. *Anesthesiology* 1994;**81**:A628 (Abstract).

30 Wilson IG, Eastley R. A modification of the laryngeal mask airway. *Anesthesiology* 1991;**74**:1157 (Abstract).

31 Brain AIJ. *The Intavent laryngeal mask – instruction manual.* London: Intavent, 1991;1–58.

32 Brimacombe J, Berry A. Translucent vinyl tubing – an alternative bite guard for the LMA. *Anaesth Intens Care* 1993;**21**:893–894.

33 Brimacombe J. The laryngeal mask airway – fixation, gags and stability. *Anaesthesiol Intensivmed Notfalmed Schmerzther* 1995;**30**:129.

34 Marks LF. Protection of the laryngeal mask airway. *Anaesthesia* 1990;**45**:259.

35 Sachs G, Baum J. Ein einfacher Beibschutz für die Kehlkopfmaske. *Anaesthesiol Intensivmed Notfalmed Schmerzther* 1994;**29**:309–310.

36 Townend M, Frew RM, Hoyle JR. Bite block for the laryngeal mask airway. *Anaesthesia* 1995;**50**:918.

37 Hasham F, Kumar CM, Lawler PG. The use of the laryngeal mask airway to assist fibreoptic orotracheal intubation. *Anaesthesia* 1991;**46**:891.

38 Carey MF, Smith J, Cooney CM. Laryngeal mask to aid tracheal intubation. *Anaesthesia* 1991;**46**:1083.

39 Loken RG, Moir CL. The laryngeal mask airway as an aid to blind orotracheal intubation. *Can J Anaesth* 1992;**39**:518.

40 Brimacombe J, Berry A. Placement of the Cook Airway Exchange Catheter via the laryngeal mask airway. *Anaesthesia* 1993;**48**:351–352.

41 Kadota Y, Oda T, Yoshimura N. Application of a laryngeal mask to a fiberoptic bronchoscope-aided tracheal intubation. *J Clin Anesth* 1992;**4**:503–504.

42 Logan S, Charters P. Laryngeal mask and fibreoptic intubation. *Anaesthesia* 1994;**49**:543–544.

43 Iwasaka T. Tracheal intubation through the LM. *J Clin Anesth (Rinsho-Masui)* 1991;**15**:1397–1398.

44 Miyawaki H. LM-aided tracheal intubation. *J Clin Anesth (Rinsho-Masui)* 1992;**16**:1588–1589.

45 Hornbein TF, Turnquist K, Freund P. Another way through a laryngeal mask airway. *Anesthesiology* 1995;**83**:880

46 Heard CMB, Caldicott LD, Fletcher JE, Selsby DS. Fiberoptic guided endotracheal intubation via the laryngeal mask airway in paediatric patients. A report of a series of cases. *Anesth Analg* 1996;**82**:1287–1289.

47 Ravalia A, Steele A. Reinforced laryngeal mask airway and nasal surgery. *Anaesthesia* 1996;**51**:286.

48 Lewis RP, Porter M. Supplementary oxygen and the laryngeal mask airway. *Anaesthesia* 1991;**46**:70.

49 Broadway PJ, Royle P. Supplementary oxygen and the laryngeal mask airway. *Anaesthesia* 1990;**45**:792–793.

50 Kennedy R, Meyer M, Joyce C. Supplemental oxygen using an LMA. *Anaesth Intens Care* 1992;**20**:118.

51 Goodwin APL. Postoperative oxygen via the laryngeal mask airway. *Anaesthesia* 1991;**46**:700.

52 Kumar CM. Supplementary oxygenation and laryngeal mask airway: use of paediatric breathing circuit. *Today's Anaesthetist* 1995;**10**:68.

53 Kumar CM. Supplementary oxygenation and the laryngeal mask airway. *Today's Anaesthetist* 1995;**10**:104–105.

54 Johnston DF, Wrigley SR, Robb PJ, Jones HE. The laryngeal mask airway in paediatric anaesthesia. *Anaesthesia* 1990;**45**:924–927.

55 Goldie AS, Hudson I. Fibreoptic tracheal intubation through a modified laryngeal mask. *Paed Anaesth* 1992;**2**:344.

56 Lumb AB, Wrigley MW. The effect of nitrous oxide on laryngeal mask cuff pressure. In vitro and in vivo studies. *Anaesthesia* 1992;**47**:320–323.

★ **57** Brimacombe J, Berry A. Laryngeal mask airway cuff pressure and position during anaesthesia lasting 1–2 hours. *Can J Anaesth* 1994;**41**:589–593.
Study of 24 patients looking at intracuff pressures and fiberoptic stability during N_2O/O_2 anesthesia. Showed that intracuff pressures plateau after 90 min and that the device is stable.

58 Brimacombe J. Spontaneous reinflation characteristics of the laryngeal mask airway. *Can J Anaesth* 1994;**41**:873.

59 Brimacombe J, Berry A. Laryngeal mask airway cuff pressure and position: the effect of adding nitrous oxide to the cuff. *Anesthesiology* 1994;**80**:957–958.

60 Marjot R. Pressure exerted by the laryngeal mask airway cuff upon the pharyngeal mucosa. *Br J Anaesth* 1993;**70**:25–29.

61 O'Kelly SW, Heath KL, Lawes EG. A study of laryngeal mask inflation. Pressures exerted on the pharynx. *Anaesthesia* 1993;**48**:1075–1078.

62 Gursoy F, Algren JT, Skjonsby BS. The effect of nitrous oxide (N_2O) on laryngeal mask airway (LMA) volume and pressure in children. *Anesthesiology* 1994;**81**:A1319 (Abstract).

63 Ri J, Iwasaki H, Yamakage M, Yamasaki Y, Kirita A, Namiki A. Intracuff pressure of the laryngeal mask during anaesthesia. *J Clin Anesth (Rinsho-Masui)* 1991;**15**:1424–1426.

64 Hamakawa T, Nakamura S, Kawasaki Y. Intracuff pressure of the LM and pressure on the pharynx. *J Clin Anesth (Rinsho-Masui)* 1993;**17**:1165–1167.

65 Epstein RH, Ferouz F, Jenkins MA. Airway sealing pressures of the laryngeal mask airway in pediatric patients. *J Clin Anesth* 1996;**8**:93–98.

66 Burgard G, Mollhoff T, Prien T. The effect of laryngeal mask cuff pressure on postoperative sore throat incidence. *J Clin Anesth* 1996;**8**:198–201.

67 Jung K, Cho C, Yang H. Clinical investigation of the laryngeal mask airway in children. *J Kor Soc Anesthesiol* 1993;**26**:763–769.

68 Jeong J, Yang H, Cho H. Clinical investigation of laryngeal mask airway. *J Kor Soc Anesthesiol* 1993;**25**:708–718.

69 Lacroix O, Billard V, Bourgain JL, Debaene B. Prevention of postoperative sore throat during use of the laryngeal mask airway. *European Society of Anaesthesiologists Annual Congress, London, 1–5 June 1996,* A51 (Abstract).

70 Pennant JH, White PF. The laryngeal mask airway. Its uses in anesthesiology. *Anesthesiology* 1993;**79**:144–163.

71 Revenas B, Lindhold C. Pressure and volume changes in tracheal tube cuffs during anaesthesia. *Acta Anaesthesiol Scand* 1976;**20**:321.

72 Brimacombe J, Berry A, Brain AIJ. Optimal cuff pressures with the laryngeal mask. *Br J Anaesth* 1996;**77**:295–296.

73 Menon DK, Peden CJ, Hall AS, Sargentoni J, Whitwam JG. Magnetic resonance for the anaesthetist. *Anaesthesia* 1992;**47**:240–255.

74 Langton JA, Wilson I, Fell D. Use of the laryngeal mask airway during magnetic resonance imaging. *Anaesthesia* 1992;**47**:532.

75 Fairfield JE. Laryngeal mask and magnetic resonance – a caution. *Anaesthesia* 1990;**45**:995.

76 Stevens JE, Burden G. Reinforced laryngeal mask airway and magnetic resonance imaging. *Anaesthesia* 1994;**49**:79–80.

77 Hayes DM, Gaba DM, Goode RL. Incendiary characteristics of a new laser-resistant endotracheal tube. *Otolaryngol Head Neck Surg* 1986;**95**:37–40.

78 Pennant JH, Gajraj NM, Miller JF. Resistance of the laryngeal mask airway to the CO_2 laser. *Anesthesiology* 1993;**79**:A1055 (Abstract).

★ 79 Brimacombe J, Sher M, Laing D. The incendiary characteristics of the laryngeal and reinforced laryngeal mask airway. *Anaesthesia* 1994;**49**:171.
Laboratory study comparing the incendiary characteristics with respect to the CO_2 laser of the LMA, FLMA and PVC tracheal tubes. Showed that the LMA/FLMA was relatively laser resistant at clinically useful power densities.

80 McCulloch T, Jones MR, O'Neill A. Safety of the laryngeal mask with the flash-pumped dye laser. *11th World Congress of Anesthesiology, Sydney, 14–20 April 1996, Abstract Handbook* p.615 (Abstract).

81 Sher M, Brimacombe J, Laing D. Anaesthesia for laser pharyngoplasty – a comparison of the tracheal tube versus reinforced laryngeal mask airway. *Anaesth Intens Care* 1995;**23**:149–154.

82 Sosis MB. Which is the safest endotracheal tube for use with the CO_2 laser? A comparative study. *J Clin Anesth* 1992;**4**:217–219.

83 Biro P. Damage to laryngeal masks during sterilisation. *Anesth Analg* 1993;**77**:1079.

84 Leach AB, Alexander CA. The laryngeal mask – an overview. *Eur J Anaesthesiol* 1991;**4**:19–31.

85 Wat LI, Templin PA, Lynch ME, Hammamura RK, White PF. Use of the laryngeal mask airway for ambulatory anesthesia: utilization, longevity and cost. *American Society of Anesthesiologist's Annual General Meeting, New Orleans, October 1996* (Abstract).

86 Maroof M, Khan R. LMA and the stylet: a source of new strength for the laryngeal mask airway. *Anesth Analg* 1993;**76**:1162.

87 Brimacombe J, Berry A. Use of a stylet with the aged laryngeal mask airway? *Anesth Analg* 1994;**78**:190.

88 Maroof M, Khan RM. Use of a stylet with the aged laryngeal mask airway? (a reply). *Anesth Analg* 1994;**78**:190–191.

89 McLure HA. Dental damage to the laryngeal mask. *Anaesthesia* 1996;**51**:1078–1079.

90 Moller JT, Pedersen T, Rasmussen LS, et al. Randomised evaluation of pulse oximetry in 20 802 patients I. Design, demography, pulse oximetry failure rate, and overall complication rate. *Anesthesiology* 1993;**78**:436–444.

91 Moller JT, Johannessen NW, Espersen K, et al. Randomised evaluation of pulse oximetry in 20 802 patients II. Perioperative events and postoperative complications. *Anesthesiology* 1993;**78**:445–453.

92 Van Damme E. Die Kehlopfmaske in der ambulanten Anasthesie – Eine Auswertung von 5000 ambulanten Narkosen. *Anaesthesiol Intensivmed Notfalmed Schmerzther* 1994;**29**:284–286.

93 Mollhoff T, Burgard G, Prien T. Low-flow and minimal flow anesthesia and the laryngeal mask airway. *Anesthesiology* 1995;**83**:A499 (Abstract).

94 Fung ST, Cheung HK, Jawan B, Tsai PS, Chen CC, Lee JH. Use of the laryngeal mask in off-floor anesthesia for hepatic angiography in pediatric liver transplant candidates. *Transplant Proc* 1996;**28**:1723–1724.

95 Swann DG, Spens H, Edwards SA, Chestnut RJ. Anaesthesia for gynaecological laparoscopy – a comparison between the laryngeal mask airway and tracheal intubation. *Anaesthesia* 1993;**48**:431–434.

96 Cork RC, Depa RM, Standen JR. Prospective comparison of use of the laryngeal mask and endotracheal tube for ambulatory surgery. *Anesth Analg* 1994;**79**:719–727.

97 Langenstein H, Moller F, Krause R, Kluge R, Vogelsang H. Die Handhabung der Larynxmaske bei Augenoperationen. *Congress on Anaesthesia in Eye Surgery, Congress-Centrum Stadtpark, Hannover, 10–11 May 1996* (Abstract).

98 Joshi GP, Smith I, Watcha MF, White PF. A model for studying the cost-effectiveness of airway devices: laryngeal mask airway vs tracheal tube. *Anesth Analg* 1995;**80**:S219 (Abstract).

★ **99** Macario A, Chang PC, Stempel DB, Brock Utne JG. A cost analysis of the laryngeal mask airway for elective surgery in adult outpatients. *Anesthesiology* 1995;**83**:250–257.
A comprehensive evaluation of four airway management techniques for healthy outpatients. Concluded that if the LMA was used more than 40 times it was the most cost-effective airway provided procedures lasted more than 40 min.

100 Mansfield MD, Miller CD. The laryngeal mask airway and resuscitation. *Anaesthesia* 1993;**48**:637–638.

101 Bapat P, Joshi RN, Young E, Jago RH. Comparison of propofol versus thiopentone with midazolam or lidocaine to facilitate laryngeal mask insertion. *Can J Anaesth* 1996;**43**:564–568.

5 Preparation for use

Cleaning and sterilizing

Cleaning

The LMA is a re-usable device and is supplied unsterile. It must be autoclaved before its first use and prior to each of its subsequent uses. Cleaning of the LMA should be carried out as soon as possible after the removal from the patient as this will enable secretions to be dislodged more easily. Cleaning should be carried out gently to avoid splashing and also because the medical-grade silicone from which the LMA is made is easily damaged by perforation or tearing. Gloves and goggles should be worn. Wash in warm water and, if required, use a soft bristled brush. A pipe cleaner brush should be used for cleaning the inside of the airway tube, inserted from the mask end, taking care not to damage the bars in the bowl of the cuff (Table 5.1). Formaldehyde,

Table 5.1 Cleaning and sterilization

- No chemicals should be used. The LMA may absorb substances causing deterioration of materials or a mucosal reaction
- On removing LMA, place in warm water and wash with simple soap
- **Wear gloves** and **use eye protection**. Rinse thoroughly
- Wash tube and cuff, using small brush upwards from the bars to clean inside
- Leave the LMA to dry before autoclaving
- Remove all air from the cuff **immediately prior** to autoclaving
- Place in autoclavable bag and **steam autoclave** at 134–138°C

glutaraldehyde, ethlylene oxide gas, iodine-containing preparations or other chemicals not specified by the manufacturer as safe should not be used to clean or sterilize the LMA. The above chemicals are absorbed by the silicone rubber, subsequently contaminating the patient. Chemicals known to attack the valve are listed in Table 5.2. Aspiration of altered cleaning chemicals may also occur. Shannon and Steel noted the presence of hard pink globules on the inner surface of the LMA tube prior to usage[1]. These contaminants were the result of accidental cleaning in 4% chlorhexidine gluconate and subsequent autoclaving which produced partial evaporation. The device should be examined carefully, paying particular attention to the inner surface of the airway tube and the area behind the two bars in the bowl of the cuff. There should be no adherent secretions or loose particles in evidence.

Table 5.2 Chemicals known to attack the valve

Chemicals resulting in severe attack	*Chemicals resulting in slight attack*
Acetic acid	Acetic acid, 3%
Bromide water, saturated	Acetone
Buffer solutions, pH 4.0	Aluminum chloride
Calcium hypochlorite	Aluminum sulfate
Chlorine	Alums
Chromic acid	Aniline
Dichloroethylene	Benzoic acid
Formic acid	Boric acid
Hydrochloric acid, 30%	Calcium bisulfate
Hydrocyanic acid	Citric acid
Hydrofluoric acid, dilute or 40%	Creosote
Hydrogen fluoride	Dimethyl formamide
Hydrogen sulfide, wet	Ethyl acetate
Nitric acid	Hydrogen, dry
Nitrogen oxides	Lactic acid
Nitrous acid	Malic acid
Oxalic acid	Methylene chloride
Phenol	Nitrobenzene
Phosphoric acid, 25%	Oleic acid
Sodium hypochlorite	Palmitic acid
Sulfate liquors	Petroleum oils
Sulfur chloride	Picric acid
Sulfuric acid, 10%	Pyridine
Sulfurous acid	Sodium thiosulfate
	Stearic acid
	Succinic acid
	Sulfur dioxide
	Tannic acid
	Tartaric acid
	Tetrahydrofurane
	Tetralin
	Thiophane
	Trichloroethylene
	Vinegar

Sterilization

After cleaning, the device should be sterilized by steam autoclaving, following the standard procedure for porous loads (Table 5.3) . LMAs should be placed in pouches and stored only with other LMAs to avoid damage by contact with sharp instruments. The temperature should be 134–138°C. At higher temperatures the tube may become brittle and prone to fragmentation[2,3]. The cuff must be completely deflated immediately prior to sterilization using a dry, clean syringe. Ensure the valve port is dry before inserting the syringe into it. Any nonresidual air left in the cuff will expand in the high temperature and low pressure of the autoclave, causing damage to the cuff and/or pilot balloon[4]. The volume at which damage occurs is unknown. Biro considers that a residual volume of 2 ml may be sufficient to damage the size 4 LMA cuff[5]. However, using a gas dilution technique, Brimacombe has shown that when the size 4 cuff is evacuated to –25 mm Hg it has a residual volume of 1.2–2 ml[4] decreasing still further to 0.6–1.1 ml at –40 mm Hg[6]. Furthermore, Brain has demonstrated that at room temperature a new size 4 cuff can be inflated with 1.6 l of air before rupture occurs. It would appear that a residual volume of 2 ml is easily avoided by careful evacuation and is probably insufficient to produce rupture unless the LMA is already defective[7]. Biro suggests omitting the vacuum phase or leaving the valve open during sterilization by priming it with an open syringe. A better solution may be to limit the low pressures used during the vacuum phase of the autoclave cycle[4]. There are two main hazards to leaving the valve open: (1) moisture will be introduced into the cuff which may not fully escape during drying; (2) the priming syringe may occasionally fall off during sterilization leaving the cuff with a large residual volume which will inevitably lead to damage. Moisture may be inadvertently introduced if the cuff is inflated using a syringe which contains fluid, commonly the syringe used for the induction agent. It must also be emphasized that the LMA cuff must be deflated immediately prior to autoclaving[6]. If the LMA cuff is deflated prematurely, the residual volume increases by slow diffusion of air along the pressure gradient[6]. The size 4 LMA cuff spontaneously re-inflates by 1 ml at 2 h, 2.4 ml at 6 h and 5.5 ml after 24 h (see Figure 4.6).

Table 5.3 Sterilization hints

1. The LMA must be autoclaved on the first and all subsequent uses.
2. Use a standard autoclave cycle after thoroughly cleansing the device. Most institutions will find it more efficient to autoclave LMAs in batches, for example every 24 h.
3. Avoid chemical disinfectants: they penetrate the silicone material and are difficult to dislodge. Aldehydes such as glutaraldehyde are hazardous. Chemicals releasing free halogens attack the silicone with rapid loss of elasticity and strength. Even one exposure may be enough to cause unpredictable failure such as tube fracture.
4. The cuff of the LMA may rupture during autoclaving if moisture and/or air are present. To avoid this problem:

- check the valve keeps the device fully deflated after withdrawing air from the cuff; older valves may be defective
- deflate immediately prior to autoclaving
- use a clean, dry syringe (label 'for LMA use')

Following autoclaving the LMA is allowed to cool. Autoclaving alters the smooth folding of the deflated LMA and it is necessary to re-inflate the LMA prior to deflating to form the correct shape for insertion. After autoclaving, handle with fresh disposable gloves. Strict adherence to cleaning guidelines[8] should optimize the structural integrity of the LMA, increase its useful life and increase patient safety[6].

Pre-use tests

A number of tests should be carried out before re-use of the device. These tests should be carried out regularly – ideally immediately before each use. Essentially, the tests are designed to ensure patency and integrity of the tube and proper functioning of the cuff and valve. Failure on any one test indicates that the device is not safe to use (Tables 5.4

Table 5.4 Pre-use tests

Test 1 Tube structure	Examine the interior of the tube to ensure it is free from blockage or loose particles. Then, holding the device at each end, flex the tube to increase its curvature. Kinking of the tube should not occur when it is bent around 180 degrees. Do not bend beyond 180 degrees to avoid permanent damage to the tube.
Test 2 Tube transparency	The tube should be transparent in order that any fluids or contaminants within it are readily apparent. Discoloration of the tube usually indicates considerable use beyond the warranty usage and impairs the ability to detect potential airway problems.
Test 3 Connector check	This test does not require cuff inflation. Examine the polysulphone 15 mm connector. It should fit tightly into the outer end of the breathing tube and it should not be possible to pull it off. The breathing tube should never be shortened.
Test 4 Aperture bars check	Examine the aperture in the mask. It is traversed by two flexible bars, the mask aperture bars. Gently probe the bars to ensure they are not damaged or broken through. The spaces between the bars must be free from any particulate matter.
Test 5 Deflation test	Deflate the mask cuff to a high vacuum so that the cuff walls are tightly flattened against each other. Without releasing the vacuum, remove the syringe from the syringe port with a rapid twisting action. Now examine the cuff walls to ensure they remain tightly flattened against each other. Gradual re-inflation indicates there is a faulty valve or a leaking cuff.
Test 6 Inflation test	Temporarily overinflate the cuff from complete vacuum as follows: size 1, 6 ml; size 1.5, 7 ml; size 2, 15 ml; size 2.5, 21 ml: size 3, 30 ml; size 4, 45 ml and size 5, 60 ml (*note:* these values represent 50% overinflation – **never use these large volumes in patients**). Any leak present will be evident after 2 min. If no leak is apparent, place the whole device under water to check for location and extent of any leaks.
Test 7 Symmetry/shape	Keeping the device inflated as in the last part of Test 6, examine the shape of the inflated cuff for symmetry. There should not be uneven bulging of the cuff at either end or on one or other of the sides. If in doubt, measure the diameter of the inflated cuff at these three points: (1) the maximal bulge of the cuff tip; (2) the maximal bulge of the wide end of the cuff; and (3) the maximum transverse diameter of the cuff (Figure 5.1, Table 5.5).

Table 5.5 LMA inflation tests (UK only)

	Size 1	*Size 1.5*	*Size 2*	*Size 2.5*	*Size 3*	*Size 4*	*Size 5*
Maximum bulge of cuff tip (mm)	7.8	9.5	11.5	13	14.8	17	21.1
Maximum bulge of wide end of cuff (mm)	8.6	10.2	13	14.5	16.6	19	22.4
Maximum transverse diameter of cuff (mm)	26.3	32.6	39	45	51.2	58.5	68.3
50% overinflation values for this test (ml)	6	10	15	21	30	45	60

and 5.5). Attempted repair to a ruptured cuff, balloon or aperture bar is likely to result in failure of the device in use and cannot be recommended. Customization of an LMA in any form will result in loss of indemnity within the device warranty. This includes the use of 'markers' such as pens and pencils, adhesive tape, etching of component part, tube shortening or use of nonrecommended valves. Riley and Browning highlighted the importance of pre-use tests when they identified a foreign body occluding the LMA tubing post sterilization[9].

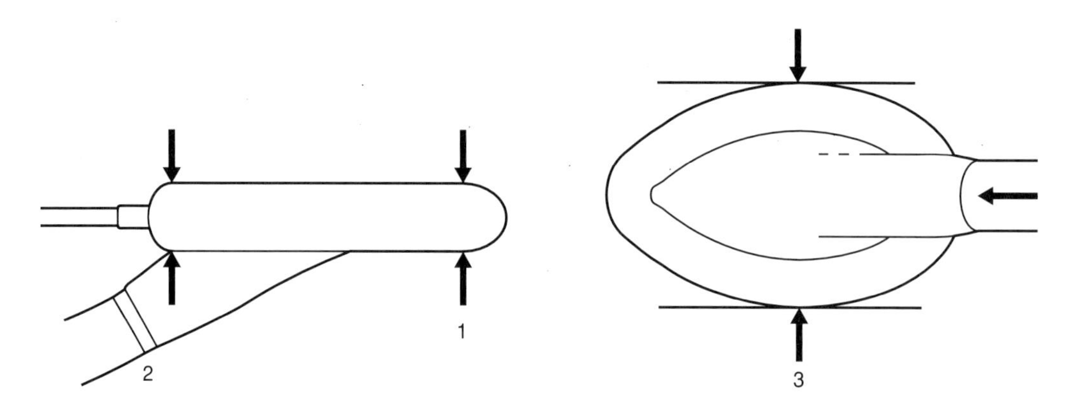

Figure 5.1 Maximum inflation tests. Location for measurement: 1 = maximum bulge of cuff tip; 2 = maximum bulge of wide end of cuff; 3 = maximum transverse diameter of cuff.

Deflation

The device is designed in such a way that when correctly deflated, it forms a smooth flat wedge, with the rim forming a concave saucer shape on its dorsal surface. Deflation should be carried out with a dry dedicated syringe (label 'LMA use only') and the cuff must be tightly deflated so that it forms an oval disk with the rim facing away from the aperture (Figure 5.2). An incompletely deflated mask may cause trauma even when correctly inserted because the tip rolls out of the way, exposing the pointed end. Try to eliminate any wrinkles on the distal edge of the rim. A completely smooth flat leading

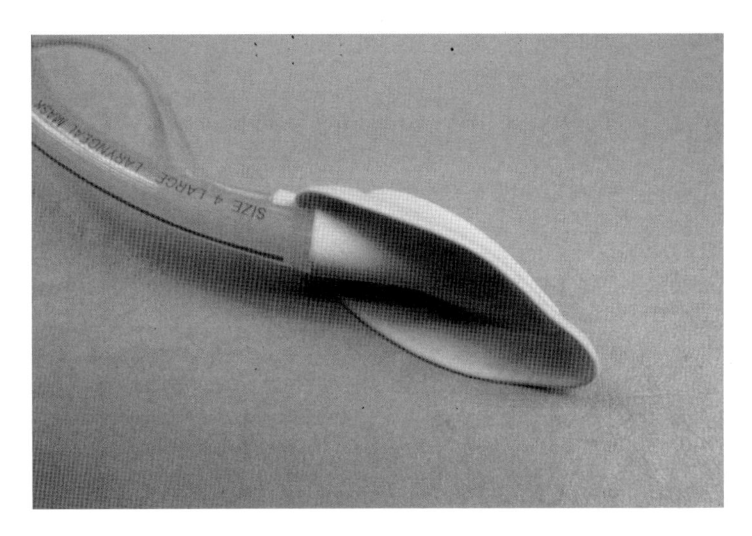

Figure 5.2 Optimal shape of deflated LMA cuff.

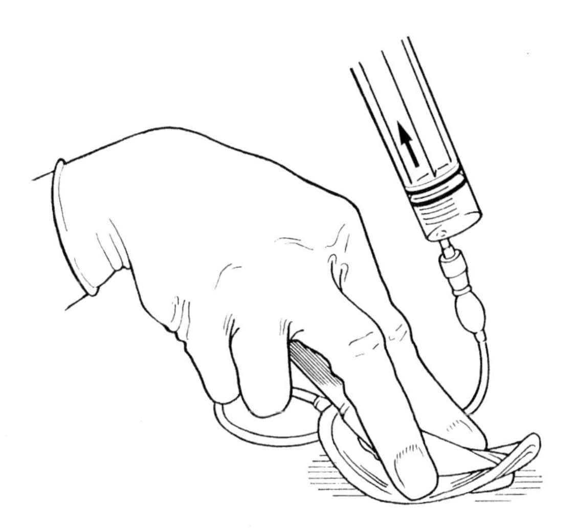

Figure 5.3 Cuff deflation can be achieved by pressing the mask with its hollow side down on a sterile, flat surface. The fingers may be used to guide cuff shape. A high vacuum should be achieved.

edge facilitates smooth insertion and avoids collision with the epiglottis. This may be achieved manually (Figure 5.3, 5.5) or with the aid of a special deflation tool available from the manufacturer (Figure 5.4, Table 5.6). The deflation tool comprises an autoclavable mold shaped like the deflated cuff of an LMA and is available in three sizes: small (LMAs 2, 2.5), medium (LMAs 3, 4) and large (LMA 5). In a randomized single blinded controlled trial the deflation tool was shown to be better than manual deflation in terms of optimal shape for insertion[10].

Table 5.6 Methods of cuff deflation

Manual method

A. Press the hollow side down onto a clean flat surface, with a finger pressing the tip flat while removing air from cuff (Figure 5.3)

or

B. Hold the hollow side down diagonally across palm of gloved hand, pressing down with thumb while deflating (inventor's method) (Figure 5.5).

Deflator device

1. The partially inflated LMA is placed in the mold with the bowl facing downwards (insert only enough air to remove wrinkles).
2. The lid of the mold is then closed and clamped while air is withdrawn from the cuff with a syringe (Figure 5.6) . Draw a vacuum with the syringe before removing.
3. When using a size 2 or 3 LMA, place the tip flush with the pointed end of the deflator cavity to ensure correct deflation (Figure 5.7).
4. Deflated masks will re-inflate slightly after even 10 min[6]. Always check for complete deflation immediately prior to insertion.

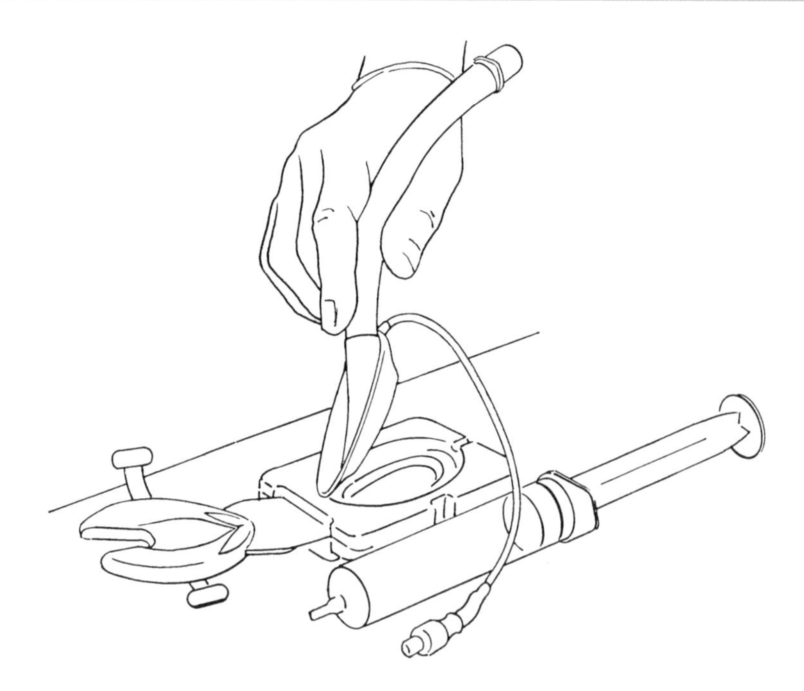

Figure 5.4 The deflation tool is available in three sizes.

Lubrication

Lubrication should be carried out just before insertion so that the lubricant does not dry out. Suitable lubricants include saline, water and water-based gels. Analgesic-containing gels or sprays have also been used[11,12], but may cause complications (see

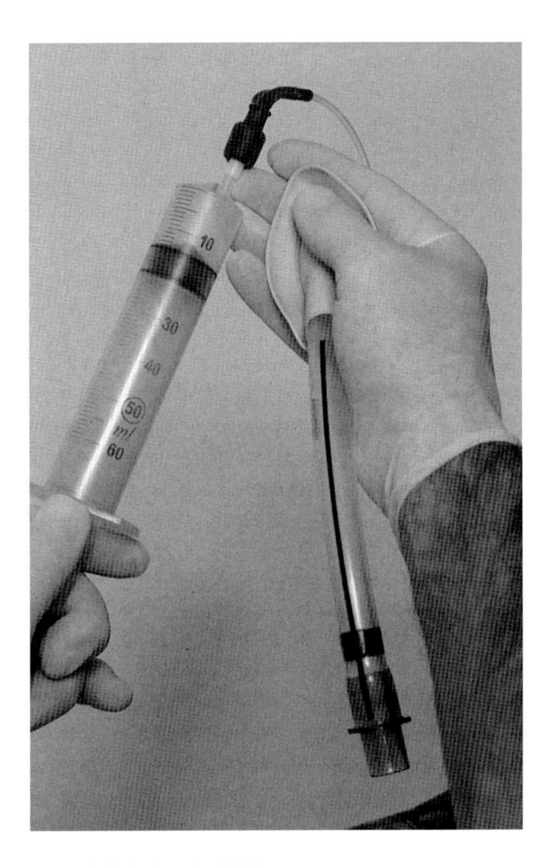

Figure 5.5 Alternative method of deflating the LMA.

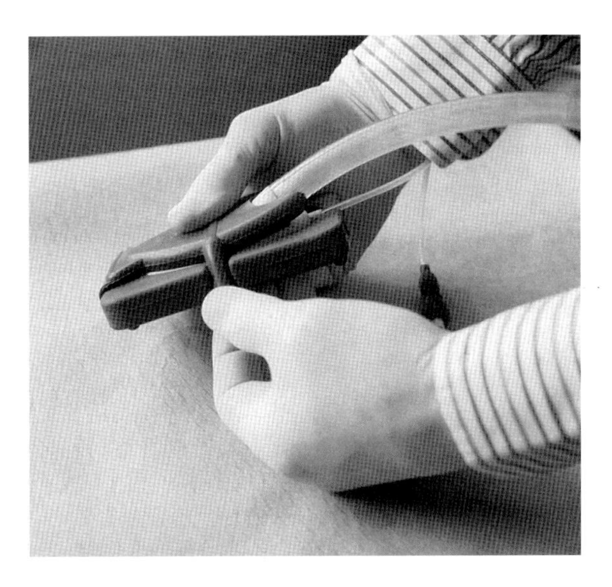

Figure 5.6 The partially inflated LMA is placed in the mold with the bowl facing downwards. The lid of the mold is then closed and clamped while air is withdrawn from the cuff with a syringe. The clamp is then opened and the LMA available for insertion.

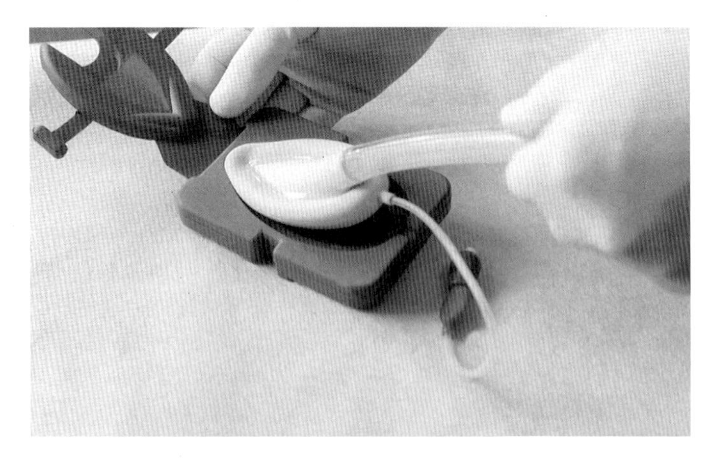

Figure 5.7 Ensure the mask tip is flush with the pointed end of the deflator tool cavity before clamping and deflating.

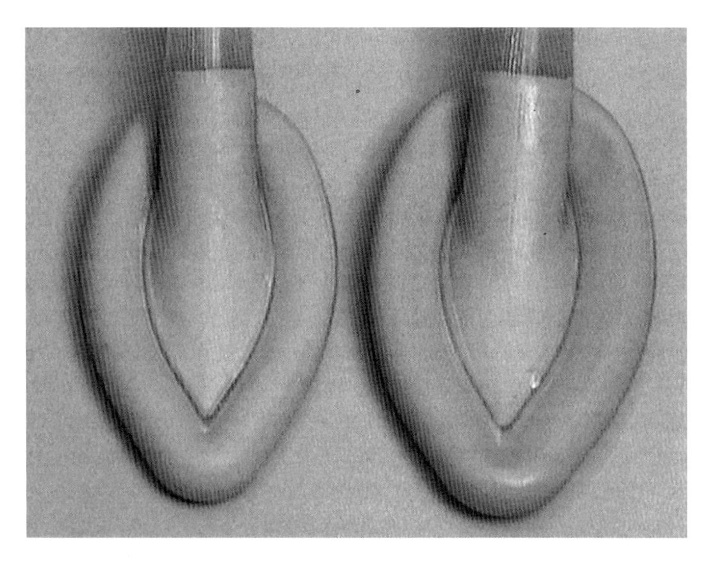

Figure 5.8 Both masks are size 4, but the larger one has been expanded by exposure to silicone-containing lubricants.

below). Avoid silicone-containing lubricants – they weaken and expand the device (Figure 5.8). Repeated exposure to silicone lubricants or other solvents makes the device harder to insert and may increase the risk of rupture or herniation causing unexpected airway obstruction. The back of the mask should be lubricated thoroughly, but it is important to avoid leaving globules of lubricant on the anterior surface of the cuff or in the bowl of the mask as this may result in blockage of the aperture or inhalation of lubricant after insertion, causing laryngeal spasm, coughing or obstruction[13]. It is not necessary to smear the whole back surface – place a bolus in the saucer-shaped depression in the dorsal tip prior to induction (don't let this dry out). As you flatten the mask tip into the palate and then move it back towards the pharynx, the mask will slide over the lubricant. Try to avoid getting lubricant on your index finger since this will make it difficult to grip the LMA tube during insertion.

There are data to suggest that inclusion of local anesthetic in the lubricant, 2% lidocaine gel[11] or 10% lidocaine spray[12], may reduce the incidence of retching during emergence following procedures lasting less than 30 min. It should be remembered that when patients are left undisturbed during recovery the incidence of retching is less than 2% in experienced hands[14,15]. Keller et al have shown that lidocaine gel does not reduce the incidence of postoperative sore throat compared with water-based lubricant (C. Keller, personal communication, 1996). Analgesic lubricants may cause several problems. Some patients complain of numbness postoperatively, reactions to the analgesic may occur, and reflex integrity on recovery may be impaired[16]. Analgesic lubricant has been implicated in nerve damage following LMA use[17]. The effect of analgesic-coated masks on the lower esophageal sphincter pressure (LOSP) has not been studied. The pharynx contains chemoreceptors known to influence LOSP[18,19]. Malpositions of the mask, which usually provoke patient reaction, may go undetected because areas subjected to excessive local pressure are anesthetized[20].

Bite blocks

The silicone tube of the LMA is easily obstructed by biting and an appropriate bite block should always be used with the LMA to prevent tube occlusion or damage. Never attempt to pull the LMA out from between clenched teeth. This may damage the teeth, but it is also likely to damage the tube, which may be torn close to its junction with the mask by the lower incisor teeth. The tube may subsequently shear through at this point when used in another patient. There is also a potential for tube damage if a rotating insertion technique is used since this imparts a twisting force to the tube. In some situations, such as in the edentulous patient, a bite block may improve stability. Suitable bite blocks can be prepared by rolling a wad of gauze swabs into a cylindrical shape thick enough to prevent occlusion of the tube if the patient bites down on it. Secure each roll tightly with adhesive tape ensuring a minimum thickness of 2.5 cm. This bite block does not damage capped or fragile teeth, is easily prepared, economical, does not irritate the posterior pharyngeal wall during recovery (unlike the Guedel airway) and supports the LMA tube when taped to it (Figure 5.9) . Gently rotate one end of the cylinder between the teeth after insertion and inflation of the LMA. Leave enough protruding to attach adhesive tape.

Translucent surgical vinyl tubing (TPVT) can be used as an alternative to gauze swabs, is available in a wide range of diameters and hardness and can be cut to any length (Portex, UK)[21]. It is also smooth, kink resistant and can be autoclaved. A tray with a selection of sizes and lengths can be made available in each operating room and allows the swift selection of a customized bite guard. TPVT has been used as a bite guard for the LMA in over 3000 patients with no untoward effects[22]. Several other bite guards have been suggested including: (1) an Olympus bite guard[23]; (2) a tracheal tube holder[24]; (3) a simple U-shaped plastic coated aluminum rod[25]; and (4) two silicone rubber cylinders[26]. The first two encircle the LMA tube, the third rests on the molar teeth and the fourth sits on either side of the LMA tube. The best choice of bite guard

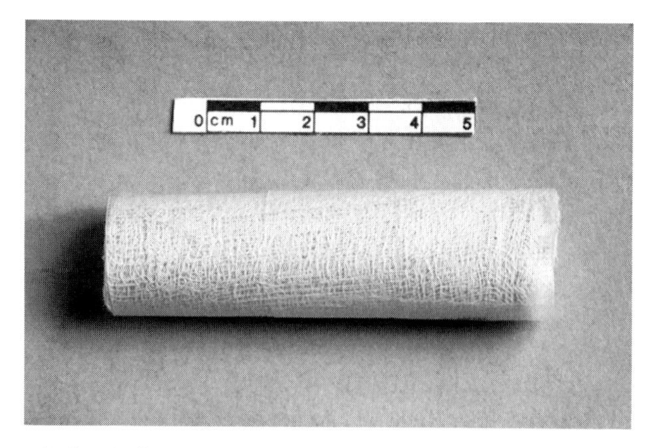

Figure 5.9 An economical and effective bite block which does not damage fragile teeth is a roll of gauze swabs 2–3 cm thick.

may vary from patient to patient according to the state of dentition, the surgical procedure and the fixation technique (see Chapter 6, *Fixation and stabilization*). The Guedel airway is not a suitable bite block for the LMA since: (1) the tip of the Guedel airway may compromise the LMA cuff; (2) both devices are intended to sit in the midline; (3) the Guedel airway is hard and may put teeth at risk; and (4) the Guedel airway may increase the incidence of sore throat[27]. Any bite block with the standard LMA should be designed to take account of the intended position of the tube, which should be pressed into the curvature of the hard palate and emerge from the mouth pointing caudad.

Size selection

There is a low probability that the mask will be exactly the right size for a given patient, but a high probability that appropriate size selection combined with optimal cuff inflation will produce a near-perfect fit[28]. Originally there was a choice of four sizes[29] and recently sizes 1.5, 2.5 and 5 have been added to the range. Judging the correct size of LMA can be difficult since the relationship between gender, weight and upper airway geometry appears inconsistent[30]. No factors have yet been identified permitting an easy measurement of potential pharyngeal volume that directly correlates with appropriate LMA size.

In lieu of an accurate predictive test, the current choice of LMA size is based on weight. The traditionally held view that a size 3 is suitable for adult females and a size 4 for adult males was never recommended by the manufacturer and now appears to be erroneous. However, the use of a size 5 for men and size 4 for women may be more suitable. Voyagis et al compared the standard method for size selection in adults based on weight and compared it with a formula based on gender. The formula was to use a size 5 for all males, a size 4 for all females and to fall back to a smaller size whenever insertion failed[31]. The mean peak inspiratory pressure at which oropharyngeal leak occurred was significantly greater using the sex-related formula compared with the conventional weight-related method (27 versus 23 cm H_2O). Brimacombe et al suggested that further evidence was needed before moving away from the weight-based recommendations[32].

Current European practice is to use the size 4 routinely for all normal sized adults, and size 5 in large adults, particularly where PPV is employed electively or reverted to during the course of an anesthetic. Insertion of too small a size will result in a leak, an increased risk of failure to align glottic and mask apertures, and possibly an increased risk of glottic impaction, although the latter is conjectural. Overinflation of the cuff rarely solves the problem of inappropriate LMA size and tends to cause loss of seal as tension in the overexpanded cuff is too rigid to follow the contours of the glottic perimeter[33]. If after full insertion it is found necessary to draw back the LMA to obtain a clear airway, this implies that the LMA is too small. It appears that it is better to choose a larger cuff size which will not encounter a Hook's Law phenomenon and which will maintain a soft low tension mass in the pharynx. The implications are that, for optimal use of the LMA, as large a sized LMA as possible should be chosen, and that cuff volume should be carefully adjusted to obtain an adequate seal. Auscultation of the neck and manual ballotting of the pilot balloon to assess cuff pressure are useful clinical guides in achieving optimal cuff inflation. The effectiveness of pilot balloon feel has been contested[34]. To avoid possible nerve damage associated with inadvertant malposition, the inventor recommends limiting cuff pressures to approximately 60 cm H_2O[35].

The current manufacturer's weight recommendations, cuff volumes, tracheal tube and fiberoptic scope sizes for the seven LMAs are given in Table 5.7.

Table 5.7 Description of different sizes of laryngeal mask airway devices

Mask size	Patient weight (kg)	ID/OD (mm)	Length (cm)**	FLMA ID (mm)	FLMA length (cm)**	Cuff volume (ml)	Largest TT (ID, mm)	FOB size LMA (mm)	FOB size FLMA (mm)
1	<5	5.25/8.2	8	–	–	<4	3.5	2.7*	–
1.5	5–10	6.1/9.6	10			<7	4.0	3.0	–
2	10–20	7.0/11.0	11.0	5.1	13	<10	4.5	3.5	2.7
2.5	20–30	8.4/13.0	12.5	6.1	16.5	<14	5.0	4.0	3.5
3	30–50†	10/15.0	16	7.6	21	<20	6.0 cuffed	5.0	4.0
4	50–70†	10/15.0	16	7.5	21	<30	6.0 cuffed	5.0	4.0
5	>70†	11.5/16.5	18	8.7	24	<40	7.0 cuffed	7.3	5.0

* A 2.2 mm fiberoptic laryngoscope is available[37].
** Approximate visible tube length.
† Very approximate guide.
Key: ID/OD = internal diameter/external diameter; FOB = fiberoptic bronchoscope.

Anesthetic breathing systems

The LMA may be used in conjunction with standard anesthetic breathing systems, including low flow or closed circuit systems[36]. The T-piece is suitable for use in small children and neonates. It is important to ensure that the anesthetic breathing system does not reduce the stability of the LMA, particularly in infants and small children.

References

1 Shannon PE, Steel D. Potential hazard from incorrect cleaning of laryngeal mask airway. *Anaesthesia* 1996;**51**:603–604.

2 Squires SJ, Woods K. Fragmented laryngeal mask airway. *Anaesthesia* 1992;**47**:274.

3 Crawford M, Davidson G, Woods K. A problem with a laryngeal mask airway. *Anaesthesia* 1992;**47**:76.

4 Brimacombe J. Laryngeal mask residual volume and damage during sterilisation. *Anesth Analg* 1994;**79**:391.

5 Biro P. Damage to laryngeal masks during sterilisation. *Anesth Analg* 1993;**77**:1079.

6 Brimacombe J. Spontaneous reinflation characteristics of the laryngeal mask airway. *Can J Anaesth* 1994;**41**:873.

7 Brain AIJ. Autoclaving laryngeal masks. *Anesth Analg* 1994;**79**:199.

8 Brain AIJ. *The Intavent laryngeal mask – instruction manual.* London: Intavent, 1991;1–58.

9 Riley RH, Browning FS. Another foreign body in a laryngeal mask airway. *Anaesthesia* 1996;**51**:286–287.

★ 10 Brimacombe J, Brain AIJ, Branagan H, Spry M, Schofield J. Optimal shape of the laryngeal mask cuff: the influence of three deflation techniques. *Anaesthesia* 1996;**51**:673–676.
Randomized single blinded trial showing that the deflator tool produces a more ideal shape for the LMA cuff on deflation than manual or free deflation.

11 Chan ST, Med M, Tham CS. The effects of 2% lignocaine gel on incidence of retching with the use of the laryngeal mask airway. *Anaesthesia* 1995;**50**:257–258.

12 Millett SV, Allman KG. Lignocaine gel and the laryngeal mask airway. *Anaesthesia* 1995;**50**:747.

13 Thomas DG, Moloney JT. Stridor after removal of the laryngeal mask. *Anaesth Intens Care* 1991;**19**:300–301.

14 Brimacombe J. Analysis of 1500 laryngeal mask uses by one anaesthetist in adults undergoing routine anaesthesia. *Anaesthesia* 1996;**51**:76–80.

15 Lopez-Gil M, Brimacombe J, Alvarez M. Safety and efficacy of the laryngeal mask airway – a prospective survey of 1400 paediatric patients. *Anaesthesia* 1996;**51**:969–972.

16 Edwards ND. Lignocaine gel and the laryngeal mask airway. *Anaesthesia* 1995;**50**:746–747.

17 Inomata S, Nishikawa T, Suga A, Yamashita S. Transient bilateral vocal cord paralysis after insertion of a laryngeal mask airway. *Anesthesiology* 1995;**82**:787–788.

18 Storey AT. A functional analysis of sensory units innervating epiglottis and larynx. *Exp Neurol* 1968;**20**:366–383.

19 de Larminat V, Dubreuil B. Modification du reflexe de deglutition au cours de la periode perioperatoire. *Ann Fr Anesth Reanim* 1994;**13**:49–56.

20 Morikawa M. Vocal cord paralysis after use of the LM. *J Clin Anesth (Rinsho-Masui)* 1992;**16**:1194.

21 Brimacombe J, Berry A. Translucent vinyl tubing – an alternative bite guard for the LMA. *Anaesth Intens Care* 1993;**21**:893–894.

22 Brimacombe J. The laryngeal mask airway – fixation, gags and stability. *Anaesthesiol Intensivmed Notfalmed Schmerzther* 1995;**30**:129.

23 Worsley MH, Howie CC. Fixation of the laryngeal mask airway. *Anaesthesia* 1990;**45**:1001.

24 Marks LF. Protection of the laryngeal mask airway. *Anaesthesia* 1990;**45**:259.

25 Sachs G, Baum J. Ein einfacher Beibschutz für die Kehlkopfmaske. *Anaesthesiol Intensivmed Notfalmed Schmerzther* 1994;**29**:309–310.

26 Townend M, Frew RM, Hoyle JR. Bite block for the laryngeal mask airway. *Anaesthesia* 1995;**50**:918.

27 Brimacombe J. The Guedel airway and the laryngeal mask airway? *Anaesthesia* 1994;**49**:643.

28 Brimacombe J, Berry A. Size selection and the sixth LMA. *J Clin Anesth* 1995;**7**:265–266.

29 McEwan AI, Mason DG. The laryngeal mask airway. *J Clin Anesth* 1992;**4**:252–257.

30 Tham LCH. Children and size of laryngeal masks. *Can J Anaesth* 1994;**41**:354.

★ 31 Voyagis GS, Batziouulis PG, Secha-Doussaitou PN. Selection of the proper size of laryngeal mask airway in adults. *Anesth Analg* 1996;**83**:663–664.
Pilot study of 300 patients suggesting that the first choice size for LMA in adults should be a size 5 for males and a size 4 for females.

32 Brimacombe J, Berry A, Campbell RC, Verghese C. Selection of the proper size of larngeal mask airway in adults (reply). *Anesth Analg* 1996;**83**:664.

33 Welsh BE, Martin DW. Will we ever learn? *Anaesthesia* 1990;**45**:892.

34 Marjot RM, Morris G. Optimal intracuff pressures with the laryngeal mask (reply). *Br J Anaesth* 1996;77:296.
35 Brimacombe J, Berry A, Brain AIJ. Optimal cuff pressures with the laryngeal mask. *Br J Anaesth* 1996;77:295–296.
36 Mollhoff T, Burgard G, Prien T. Low-flow and minimal flow anesthesia and the laryngeal mask airway. *Anesthesiology* 1995;83:A499 (Abstract).
37 Wrigley SR, Black AE, Sidhu VS. A fibreoptic laryngoscope for paediatric anaesthesia. A study to evaluate the use of the 2.2 mm Olympus (LF-P) intubating fibrescope. *Anaesthesia* 1995;50:709–712.

6 Anesthetic management

Preoperative visit

The decision to use the LMA begins at the preoperative visit. It is important to take a history and to examine the airway, looking for factors which would make LMA insertion difficult (e.g. limited mouth opening, palatal defects, oropharyngeal masses, hard palate crib for thumb sucking, sharp edges in the mouth[1]) or contraindicated (e.g. reflux or low compliance lungs). Other surgical or patient factors (surgical access, unreliable history, known airway problems) may make LMA usage more or less desirable. When using the LMA in the awake patient this should be discussed at the preoperative visit.

Premedication

Premedication is not necessary for LMA insertion, but will probably reduce the dose of induction agent required. The efficacy of most premedicant drugs has not been assessed with respect to LMA usage in adults. Martlew et al have shown that premedication with midazolam reduces the induction dose of propofol in children[2]. It has been suggested that an antisialagogue may also improve conditions for insertion in children, but this has not been proven[3–6].

Preinduction

It is important to check that the size of the LMA is correct for the patient and that it is appropriately deflated and lubricated and has passed the pre-use checks. Spare LMAs (of the same and different sizes) should be ready and prepared for immediate use. The facility for intubation and face mask ventilation should always be available when conducting any LMA anesthetic.

Induction

The patient is preoxygenated and the preinduction agent of choice administered. Fentanyl 1–1.5 μg kg^{-1}, alfentanyl 10 μg kg^{-1}, and/or midazolam 0.05–0.1 mg kg^{-1} is commonly given. This is then followed by an induction dose of propofol 2.5 mg kg^{-1} given over 30 s (a lesser dose is recommended for the elderly and premedicated; children and those with induced liver enzymes may require a higher dose) until there is apnea, loss of eyelash reflex and no resistance to manipulation of the lower jaw. Low resistance to lung inflation with the face mask is also a test commonly employed. Placement should be timed with peak cerebral concentrations of propofol and this will vary with speed of injection and the arm–brain circulation time[7]. Delayed insertion (up to 2 min) may be associated with fewer airway complications provided that face mask ventilation with nitrous oxide, oxygen and a volatile agent[8] or possibly total intravenous anesthesia is continued. If muscle relaxants are used, timing of insertion is less critical. The depth of anesthesia required is a little more than that required for insertion of a Guedel airway, but the inexperienced should attempt insertion at a level closer to that of surgical anesthesia. If adequate conditions for insertion are not achieved, additional 30 s boluses of propofol 0.5 mg kg^{-1} may be given until a satisfactory end point is reached[9]. This is due to the high variability in the effect of a given dose of propofol on individual patients[10]. No muscle relaxing agent is required for LMA insertion, but one can be given with the induction agent if PPV is planned. Suxamethonium is not required for insertion and does not improve insertion conditions provided an adequate anesthetic depth is achieved[11]. Uchiyama et al showed that suxamethonium 0.5 mg kg^{-1} improved insertion conditions compared with saline or suxamethonium 0.25 mg kg^{-1}, but myalgia was more common with the higher dose[12]. Thiopentone was used as the induction agent, but no mention was made of the dosages involved.

Propofol depresses pharyngeal and laryngeal activity more than thiopentone for a given induction dose and was generally considered to be the agent of choice even prior to the completion of comparative trials[13–15]. Brain was the first to investigate the suitability of propofol for LMA insertion. This work was conducted in 1987, but remained unpublished until 1991. Brain found that insertion conditions were close to ideal within 20 s in 100 consecutive patients and obviously superior to his previous experience with thiopentone[16]. There have been three randomized controlled studies comparing LMA insertion using propofol or thiopentone. Brown et al compared propofol 2.5 mg kg^{-1} with thiopentone 4 mg kg^{-1} and found the incidence of coughing and gagging significantly less in the propofol group. Additional thiopentone, however, resulted in no difference between the groups[17]. Scanlon et al compared propofol 2.5 mg kg^{-1} with a higher dose of thiopentone (5 mg kg^{-1}) and found that propofol continued to provide superior insertion conditions[18]. Glaush-Wild et al compared propofol 2.5–3 mg kg^{-1} with thiopentone 5–6 mg kg^{-1} in 60 patients and found fewer failed insertions, higher seal pressures and less bronchospasm/laryngospasm with propofol[19]. A propofol blood level of 6–9 μg ml^{-1} has been recommended as providing suitable conditions for insertion[9].

It has been suggested that pretreatment with intravenous lidocaine 1.5 mg kg^{-1} improves conditions for LMA insertion with propofol[20,21]. Driver et al have shown that midazolam 0.04 mg kg^{-1} combined with alfentanyl 10 μg kg^{-1} significantly reduces the dose of propofol required for LMA insertion in adults[22,23]. When combined with this dose of midazolam and alfentanyl, propofol 1.25 mg kg^{-1} provided better conditions than 2.5 mg kg^{-1}. Although thiopentone alone does not produce ideal conditions for insertion of the LMA, it can be used if anesthesia is deepened with an inhalational agent for several minutes before insertion. Chan et al suggested that topicalization of the pharynx may facilitate LMA placement with thiopentone[24]. This has been confirmed by Seavell et al, who compared thiopentone 5 mg kg^{-1} preceded by 40 mg topical lidocaine spray to the posterior pharyngeal wall with propofol 2.5 mg kg^{-1} and found that insertion conditions were similar, but that the period of apnoea and drop in blood pressure were less with thiopentone[25]. Cook et al have also shown that topical lidocaine 40 mg provides superior insertion conditions compared to intravenous lidocaine 0.5 and 1.5 mg kg^{-1} when patients are induced with thiopentone 5 mg kg^{-1} and fentanyl 1 μg kg^{-1} [26]. The authors, however, did not assess patient discomfort during topicalization or the immediate postoperative period in either study[25,26]. Bapat et al have shown that fentanyl 1 μg kg^{-1}, midazolam 0.1 mg kg^{-1} and thiopentone 5 mg kg^{-1} produces equally good conditions for LMA insertion as fentanyl 1 μg kg^{-1} and propofol 2.5 mg kg^{-1} [27]. There is tentative evidence that metoclopramide 0.3 mg kg^{-1} may improve LMA insertion conditions following a slow dose of propofol (2.5 mg s^{-1})[28]. The LMA may also be inserted under deep volatile anesthesia.

Taguchi et al have shown that placement of the LMA requires a lower MAC of sevoflurane than placement of a tracheal tube in children[29]. Successful LMA insertion has been reported following induction with etomidate, but in this study the patients had been paralyzed prior to LMA insertion[30]. Etomidate 0.3 mg kg^{-1} combined with alfentanyl 15 μg kg^{-1} does not provide suitable conditions for LMA placement[31]. Other authors have found induction with etomidate to be more acceptable in combination with alfentanyl or sufentanyl[32,33]. In children, ketamine followed by halothane-enriched air has been used to facilitate LMA insertion in a remote hospital[34] and also in combination with fentanyl and midazolam[35]. There are no published reports of LMA insertion with methohexitone. Dasey and Mansour have suggested using a superior laryngeal nerve block to aid placement[36]. This may be useful for awake placement, but would seem unnecessary for placement under general anesthesia and is probably rarely used[37].

Head and neck position

The ideal position for placement is extension of the head with flexion of the neck, the classical 'sniffing the morning air position', as for tracheal intubation[38]. This can be achieved by pushing the head from behind with the nondominant hand during the movement of insertion. If necessary, an extra pillow can be used to keep the neck flexed. By adopting this position the angle between oral and pharyngeal axes is normally greater than 90 degrees[39], and the epiglottis is lifted away from the posterior pharyngeal wall[40,41], thus facilitating smooth passage of the mask into the oropharynx (Figure 6.1). Although neck flexion/head extension provides the best conditions for placement, insertion is also possible with the head maintained in the neutral position by halo[42] or manual in-line traction[43], in patients with abnormal cervical spines[44,45], and in the prone[46] and lateral positions[47]. Fukutome recommends jaw thrust to maximize clearance behind the tongue and larynx[48].

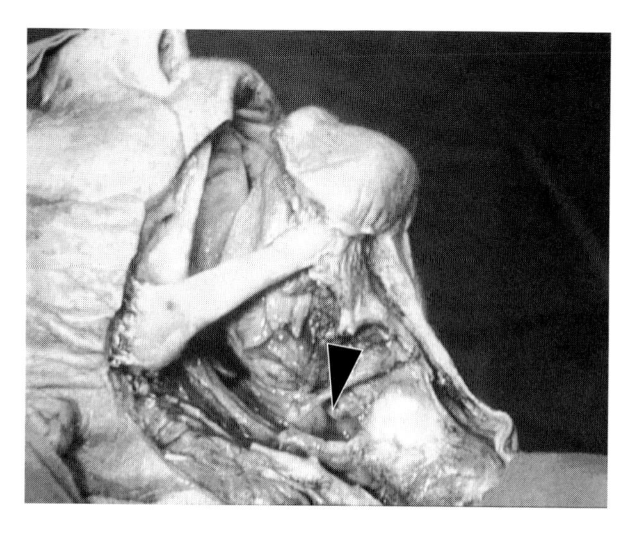

Figure 6.1 Lateral dissection of cadaver with head extended and neck flexed to show effect of oropharyngeal axis on position of epiglottis (arrowed).

Standard insertion technique

The standard insertion technique involves insertion using a midline or slightly diagonal approach with the cuff fully deflated into a flattened oval saucer shape and has evolved through many different stages. Brain's first prototype was inserted facing backwards and then rotated through 180 degrees[49]. Later prototypes used an introducer designed to prevent epiglottic downfolding during insertion[50]. This was phased out in favor of a more refined insertion technique[16]. LMA insertion can be considered in the context of swallowing and combines the ability to insert blindly, and without muscle relaxation, while avoiding collision with highly innervated anterior pharyngeal structures[16] such as the epiglottis[51], larynx[52] and arytenoids[51]. In swallowing, the tongue sweeps and flattens the food bolus around the curved wall formed by the palate and posterior aspect of the pharynx[53]. LMA insertion is achieved by a similar action with the index finger pressing the mask upwards, imitating the action of the tongue pressing the food bolus into the palate. This requires the person to point his or her finger towards his or her own umbilicus during the whole insertion maneuver[54] (Table 6.1). Insertion is relatively unstimulating because it does not require the use of a laryngoscope and avoids manipulation of structures associated with noxious reflex responses[55]. To obtain optimal placement in the laryngopharynx with its surrounding musculature, the LMA is inserted with reflexes obtunded by either general or topical anesthesia, and with the cuff fully deflated and flattened into the posterior pharynx[56]. Full insertion is indicated by definite resistance as the mask tip encounters the upper esophageal sphincter.

First time successful insertion rates vary with experience and technique, but should reach over 96% as the short-term learning curve is achieved[57]. In experienced hands, the LMA is inserted and functions well at the first attempt in 98% of patients within 20 s[58]. There is also a long-term 'learning curve' to optimal use of the LMA[59]. Experienced users have overall success rates greater than 99.5%[59–61]. Recent large-scale studies have reported failure rates of between 4.7%[62] and 0.2%[60]. The majority of

Table 6.1 Parallels between LMA insertion and deglutition

Deglutition function	*LMA insertion function*
Lubrication of food bolus with saliva	Mask lubrication prior to insertion
Formation of soft, flat bolus of appropriate size by mastication	Deflation of mask to form thin flat wedge shape
Mastication causes stimulation of palate, initiating swallow reflex	Stimulation of hard palate by pressing mask tip upwards against it
Upward and backward sweeping action of tongue flattens bolus against palate and posterior pharyngeal wall while forcing it into hypopharynx	Index finger imitates tongue action by pressing flattened mask upwards and backwards
Simultaneous neck flexion with head extension opens space behind larynx to allow passage of food bolus	Operator's free hand pushes occiput to flex neck and extend head to permit mask to pass behind larynx

Reproduced from reference 54 with kind permission from the International Anesthesia Research Society, *Anesthesia and Analgesia*.

failures are likely to be related to poor technique or inadequate anesthetic depth. The diagrams and text accompanying Figure 6.2 should be carefully studied to fully understand the correct technique of LMA insertion.

Insertion problems

The commonest error during insertion is failure to maintain a constant centrifugal force with the index finger against the curve of the hard palate and posterior oropharynx until the LMA passes down into the hypopharynx. The commonest problems encountered during insertion are failure to pass the cuff over the back of the tongue due to the tip folding over against the posterior oropharyngeal wall during placement or due to light anesthesia causing increased tone in the surrounding musculature (Table 6.2).

During normal swallowing the vocal cords transiently close. This may occur during placement of the LMA and will be associated with an inability to inflate the lungs until the glottic sphincter relaxes, usually about 20 s later. It is important to recognize transient glottic closure because it is otherwise easily mistaken for misplacement of the LMA or laryngeal spasm. It is also important to make the distinction between malposition and inadequate anesthetic depth when the airway is clinically obstructed, so that appropriate action may be taken. Problems at insertion become progressively less as experience is gained if the recommended insertion technique is carefully followed[57].

Placement of the LMA may be difficult or impossible in patients with limited mouth opening or pharyngeal pathology. Maltby et al have reported successful insertion in patients with mouth opening of 12–18 mm[63] and one of the authors (AB) has inserted a size 3 LMA through an interdental gap of 8 mm. Tonsillar hypertrophy[4,64] and a high arched palate[65] may also make insertion difficult. Occasionally anatomical abnormalities, such as a large, floppy epiglottis, may be responsible for failure to function

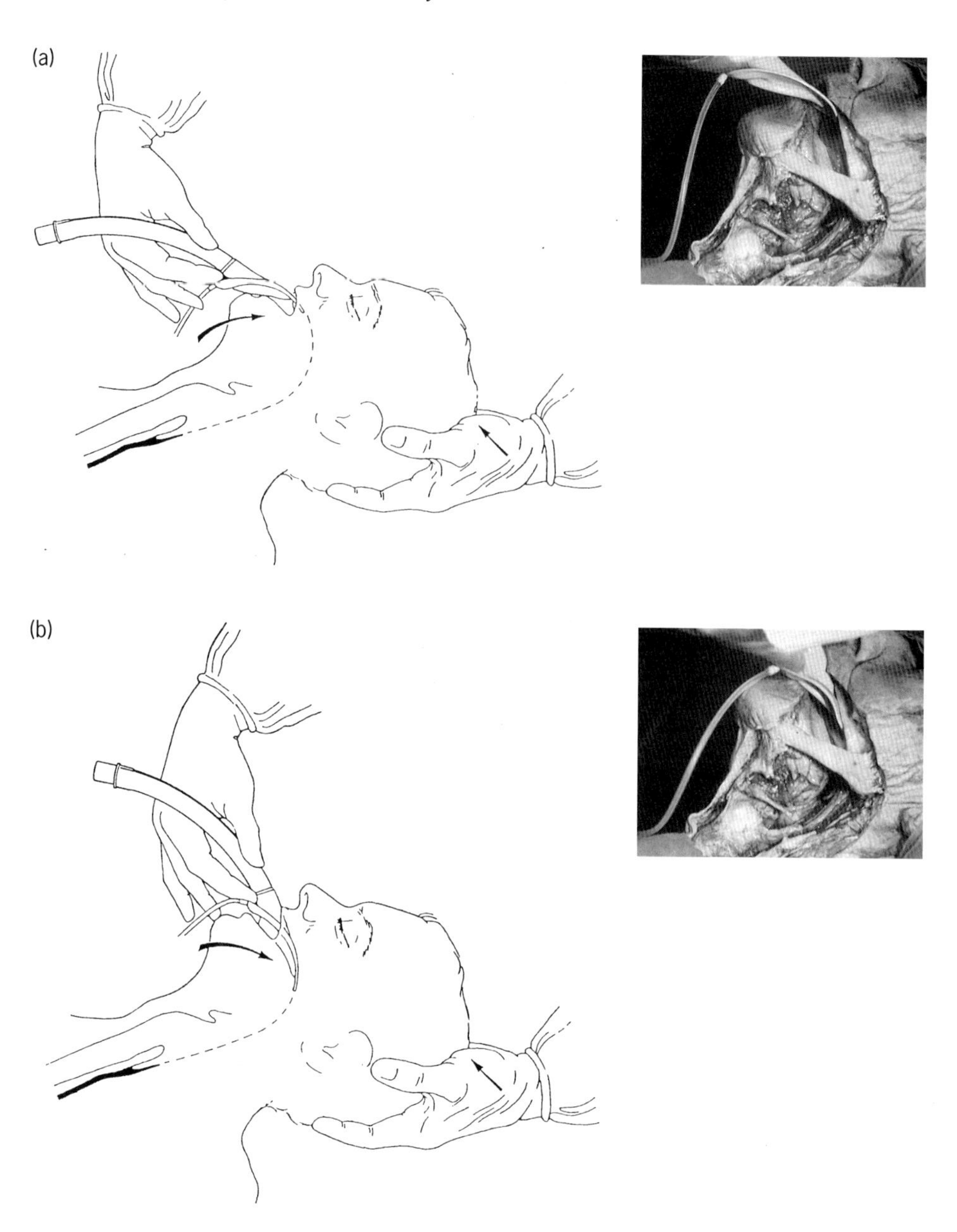

Figure 6.2 Illustration sequence for LMA insertion.

(a) To obtain optimal placement in the hypopharynx with its surrounding musculature, the appropriate sized LMA should be inserted with reflexes obtunded by either general or topical anesthesia with the head and neck in the standard intubating position. The cuff should be fully deflated and lubricated on its posterior surface. The intention is to follow the line of the palatopharyngeal curve as indicated.

(b) Under direct vision and holding the LMA at the mask–tube junction between the index finger and thumb, press the mask tip upwards against the hard palate to flatten it out. The mask aperture must face forward and the black line on the tube should be facing the upper lip. Use your middle finger to push the lower jaw downwards at this point. This makes it easier to see into the mouth and verify the position of the mask. It will also enable you to insert the index finger further into the mouth during insertion. Alternatively, instruct a nurse or assistant to pull the lower jaw downwards. A high arched palate may require a slightly lateral approach. Do not continue to hold the jaw open once the mask is inside the mouth because this action allows the epiglottis to fall back against the posterior pharyngeal wall.

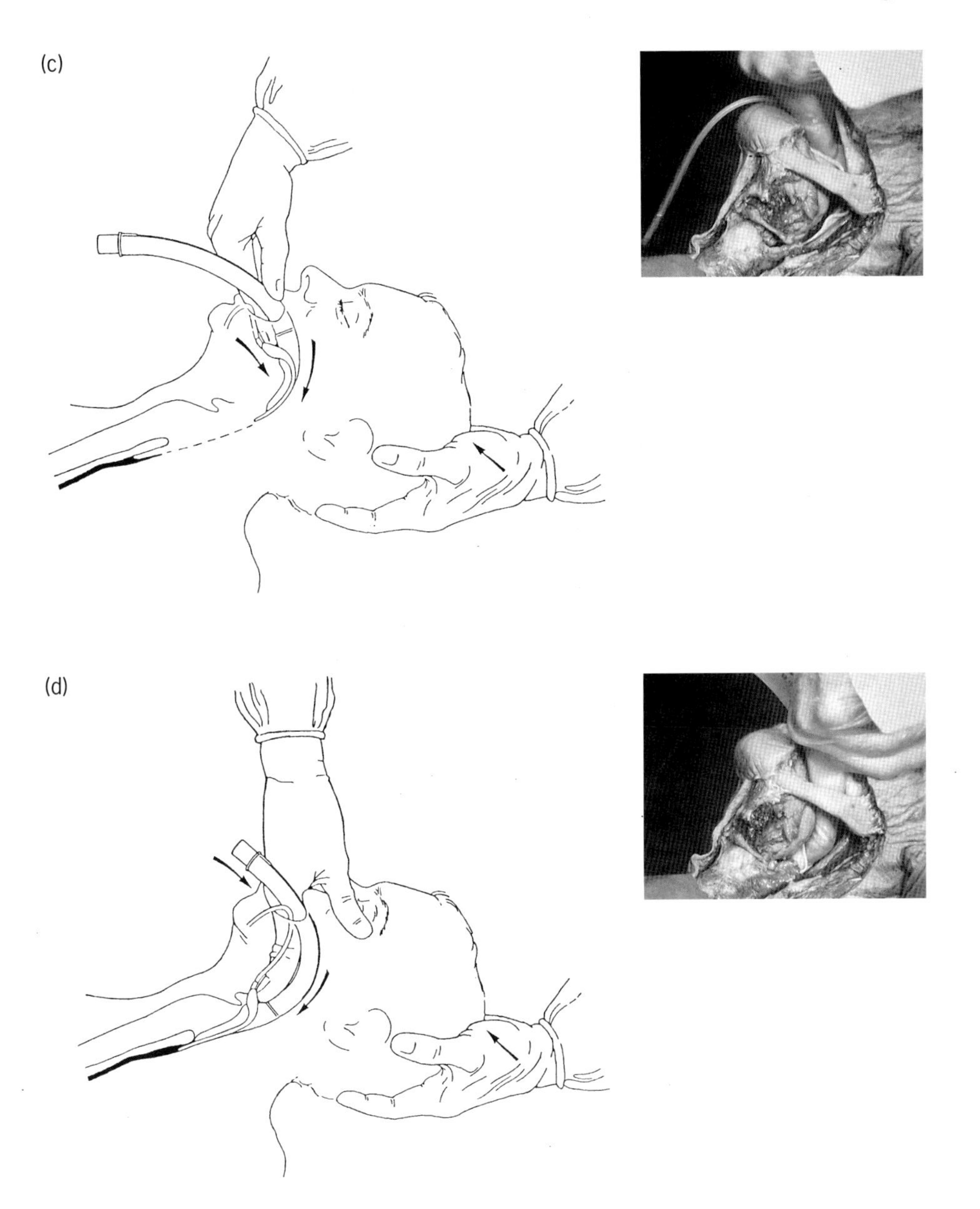

Figure 6.2 *(continued)*
(c) Keeping the neck flexed and head extended, press the mask into the palatopharyngeal curve and advance the mask into the oropharynx and along the posterior pharyngeal wall using the index finger. It is important as you advance the mask into the pharynx to ensure that the tip remains flattened and avoids the tongue.
(d) Continue pushing with the index finger until the mask is guided into position. Do not use force. A definite resistance is felt as the tip enters the hypopharynx. If required the LMA can be pushed into final position by pressing along the shaft with the other hand once the mask has circumvented the oropharyngeal inlet. Depending on patient size, this may mean that the finger is inserted to its fullest extent into the oral cavity before resistance is encountered.

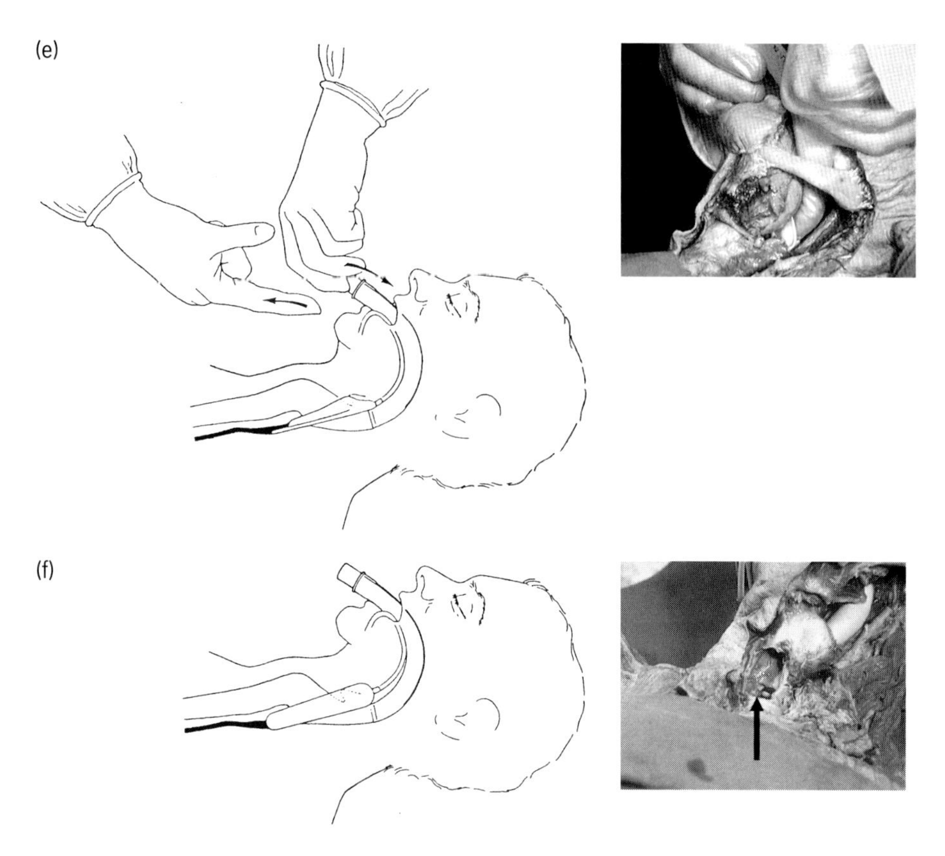

Figure 6.2 (*continued*)
(e) Now grasp the tube firmly with the other hand and then withdraw the index finger from the pharynx. Press gently downward with this other hand to ensure the mask is fully inserted. At this point the LMA should be correctly located with the tip resting against the upper esophageal sphincter.
(f) Check to ensure that the black line on the airway tube faces the upper lip. Inflate the mask with the recommended volume of air. Never overinflate the cuff. Do not touch the LMA while inflating unless the position is obviously unstable (this may be the case in elderly edentulous patients with slack tissues). Normally the mask should be allowed to rise up slightly out of the hypopharynx as it is inflated, to find its correct position. Taking care to avoid dislodgment, connect the LMA to the anesthetic circuit and employ gentle manual ventilation to airway pressures of less than 20 cm H_2O. Capnography should be used to confirm the presence of an adequate airway. Check for airway patency by inflating the lungs and auscultate for breath sounds. Auscultate in the anterolateral neck region to check for the presence of any wheezing that might indicate the presence of mild laryngeal spasm and light anesthesia. In addition, ausculate over the left hypochondrium to check for gas entering the stomach. The mask may leak slightly for the first three or four breaths before settling into position in the pharynx. If the leak persists, check that the inflation pressures are low and there is adequate depth of anesthesia before assuming that there is a malposition requiring re-insertion of the LMA or selection of a larger size. The cadaveric picture shows the mask tip (arrowed) seated in contact with the upper esophageal sphincter

following successful placement[59]. Recent cadaver studies have shown that adoption of the correct head position for insertion, smooth deflation of the LMA with a posterior tip and adherence to the swallowing principle of insertion will cause the LMA to follow the ideal posterior pathway to its final position. In contrast the semi-inflated, anterior tip and 'midshaft push' or 'spear' techniques do not (Figure 6.3). Important practical points are to avoid force and to ensure an adequate depth of anesthesia. The largest

Table 6.2 Aetiology of LMA related adverse events

Event	*Consider*
Unable to push LMA past the back of the tongue	1. Inadequate anesthetic depth 2. Need to increase neck flexion and/or head extension 3. Need to change angle of approach 4. Incorrect mask deflation 5. Inadequate lubrication 6. Anatomical problem
LMA inserted, unable to hand ventilate (no thoracoabdominal movement, no capnograph trace)	1. Inadequate anesthesia (glottic closure) 2. Epiglottis downfolded (can be due to large floppy epiglottis in elderly men) 3. Wrong LMA size 4. Mask doubled over 5. Mask folded back 6. Mask facing backwards/lateral
Poor seal (audible mask leak, poor lung inflation, low end-tidal CO_2)	1. Inadequate depth of anesthesia 2. Wrong size LMA 3. Incorrect LMA position 4. Leaking cuff (device failure) 5. Not enough air in cuff 6. Laryngeal or pharyngeal pathology
Gastric insufflation (visible abdominal distension, gas entering stomach detected by stethoscopy)	1. Inadequate depth of anesthesia 2. Mask folded backwards 3. Excessive flow/tidal volume 4. Mask not fully inserted 5. Relaxant wearing off 6. LMA too small 7. Prior difficult face mask ventilation
Reflux of gastric contents (gastric contents seen in pharynx or LMA tube)	1. Inadequate depth of anesthesia 2. Unsuspected full stomach 3. Surgical manipulation 4. Gastric insufflation 5. Autonomic neuropathy 6. Drug induced 7. Intestinal obstruction 8. ?Extreme preoperative anxiety
Aspiration has occurred (bronchospasm, coughing, gastric contents present on tracheal suction, chest X-ray changes)	1. Massive reflux 2. ?Removal of LMA during reflux 3. ?Suxamethonium administration 4. ?Laryngoscopy 5. Failure to tilt head down 6. Mask lying in upper pharynx

LMA for the patient's size should be used and the mask fully and correctly deflated. If insertion failure occurs, the LMA may be removed and quickly prepared again for re-insertion or a second LMA used. Alternative techniques may be useful where the standard technique fails or is inappropriate. The thumb technique is useful when an operator cannot gain access to the head from behind (see Quick Reference, *Thumb insertion technique*, page 285).

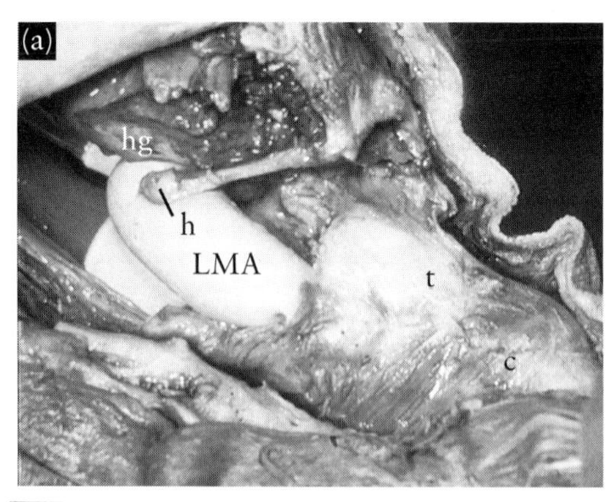

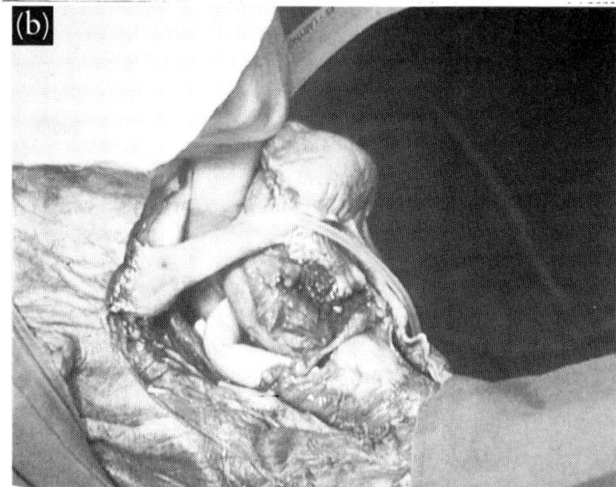

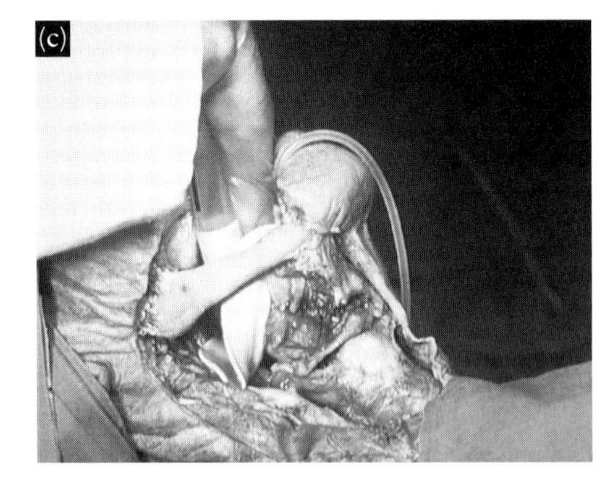

Figure 6.3 Cadaver, lateral neck dissection.

(a) The LMA optimally positioned in the pharynx. hg, hypoglossal nerve; h, hyoid bone with muscle attachments removed; LMA, laryngeal mask airway; t, thyroid cartilage; c, cricoid cartilage.

(b) Insertion of the LMA with the cuff fully inflated increases the chances of impaction with anterior pharyngeal structures such as the glottic inlet.

(c) Failure to press the LMA into the hard palate frequently results in impaction with the oropharyngeal wall since the oropharyngeal curve is not followed.

INSERTION HINTS

1. To imitate the action of the tongue, the index finger must be placed at the junction of the tube and mask in line with the central mask aperture, tucking the finger behind the deflated upper rim of the mask (Figure 6.4). The finger remains in this position until the mask is fully inserted.

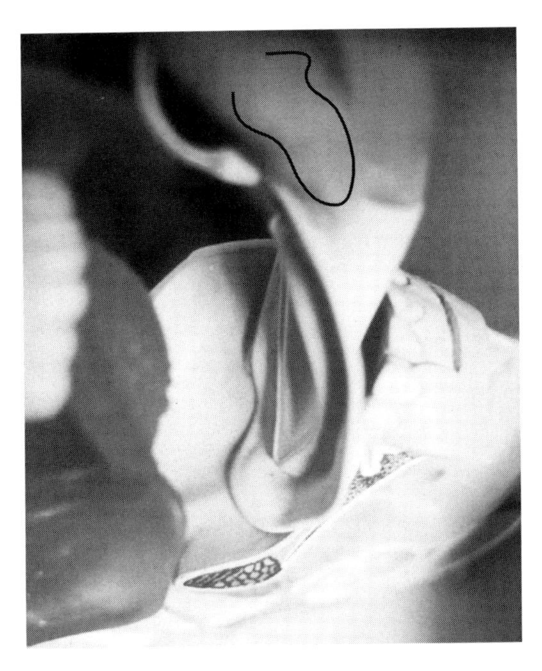

Figure 6.4 The position of the index finger shown here is critical, enabling the tube to be pressed up into the palate as the mask slides inwards.

2. The index finger may slip off to one side during insertion if it is not positioned centrally or gets slippery. The LMA should be held comfortably as though it were a pen, with the index finger flexed. However, during the actual insertion, the index finger is straightened out, while the other fingers and thumb are drawn away to permit the extended index finger to be inserted to the fullest extent into the oral cavity. This involves fully extending the thumb at right angles to the index finger and flexing the second, third and fourth fingers to make a right angle with their metacarpals (Figure 6.5). Slight pronation of the forearm helps full insertion of the index finger.

   Hold the mask with its tip pointing towards your own umbilicus and the bowl of the mask facing downwards. Your other hand should be positioned with the palm facing upwards to cup the patient's head in the region of the occiput. By pushing forwards with this hand, the head is extended and the neck flexed (Figure 6.6). This 'sniffing' position is held until the mask has passed behind the larynx. Otherwise the mask may not pass into the hypopharynx, especially if the neck is mobile and falls back, creating a convex curve on the posterior pharyngeal wall which tends to obliterate the pharyngeal space. In cadavers, the epiglottis can be held approximately 2 cm away from the posterior pharyngeal wall by occipital pressure as described, but falls back to block the airway when this pressure is released (Figure 6.7).

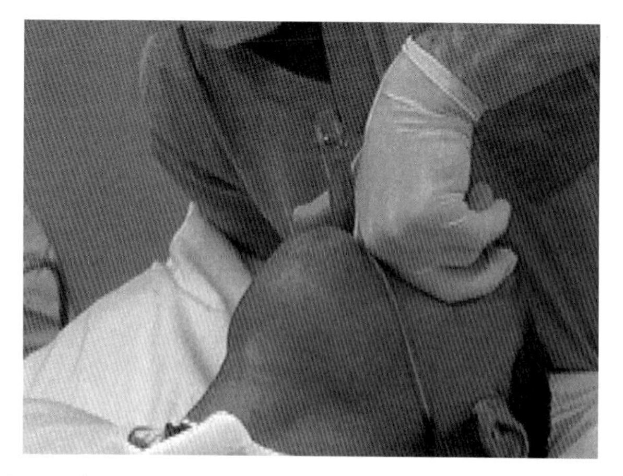

Figure 6.5 The thumb must be extended and the second, third and fourth fingers flexed to permit full insertion of the index finger.

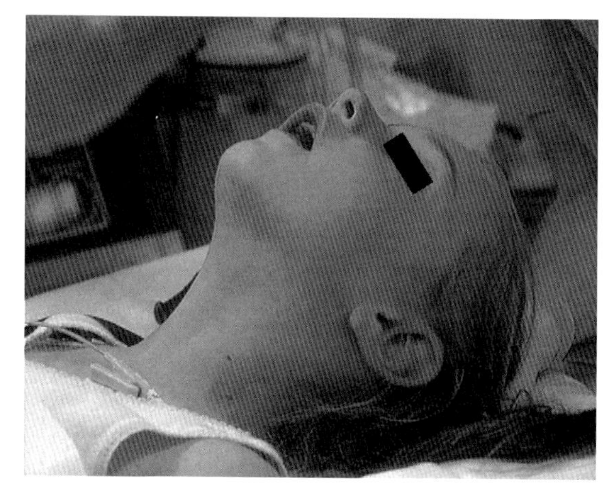

Figure 6.6 The 'sniffing position' is achieved by pushing the supported head up from behind so that the chin juts forward.

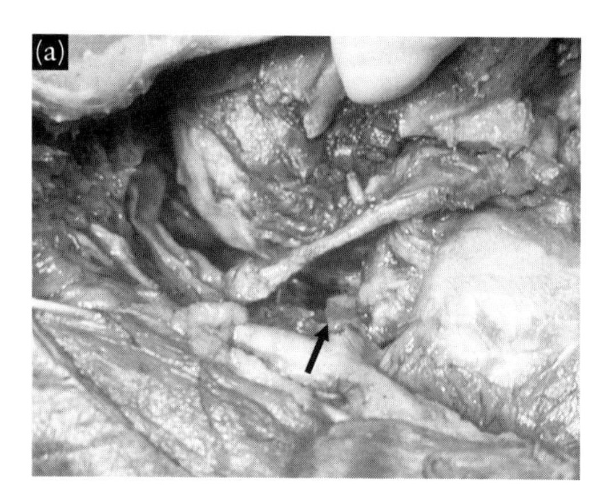

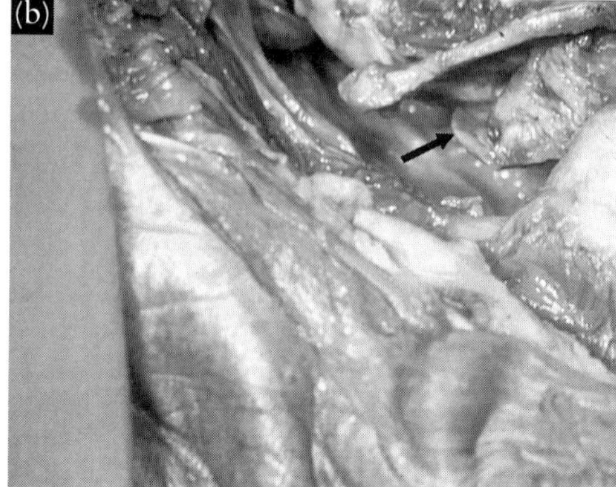

Figure 6.7 Cadaveric preparations demonstrating the increased space created between the epiglottis (arrowed) and posterior pharyngeal wall when the head is extended and the neck flexed. (a) Neutral position, head supported to flex neck, (b) head extended with neck flexed.

3. At the start of insertion, the LMA tube should be held parallel to the patient's chest. Advancing from this angle, the extreme tip of the mask is carefully introduced between the teeth.

   Explanatory note: food is normally brought to the mouth at a similar angle. The upper incisors usually protrude beyond the lower, so the maximal gap between them lies perpendicular to this line of approach at moderate degrees of mouth opening.

4. When the leading edge of the mask has passed between the teeth, press it upwards and gently massage the front of the hard palate (Figure 6.8). Only proceed when you are sure that the mask is not folded.

   Explanatory note: massaging the palate provokes the swallowing reflex and therefore is likely to inhibit the reflex associated with retching.

5. The next movement is rapid but gentle (see Figure 6.2).
6. A diagonal approach is helpful when the tonsils are hypertrophied or when the midline approach fails.
7. When the palate is narrow and vaulted, the mask should be flattened into one or other sides of the arch, to prevent it losing contact with the mucosa and folding back on itself. Look into the mouth to ensure this has not happened.
8. The direction of pressure of the index finger **never** corresponds with the direction of passage of the mask. The inserting finger must always press in a cephalad direction.

   Explanatory note: this is because the finger has to keep the mask flattened out against the posterior pharyngeal wall. It is the anteroposterior curvature of this wall which guides the mask into place, not the inserting finger. The finger is providing a centrifugal pressure to keep the mask in contact with the wall, just as the tongue presses the food bolus backwards during swallowing.

9. Do not adjust the finger position during insertion. This allows the mask to spring away from the posterior pharynx, so it loses its flattened out shape and begins to double back on itself or collide with the larynx.
10. Do not point the inserting finger in the direction of the lower pharynx when making the insertion attempt (Figure 6.9).

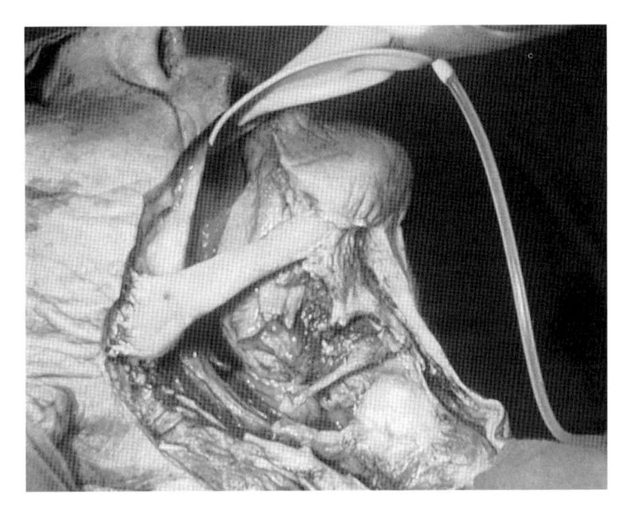

Figure 6.8 When the leading edge of the mask has been passed between the teeth, press it upwards to flatten out the saucer-shaped mask tip, so distributing pressure evenly over the palatal surface while gently massaging the palate to distribute the lubricant.

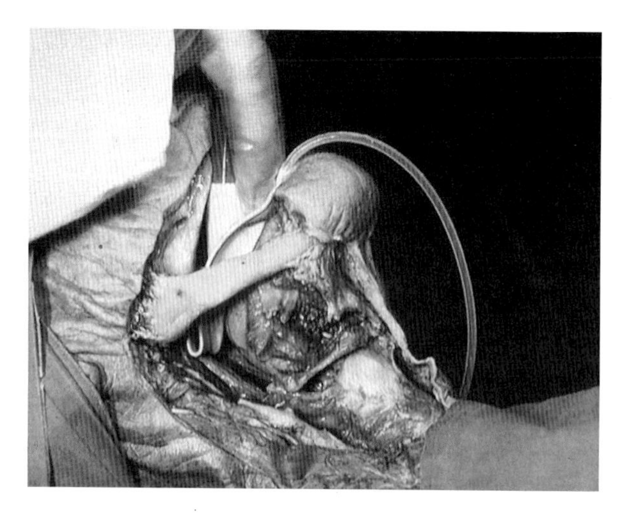

Figure 6.9 Do not point the index finger in the direction of the lower pharynx when making the insertion attempt.

Explanatory note: this results in the mask being driven into the tongue, which is forced backwards, allowing the epiglottis to get in the way.

11. When the leading edge of the cuff reaches the arytenoid cartilages it should pass posterior to them. The pointed end of the mask bowl then comes in contact with the interarytenoid area and slight resistance can be felt as the larynx is displaced forwards.
12. With a normal length of index finger, a second, definitive resistance is felt when the leading edge of the cuff reaches the base of the hypopharynx. A short finger may not reach this far. This does not matter provided that the other hand exerts pressure on the LMA tube, again in a cephalad direction, before the index finger is removed. This will ensure insertion to the correct depth, and also prevents accidental dislodgment of the mask as the finger is withdrawn. Always stabilize the device in this way before removing the inserting finger.
13. The identical technique is effective for insertion of the flexible LMA. However, because the tube is more flexible, when the second hand is used to complete insertion, the tube should be fed inwards 2–3 cm at a time holding it close to the teeth and feeding it cephalad using the vault of the hard palate to prevent it bending.

Cuff inflation

General

It is important to distinguish between pressure in the cuff, pressure exerted by the cuff on the mucosa and the pressure in the airway at which leaks occur[66]. Unfortunately, because of the nature of the anatomy surrounding the mask and the low probability that the mask will be exactly the right size for any given patient, there can be no fixed relationship between these three variables. It is therefore logical to determine an intracuff pressure which will provide an effective seal empirically, a 'just seal' pressure. This value will be higher if the mask is small relative to the anatomical space available and lower if the mask is large relative to the available space. For this reason it is sensible to choose as large a size of mask as possible in order to ensure the 'just seal' pressure is as low as possible. The smaller the mask relative to the patient, the weaker the relationship between intracuff pressure and average pressure on the mucosa, since the elastic material of the cuff is being stretched relatively more than the tissues surrounding it. On the other hand, because the cuff surface becomes more rigid with increasing intracuff pressure, local high pressure points may develop if excessive stretching of a small mask is resorted to as a means of achieving a seal in a large patient.

Morris and Marjot demonstrated that LMA cuff pressures can be reduced to 22 mm Hg without significantly affecting tidal ventilation in spontaneously breathing anesthetized patients[67,68], but perioperative cuff deflation to such low pressures may be potentially hazardous. A major function of the LMA cuff during spontaneous breathing is to protect the larynx from oropharyngeal saliva. To perform this function an oropharyngeal leak pressure of up to 10 cm H_2O may be required (the approximate pressure of fluid at the posterior pharyngeal wall if the oral cavity is flooded). An intracuff pressure of 22 mm Hg may or may not be adequate to ensure an adequate seal to prevent flooding of the larynx with oropharyngeal secretions depending on the factors outlined above. We would therefore suggest that in spontaneously ventilating patients a leak pressure of greater than 10 cm H_2O is a more useful guide to airway safety than intracuff pressure alone. When positive pressure ventilation is used, it is found empirically that using an adequate size of LMA a sufficient seal may be achieved without exceeding the maximum recommended value in the cuff if it is inflated to a pressure of 60 cm H_2O.

Once in place, the cuff should be inflated with the correct amount of air defined as that volume within the recommended maximum volume which provides an adequate seal and lung inflation without leak. Inflation of the cuff should be done gradually. One of the authors (JB) has noted that rapid inflation of the cuff may occasionally trigger hiccups. The maximum recommended volume should not be exceeded or the seal may worsen. The tension in the pilot balloon reflects cuff tension and should be noted by manual ballotting or direct measurement after inflation. The tension in the cuff should be checked at regular intervals. It may be necessary to remove small volumes of air as the pressure in the cuff rises due to nitrous oxide diffusion.

Whilst there is a low probability that the mask will be exactly the right size for a given patient, there is a high probability that appropriate size selection combined with optimal cuff inflation will produce a near-perfect fit[69].

Hints on cuff inflation

1. The cuff should be inflated as soon as the mask has been fully inserted.
2. **Do not hold the tube while inflating the cuff.**
3. Use only a marked, dry, clean syringe of adequate size filled with ambient air. (Contaminated syringes may introduce moisture into the cuff resulting in device rupture during autoclaving. Organic substances, such as propofol, will form a sticky residue after autoclaving and may cause valve failure.)
4. The pharyngeal muscles adapt to mask volume. Inflate over 3 to 5 s. By gently holding the pilot balloon with the other hand, you can feel the muscular sack accommodating to

the mask. Too rapid inflation might provoke generalized laryngopharyngeal reaction in the unparalyzed subject. In awake subjects, volume and rate should be lower.

5. The maximum inflation volumes are given in Table 5.7. In practice it is rarely necessary to inflate with the full amount and a 'just seal' volume should be sought[66].
6. Inexperienced or untaught users frequently provoke a greater stimulus when inserting the device and may find leaks occurring even when they exceed the maximum inflation value. This is due to glottic closure provoked by the stimulus of insertion. Do not remove the device or exceed the maximum inflation volume if this occurs. (This is likely to worsen the problem by increasing the stimulus.) The appropriate action is to deepen the anesthetic.

Assessment of position

General

Anatomical and functional signs of correct placement are listed in Table 6.3. It is important to ensure that the LMA tubing does not press against the side of the tongue or third molar since this has been implicated in transient lingual nerve injury[70]. The LMA tubing should lie in contact with and following the sagittal contour of the hard palate. Fiberoptic laryngoscopy is a noninvasive method of assessing the position of the LMA in relation to the glottis and determining whether the vocal cords are open or closed[71], but does not give useful information on the position of the mask tip in relation to the esophageal sphincter. The esophageal detector device[72] has been used to confirm placement of the LMA[73,74], but is probably a less reliable test than for tracheal intubation since air may be drawn in from the oropharynx and it cannot distinguish between malposition and a closed larynx[75].

Once placed in the laryngopharynx, light anesthesia may cause laryngeal spasm, coughing, breath holding or failure to manually ventilate, all of which are usually treatable with additional doses of induction agent or volatile agent. If the adverse event does not settle, it is possible there is a malposition and the LMA should be removed and

Table 6.3 Anatomical and functional signs of correct placement

Anatomical	*Functional*
Oval swelling extending over thyroid and cricoid regions at cuff inflation	Observation of reservoir bag movement
Slight outward movement of LMA tube at inflation	Gentle hand ventilation possible
Cuff not visible in mouth	Normal breath sounds heard on auscultation of lungs and side of neck
Tube protruding approximately 8 cm above teeth (size 3 and 4 LMA)	No gas leak heard on auscultation of left hypochondrium*
Black marking on tube facing cranially (not FLMA)	Normal capnograph trace
Fiberoptic laryngoscopy via LMA shows normal view of larynx	(Esophageal detector device)

*During PPV to detect gastric insufflation.

replaced by face mask ventilation until the patient is re-stabilized under deep anesthesia and the LMA correctly prepared for a second attempt.

Hints on assessment of position

1. Premature resistance to insertion may be felt at uvular level (incorrect angle of insertion), at epiglottic level (mask tip impacted in valleculae) or at arytenoid level. The first two are usually fairly easy to diagnose, because it will be obvious, at least to trained users, that the mask has not reached its correct destination. The third case is harder to detect, the possibilities being that the mask tip has become directed anteriorly into the laryngeal vestibule, or that the stimulus provoked by downward passage of the mask has caused the inferior constrictor muscles to contract (light anesthesia).
2. For the mask to be correctly inserted, resistance must be felt as the mask tip reaches the base of the hypopharynx. To avoid confusion with resistance due to obstruction at a higher level/misplacement into the laryngeal vestibule, look at the front of the neck to see if the cricoid cartilage has become more prominent. If only the thyroid cartilage is seen to bulge outward, suspect incorrect placement. In the correct position, the cricoid cartilage becomes more prominent when the mask is inflated.
3. Failure to ventilate does not always mean misplacement has occurred. It may be due to laryngeal reaction if anesthesia is too light.
4. Persistent coughing in the unparalyzed patient does suggest misplacement of the mask into the larynx; in the paralyzed patient, the same misplacement may be associated with obstructed expiration and sometimes a stridor-like sound.
5. The black line is a guide to correct mask orientation for the standard LMA; for the flexible LMA its purpose is to indicate only the degree of rotation of the tube and it gives no information on orientation of the mask. It may be necessary to confirm correct depth and orientation of the flexible LMA using a laryngoscope if in doubt.

Alternative insertion techniques

Numerous alternative methods of LMA/FLMA insertion have been described since 1988[3–6,24,36,37,48–50,54,56,76–117] and there are a number of others which are widely practiced but undescribed in the literature (Table 6.4). By combining different techniques there are theoretically thousands of possible combinations. To some extent, this high figure reflects a failure to understand the basic principles of LMA insertion and to apply those principles clinically[118]. It also reflects the forgiving nature of the LMA in that some success is likely regardless of technique, as suggested in studies of inexperienced personnel[119–122]. Dingley and Asai surveyed insertion practices in Wales and found that the most popular insertion technique was the standard method, but it was only utilized by 32% of anesthesiologists[37]. Other popular methods were partially inflated (16%), back to front (10%), jaw thrust (9%), reposition head (8%), laryngoscope (7%), anteriorly deflated tip (6%), rotation back and forth (5%), extra mouth opening (5%) and lateral approach (3%).

It is generally considered that insertion of the LMA from a diagonal direction or by twisting it through 180 degrees (like a Guedel airway) are useful backup techniques, although the latter may result in some residual rotation in the sagittal plain[56]. If mouth opening is inadequate, an assistant may pull the jaw downwards during insertion into

Table 6.4 Alternative insertion techniques for the LMA

Active swallowing (awake)[110]	Magill's forceps (FLMA)[129]
Anteriorly deflated rim[84–88]	Measuring spoons[114]
Anterior traction of glottis[79]	Midshaft push or spear technique (avoiding finger in mouth)
Anterior traction of tongue[4]	Partially inflated cuff[56,89,90,113]
Digital exploration[116,126]	Partial removal and re-insertion[79]
Dingley's insertion tool[109]	Repositioning head[79]
Extra mouth opening[92,117]	Rotation back and forth[37]
Finger on posterior pharyngeal wall[4,54,95]	Skid[100,101]
Fully inflated cuff[56,91]	Stylet or bougie (FLMA)[104–108,130]
Guedel airway[97,98,49,56,76–78]	Sugar spoon[99]
Introducer[50]	Thread[115]
J-forceps[111]	Thumb technique (for insertion from the front)[112] (see Quick Reference)
Jaw thrust[92,93]	Tracheal stabilization[117]
Jaw thrust/semi-inflation/head extension[102,103]	Triple airway maneuver[48,123]
Laryngoscope[80–84,124,127,128]	Twisting[94]
Lateral approach[90,96]	
Lift and rotation[116] (to improve position once in situ)	

the mouth. The jaw should be released during further insertion through the pharynx as it causes the epiglottis to fall back into the path of the mask tip, thereby increasing the risk of epiglottic downfolding. Few of the alternative techniques have been tested in randomized controlled trials and in situations where controlled trials have been attempted the correct application of the standard technique has not been ensured. For example, in six trials comparing the standard technique with various alternatives[48,90,113,117,123,124] the success rates and fiberoptic positioning or success rates for the standard technique groups would be considered suboptimal[118,125].

Currently there are insufficient data available to know with certainty which is the optimal technique and it is possible that this will vary in different clinical circumstances. There are theoretical reasons why some techniques may be an improvement on the standard. For instance jaw thrust, by lifting the pharyngeal structures anteriorly, should make passage into the hypopharynx easier with less risk of epiglottic impaction. There is some comparative evidence to support this concept[48,123], although the standard insertion technique was probably used suboptimally in this study[125]. A lateral or laryngoscope guided approach may be more appropriate in tonsillar hypertrophy. In a study of 47 children, Elwood and Cox have shown that the epiglottis is less commonly visible fiberoptically if a laryngoscope is used for insertion[124,127]. They suggested that the technique would be suitable when LMA insertion precedes bronchoscopy or intubation via the LMA. However, jaw thrust and/or laryngoscopy can be extremely stimulating and may therefore only be appropriate in paralyzed patients with no history of ischemic heart disease[125]. There is some evidence to support the concept that insertion with the cuff semi-inflated may be easier than the standard technique for inexperienced personnel, and this is an important finding[102,103,113]. It is important to stress, however, that this does not imply that it is the best technique for experienced LMA users since it is possible that after experience is gained insertion rates may be higher than those achievable with an inflated technique, and with better fiberoptic position[131]. There is also some evidence to suggest insertion is easier in children when the Guedel[132] or partially inflated techniques[90] are used. Kondo, however, has suggested that the rotational technique is more likely to damage teeth[77]. Kumar has suggested that manual external stabilization of the trachea with the thumb on one side and index and middle fingers on the other side may help position the LMA correctly.

Further trials are clearly required to answer these questions; meanwhile clinicians should be sensible in their approach to both acquiring and then teaching LMA insertion skills[58]. Ultimately the choice of technique is made by the individual and will be based on individual skills and patient factors. It is important that individuals are exposed to the optimal learning environment to be able to make the most sensible choices.

Insertion of the FLMA

The technique for placement of the FLMA is similar to that for the standard device[133], but is more difficult since pressure cannot be transmitted along the flexometallic tube and malposition (e.g. rotation) is less easily diagnosed[134,135]. The FLMA is held at the junction of the tube and mask and pushed into position by extending the index finger. Where extension of the index finger does not push the device tip into the hypopharynx, the operator's wrist may be internally rotated so that the index and middle fingers can penetrate more deeply into the pharynx by following the oropharyngeal curve. For those with short fingers or in large patients, it may be necessary to use the other hand to achieve full insertion by pushing the tube cranially. This ensures the tube is kept in a central position by being pressed into the palatopharyngeal curve. Some force is thus transmitted to the mask without lateral tube flexion. Grasp the tube with the other hand before withdrawing the index finger. Once experience is gained there is a high success rate although placement may be slightly slower than with the standard device[136,137]. A variety of aids have been suggested to transiently stiffen the FLMA to improve insertion[104–106,108,129], but these are not necessary if the correct technique is applied[136]. None of these aids deals adequately with rotation along the sagittal plane. Fiberoptic observation of FLMA placement may be impeded by the narrower bore of the tube[138].

Fixation and stabilization

LMA

Fixation and stability are important, but frequently neglected aspects of LMA anesthesia[139–141]. Before fixing the LMA in place, insert an appropriate bite block (see Chapter 5, *Bite blocks*). Use adhesive tape for fixation rather than ties. Cotton ties may slip on silicone when wet and may cut into the tube, but may be the best option in bearded patients. Do not precut lengths of adhesive tape; instead, fix one end of the tape to the maxilla, then unwind the roll over and then under the tube and bite block, fixing down to the opposite maxilla before tearing off the roll. This way, the tube is held firmly into the arch of the palate, soft palate and pharynx (Figure 6.10). The

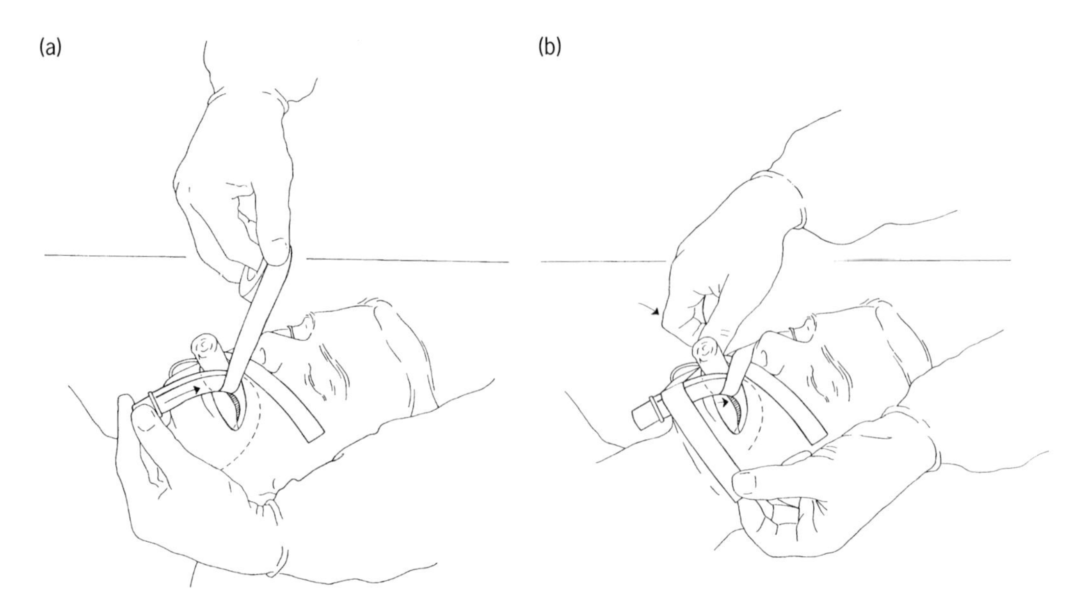

Figure 6.10 The stability of the LMA is greatly enhanced by correct fixation which holds the tube pressed into the arch of the palate, soft palate and pharynx. (a) Application of tape and correct tube orientation. (b) Additional tape to provide further support if required.

connector end of the LMA tube is designed to face caudally. Optimal stability is best achieved by ensuring that this natural caudal curve of the LMA is maintained, in effect locking it into the sagittal plane, preventing rotation and perhaps even improving the seal around the glottis[142]. To achieve this it is recommended that the LMA is fixed to the anesthetic breathing system below the chin. There should be sufficient length of tube beyond the mouth to permit it to be bent downwards towards the chin and for it to be sufficiently visible for fluids entering the tube to be detected. A popular means of achieving this is to loop the inspiratory and expiratory limbs around the side of the head to meet at a point approximately 5 cm inferoanterior to the chin[143] (Figure 6.11). An alternative is to use a short flexible silicone hose attached to the anesthetic breathing system and mounted on the forehead[144]. Several other aids to fixation have been described[145–147]. When using a Bain/Magill anesthetic breathing system the anesthetic hosing may be fixed to the LMA tube via a right angle connector. This enables the hosing to be fixed to one or other side of the patient's head (for example under a pillow) so it does not drag on the LMA. This arrangement is illustrated in Figure 6.12. Recent studies have suggested that the position of the LMA is stable under these circumstances[148,149]. The best mode of fixation may vary according to patient and surgical requirements[150]. Bending the tube against its natural curve may kink the tube or dislodge or rotate the mask, resulting in airway obstruction. Excessive traction from anesthetic breathing systems should be avoided.

FLMA

The FLMA can be taped directly to the face according to the requirements for surgical access. Where the surgeon needs to move the tube around the mouth fixation is

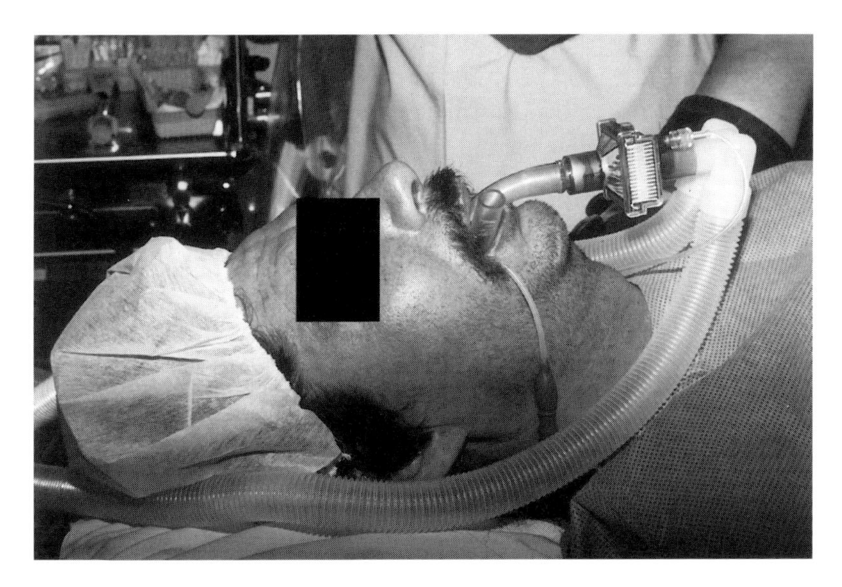

Figure 6.11 Fixation method using circle system. The bite guard in this instance is PVC tubing[143]. Reproduced with permission, *Anaesthesia and Intensive Care*.

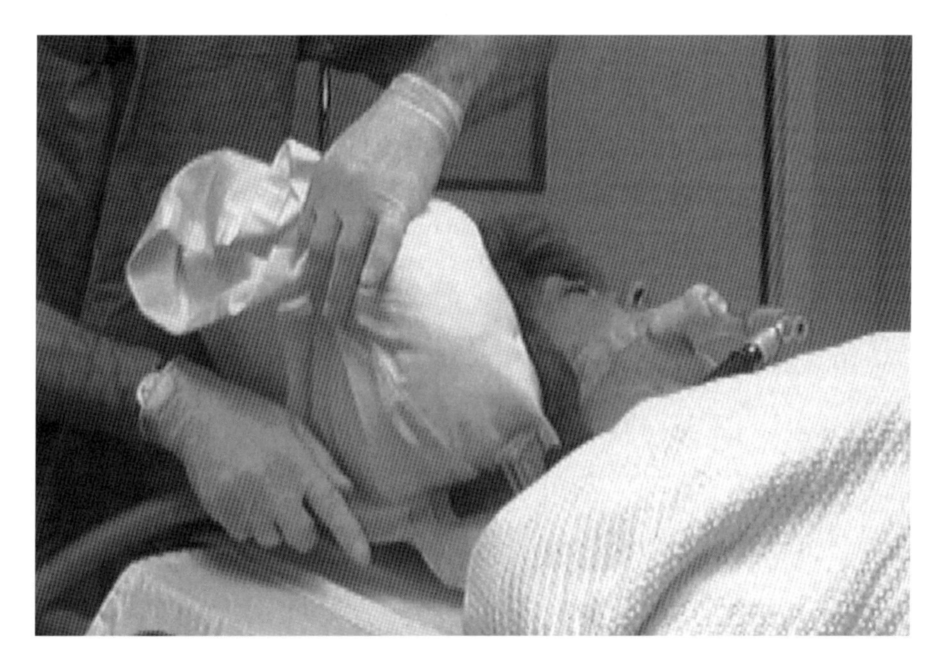

Figure 6.12 Fixation method using a right angle connector.

unnecessary, but constant vigilance is required to avoid displacement. There is no benefit in terms of stability to fixing it in a certain direction since it is a design feature that significant rotational force cannot be transmitted down the shaft. It may be dislodged by traction or the cuff compromised directly by instruments such as suction catheters passed too far into the pharynx. Although the FLMA is designed for maximum flexibility without kinking, it is not bite proof and cannot withstand strong compressive forces, particularly tangential compression forces[151,152]. When a tonsillar gag is used there is no need to fix the FLMA to the face during the procedure since it is held in position by the gag. However, it is important to remember to insert a bite guard at the end of the procedure to protect the device during recovery.

Malposition

LMA insertion is relatively easy, but fails in a small percentage of patients depending on the level of experience of the anesthesiologist. Highly experienced LMA users have a low incidence of fiberoptic malposition with the vocal cords visible from the mask aperture bars in > 97% and the esophageal inlet visible in < 1%[59]. While the incorrectly placed LMA may function well[153–155], it is more likely to be displaced or trigger airway reflexes or precipitate airway obstruction.

The most common malposition is severe epiglottic downfolding which may lead to an increased work of breathing[156] and, if sufficiently severe, to complete airway obstruction. Lesser degrees of epiglottic downfolding are common (20–30%) and should not be considered a malposition[59]. Avoidance of holding the LMA tube while inflating the device may be important in allowing a downfolded epiglottis to recover its normal position. Impaction with the laryngeal inlet (Figure 2.3b) is less common, but may result in laryngeal spasm or stridor. Impaction is further suggested by absence of swelling over the cricoid region when the device is inflated. Epiglottic downfolding and impaction with the laryngeal inlet are more likely to occur if: (1) the LMA is inserted with the cuff semi or fully inflated; (2) the rim is deflated anteriorly; (3) the LMA is not pressed into the posterior pharyngeal wall during its passage towards the hypopharynx[56]. If the LMA is not inserted far enough, either through inadequate depth of insertion, inadequate depth of anesthesia or too large a mask, the tip may press into the arytenoid cartilages, causing them to fold inwards and obstruct the airway. If the hypopharynx is seen through the fiberscope the mask is not inserted far enough or is folded back on itself. Insertion of too small a mask or with excessive force may result in penetration of the distal mask into the upper esophageal sphincter or impaction with the glottic inlet. Inflation of the cuff will then result in airway obstruction. Finally, folding of the LMA is possible if excessive force is used, the mask is inadequately lubricated or the cuff is not pressed into the hard palate. In this situation the mask may pass into the nasopharynx[155] or torsion may occur[56], particularly if the mask is rotated during insertion.

Maintenance

Less anesthetic is required to tolerate the LMA than the tracheal tube[29,55,157]. A readjustment of the operator's preconceived sense of anesthetic requirement is necessary when learning to use the LMA as anesthesia is now given for the intensity of surgical stimulus and not for airway tolerance. However, if anesthesia lightens, the patient will react to both the surgery and the LMA.

Although not shown to be associated with pharyngeal morbidity, nitrous oxide will rapidly diffuse into the cuff[158–161] and this will continue for the first 90 min of anesthesia[149,162] (Figure 6.13). To reduce the risk of postoperative pharyngeal morbidity,

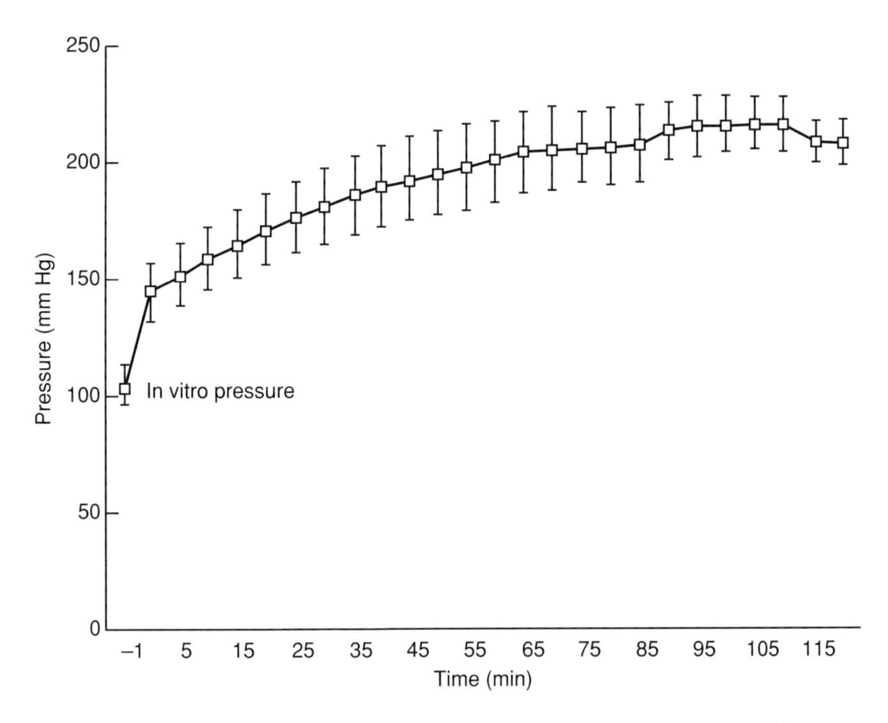

Figure 6.13 Cuff pressure increases during the first 1–2 h of nitrous oxide anesthesia[149]. Reproduced with permission, Canadian Society of Anaesthetists.

the cuff pressure should be checked at intervals either by feeling the tension in the pilot balloon, or by monitoring changes with a direct pressure transducer[163–165] (Portex Cuff Inflator, Hythe, Kent, UK). Volume may then be withdrawn to maintain values close to the initial control pressure. Avoiding nitrous oxide would minimize changes in cuff pressure. The addition of nitrous oxide to the cuff will have a variable effect on cuff pressure and is not recommended[148] (see Chapter 4, *Diffusion of gases*). Other factors, such as avoidance of lidocaine gel for lubrication, choice of correct size of LMA and ensuring that tension in the pilot balloon does not rise during nitrous oxide anesthesia may help minimize the risks of pharyngeal morbidity.

Halothane[166], enflurane[167], isoflurane[55,59,168], sevoflurane[29,169,170], desflurane (I. Smith, unpublished data), and total intravenous anesthesia with propofol[57,167,171–175] are suitable for maintenance of anesthesia with the LMA. There are currently no controlled trials comparing the different volatile agents for LMA usage. It is possible that isoflurane[176] and desflurane, which are irritant to the upper airway[176], are more suitable for use with the LMA than the face mask because most of the upper airway is bypassed.

Spontaneous breathing

The initial experience with the LMA should ideally be confined to short cases requiring the patient to remain spontaneously ventilating. This is the chosen mode of ventilation in approximately 60% of LMA uses in the UK[60,177]. Once the LMA is placed, respiration is supported initially by gentle manual ventilation and the patient allowed to gradually take over their own breathing. Even if spontaneous ventilation is planned, some initial positive pressure ventilation should be carried out by hand. This ensures ventilation, reduces atelectasis risk and gives valuable information of airway patency, adequacy of anesthesia and correctness of mask position. Using the LMA in the absence of neuromuscular block, the shape of the end-tidal CO_2 trace may give valuable information about the degree of phasic activity of the glottis. A square wave indicates that the glottis is relatively relaxed – evidence that anesthesia is adequate. A common problem is failure to maintain an adequate level of anesthesia following LMA insertion. If the induction agent is allowed to wear off before maintenance is achieved this may result in coughing, breathholding and movement[13]. This adverse reaction is particularly likely to occur following the introduction of an external stimulus such as surgery or moving the patient when the level of anesthesia has been misjudged. This situation can be corrected by administering an additional bolus of induction agent or increasing the concentration of volatile agent.

During spontaneous breathing, end-tidal carbon dioxide ($ETCO_2$) levels will tend to rise, depending on the depth of anesthesia and the plasma levels of other respiratory depressant drugs[178]. The $ETCO_2$ levels with the LMA during spontaneous breathing are not higher than with the face mask (which is prone to leaks) or with the tracheal tube (which produces a larger stimulus to respiration). A modest rise in $ETCO_2$ is acceptable provided there are no signs in the patient of impending clinical effects. The capnograph alarm limits may need to be reset for spontaneous breathing if they are normally set for controlled ventilation. However, if the $ETCO_2$ levels begin to rise above acceptable levels, anesthesia may be too deep and the amount of volatile agent should be reduced so that the tidal volume will increase accordingly. If narcotic breathing is observed, no further opioid should be given and ventilation gently assisted to maintain normocarbia. With experience, it will be found that less anesthetic agent is required during anesthesia with the LMA and patient recovery should be improved as a result. Balanced regional anesthesia with spontaneous ventilation has been used in procedures lasting up to 8 h with the LMA[179,180].

Positive pressure ventilation

Efficacy

The operator should be experienced with using the LMA in spontaneously ventilating patients before using it with PPV, as there are differences in the principles of maintenance of and recovery from anesthesia. Nonetheless ventilation via the LMA is an established technique[181] and may have particular application in some forms of elective surgery such as open eye surgery[182,183]. Data from one typical district general hospital indicate that PPV is utilized in approximately 40% of patients undergoing LMA anesthesia in the UK[60,177].

Six groups have examined either the efficacy of ventilation and/or the risk of gastric insufflation during PPV with the LMA[61,184–188]. Devitt et al demonstrated that ventilation through the LMA is adequate at ventilation pressures varying from 15 to 30 cm H_2O, and comparable to that with tracheal tube ventilation[184]. Leak fractions were consistently higher than for tracheal tube ventilation and increased with increasing airway pressures[184]. Berry and Verghese reported no leaks with tidal volumes of 10 ml kg^{-1} [185]. Graziotti studied the effects of PPV on gastric insufflation using a nasogastric tube/aspiration technique and found no difference between the LMA and the tracheal tube[186]. All patients were ventilated to mean peak airway pressure > 17 cm H_2O. Van Damme assessed leak pressures in 4866 patients and showed that a leak pressure of < 15 cm H_2O occurred in only 2.7%[61]. Epstein et al looked at leak pressures in 78 children aged 3 months to 17 years and found the initial mean leak pressure was 25.9 cm H_2O, increasing to 31.2 over 30 min of O_2/N_2O anesthesia. They concluded that seal pressure was well maintained during surgery[187,189]. There was no evidence of gastric distension or dislodgment during the leak test, suggesting that the leak test can be performed safely. Recently, Heinrichs et al showed that the mean (range) for gastric insufflation pressure was 28 (19–33) cm H_2O and that the mean (range) oropharyngeal leak was 31 (19–41) cm H_2O[188] using size 4 and size 5 LMAs. They suggested that the margin of safety with regard to gastric insufflation was essentially comparable to that of the face mask, but inherently inferior to that of a cuffed tracheal tube.

Size 5 LMA

The introduction of the size 5 LMA has increased the scope for PPV with the LMA[190,191]. Brimacombe and Berry reported its successful use in 30 patients undergoing spontaneous ventilation[190]. Van Damme compared the size 4 and 5 LMA in patients > 90 kg and showed that the size 5 provided a more effective seal[191]. In a prospective survey of 179 patients, Brimacombe has shown that PPV with the size 5 is a safe and effective technique with a high success rate and a low problem rate[192]. At tidal volumes of 10 ml kg^{-1}, 97.2% of patients could be ventilated without gastric insufflation and 98.3% without an oropharyngeal leak. At tidal volumes of 8 ml kg^{-1} no patient had gastric insufflation and 0.7% had an oropharyngeal leak.

Complications

The incidence of complications with the PPV/LMA technique appears to be similar to that for spontaneous ventilation and may be less than that for the PPV/tracheal tube technique. Haden et al reported using the LMA/PPV technique on 593 occasions with only two significant clinical problems (0.3%)[193]. Over the same period there were three serious problems with the PPV/tracheal tube technique in 187 uses (1.6%). Several large-scale studies have confirmed the safety of PPV with the LMA. In a prospective survey of 2359 LMA anesthetics, in which 41% underwent PPV, there were no cases of aspiration[177]. This study has now been extended to 11 910 patients, of whom 5236 underwent PPV, and with a similar absence of morbidity[60]. Positive pressure ventilation was unsuccessful on 14 occasions due to inadequate seal. Wainwright reported the use of the LMA in 1424 patients undergoing ophthalmic surgery without complications[183]. A meta-analysis of 547 LMA publications failed to show any link between PPV and aspiration either in patients included in LMA studies (n = 12 900) or aspiration case reports (n = 10)[194].

Practical considerations

From a practical viewpoint, most fasted patients with normal lung compliance may be mechanically ventilated through the LMA to airway pressures of approximately 20 cm H_2O. The low pressure seal implies that tidal volumes should be approximately 8 ml kg^{-1} and the inspiratory flow rates should be reduced to achieve adequate and safe ventilation. The $ETCO_2$ may be controlled by altering respiratory rate. Epigastric auscultation should be performed in all patients to ensure that gastric insufflation is not occurring. In infants a nasogastric tube should probably be placed if PPV is to be used with the LMA. Anterior neck auscultation is a valuable procedure for determining oropharyngeal leak pressure. It may give useful information on adequacy of anesthetic depth and level of neuromuscular blockade.

Factors influencing maximum leak pressure and seal around the glottis include choosing the largest LMA appropriate for the patient, placing the LMA optimally, avoiding over- or underinflation of the LMA cuff, correct fixation of the LMA and maintaining low compliance by monitoring neuromuscular blockade and depth of anesthesia. Isserles and Rozenberg describe a simple technique for reducing leak with the laryngeal mask airway (LMA) which involves flexion of the neck[195]. Neck flexion removes the longitudinal tension in the anterior structures, allowing them to settle down onto the mask. A further method is to apply gentle pressure to the front and/or sides of the neck with the palm of the hand[196]. By squeezing the periglottic tissues more firmly around the LMA cuff, the efficacy of the seal is increased and leak is reduced. Provided the glottis is open and in approximate alignment with the LMA bowl there will usually be an increase in ventilatory capability. Neck pressure should be applied gradually and gently over the thyroid region (where the cuff is often seen to bulge forward on inflation), while assessing the impact of the maneuver on leak. Care must be taken as excessive external neck pressure could lead to displacement of the LMA, airway obstruction or compression of vessels to the head and neck. Concerns about blood flow may be minimized by palpation of the carotid artery or by the intermittent application of neck pressure. Because of these restrictions, the neck pressure maneuver should be regarded as a temporary measure to improve seal with the LMA while a more lasting solution is reached.

Neuromuscular blockade

If leaks occur during maintenance this may be due to light anesthesia leading to glottic closure, inadequate neuromuscular blockade leading to increased airways resistance, displacement of the LMA, or a reduction in lung compliance related to surgery or patient factors. The most common cause is the muscle relaxant wearing off. When wheezing is heard during neck auscultation, it is usually caused by adduction of the vocal cords because of inadequate muscle relaxation or more rarely by the tip of the mask being misplaced against the glottis (Figure 2.3). Administration of muscle relaxants rather than addition of air to the cuff usually relieves the problem. It is important that whenever possible the LMA tube is always visible and accessible even during head and neck surgery. In the event of a leak around the cuff do not simply add air to the cuff as this will not always improve the seal and may make the leak worse by adding tension to the normally soft cuff, reducing its ability to conform to the perilaryngeal contours. If the leak persists, auscultation of the anterolateral part of the neck or fiberoptic laryngoscopy may be useful in differentiating between malposition or degrees of glottic closure[71]. Leaks may also be demonstrated by observation of the airway pressure waveform[195], or pressure volume loops.

When a relaxant technique is chosen, the relaxant drug may be given either before or after insertion of the LMA. The fact that paralysis is not required for insertion may be useful if there is a risk of losing airway control following induction. Alternatively when a change in the planned operation requires conversion to a relaxant technique, the anesthesiologist can simply administer the relaxant and connect the ventilator circuit, without needing to make any adjustment to the airway.

When using the LMA with PPV, reversal of neuromuscular block is best carried out under a continued level of anesthesia. There will then be smooth transition to spontaneous ventilation which avoids the problem of laryngeal spasm in the semi-reversed patient. Reversal of neuromuscular block coincidentally with discontinuation of anesthesia can cause uncoordinated reflex responses and airway obstruction[197,198]. If the airway is obstructed secondary to malposition or reflex cord closure, significant negative intrathoracic pressures may develop during inspiration and promote gastro-esophageal reflux[199,200]. Pulmonary edema may also occur, creating a radiological appearance which can be confused with that of aspiration pneumonitis[201].

Other ventilatory modes

Synchronized intermittent mandatory ventilation, continuous positive airways pressure and pressure support ventilation (PSV) may be utilized with the LMA, particularly in the intensive care or post anesthesia care unit (PACU) setting[202-206]. Capdevia et al investigated the use of PSV for general anesthesia with the LMA and found that, compared with PPV, PSV produces lower airway pressures and as such decreases leaks around the LMA[205]. Smirnova et al found pressure support in combination with extended mandatory minute volume to be useful for general anesthesia with the LMA[207].

Pollution

The concerns regarding pollution of the operating room atmosphere are often overlooked, and PACU personnel are particularly exposed to waste anesthetic gases and their concomitant effects on general health and potential mutagenic properties[208,209]. The LMA meets occupational safety requirements on nitrous oxide concentrations in the operating room environment during spontaneous ventilation and PPV[210]. Reinhart looked at operating room pollution during PPV comparing the LMA and tracheal tube with the cuff deflated and inflated and found that pollution was slightly higher with the LMA, but was within safety limits at 1 m [211]. Hoerauf et al found similar results with isoflurane and showed that all measured values at the personnel-related points were low (usually < 2 ppm)[212]. Pollution may be reduced still further by the use of low flow systems[213] and spontaneous breathing to reduce leaks[214]. Berry and Brimacombe have suggested that if the LMA is left in situ during emergence scavenging may be conducted in the PACU[215].

Emergence/removal

Awake versus deep

The LMA may be removed with the patient deeply anesthetized[216,217] or awake[218], either in the supine or lateral position[219]. It must not be removed at a halfway stage or laryngeal spasm, coughing or gagging may result. Gature et al showed that there were more complications when the LMA was removed awake versus deep[220], but removal practices were suboptimal in the awake group. Problems occurring during emergence could be avoided by removal whilst the patient is still anesthetized[217], but it seems logical to remove the LMA after airway reflexes return. In the authors' opinion, awake removal is the most common and preferred technique, at least in adults. It is important, however, to minimize cuff pressure so as to avoid overstimulation of the patient. In our combined experience of over 20 000 patients we have found the LMA is well tolerated during emergence with few serious problems. It provides a clear and 'hands free' airway, allows end-tidal gases to be monitored, facilitates positive pressure ventilation and protects the airway from oropharyngeal contamination. This view is supported by a recent comparative study of awake versus deep removal[221] and a prospective study of 600 children in which bite guards were used and the LMA was removed awake in the operating room by anesthetists trained in LMA removal[57]. The overall incidence of complications during emergence was 6% (compared with 54% in Gataure et al's study[220] and 13% by Mason and Bingham[4]). Laryngeal spasm/bronchospasm occurred on seven occasions, partial airway obstruction on 10 occasions, and coughing/gagging/ retching on 13 occasions. Interestingly, the oxygen saturation fell below 90% only once. Problems during emergence may be reduced by use of lidocaine lubricant if the procedure is brief[90,222,223]; however, protective reflexes are partially obtunded. Furthermore, the patient may complain of dysphagia or perioral numbness[223].

Recommendations

Current recommendations are that the LMA may be removed with the patient deeply anesthetized or awake, but not at a halfway stage. Guidelines for the management of the LMA in recovery are given in Table 6.5. Awake removal should take place when reflexes are fully returned and the patient is able to open their mouth to command. Disturbance of the patient during emergence with the LMA in situ and high intracuff pressures should be avoided[224,225]. The optimal position for LMA removal is unknown. It has been suggested that since the LMA prevents gastric contents from escaping through the pharynx, one key advantage of the lateral position is negated[226]. Care must be taken to maintain anesthesia during transfer of the patient.

Patients may be transferred into the PACU where the LMA may be removed by appropriately trained PACU staff or an anesthesiologist. This probably reduces operating room time in some situations. The patient should be left undisturbed until the

Table 6.5 Guidelines for management of the LMA in recovery

General principles

1. The PACU nurse requires training and certification
2. An anesthesiologist must be readily available
3. There should be minimal patient disturbance

Immediate assessment on arrival in PACU

The anesthesiologist should remain until baseline observations have been established

1. Verify a clear airway by placing the palm of the hand close to the end of the tube to feel the expired breath. Capnography may also be useful.
2. Check that the black line of the LMA is facing the upper lip of the patient. The presence or absence of a mouth gag should be noted.
3. Ensure that oxygen saturation, blood pressure and pulse are within predefined limits for the individual patient.

Recovery period

1. The patient must not be actively aroused.
2. Do not move the patient from the supine to the lateral position.
3. Administer supplementary oxygen.
4. Suction down the LMA tube should only be performed in the presence of an anesthesiologist.

Removal of the LMA

1. Watch for signs of swallowing. Remove tape fixing LMA to the face.
2. Remove the LMA when patient opens mouth to command. Deflate the cuff as the LMA is being removed.
3. Verify airway patency and respiratory depth.
4. Oral suction may now be carried out if required.
5. Administer oxygen via a clear face mask.

reflexes are restored, except to administer oxygen[227–230] and perform monitoring procedures. They should not be moved from the supine to the lateral position unless there is an urgent reason to do so, such as regurgitation or vomiting. Respiration may be assisted manually during patient transport and subsequent recovery to adequate tidal volumes by intermittently occluding the T-piece with the palm of the hand[231,232]. This has the effect of inflating the chest at a rate which is dependent on the oxygen gas flow. The volume of breath given can be judged by timing (for example, an oxygen flow of 6 l will provide a tidal volume of 500 cm^3 in 5 s) or observation of chest wall movement. The low pressure seal of the LMA ensures that barotrauma cannot easily occur[233], although gastric distension is still a possibility if the technique is used injudiciously.

It is not necessary to remove the secretions in the upper pharynx by suction since they do not enter the larynx provided that the cuff is not deflated prior to removal[234–236]. Only attempt blind suction down the LMA tubing if secretions are present within the

LMA tube and impeding respiratory function. For this it is essential to be aware of the precise length of the LMA tubing (see Table 5.7). Passage of a suction catheter beyond the mask aperture bars may trigger protective reflexes and should only be conducted in the presence of the anesthesiologist and preferably with fiberoptic guidance. Langenstein et al reported a < 1% success rate for blind passage of a suction catheter into trachea[237].

Deflation of the cuff should occur synchronously with LMA removal. If the cuff is deflated before the effective return of swallowing and cough reflexes, secretions may enter into the larynx, provoking laryngeal spasm. The LMA should certainly be left in situ during recovery from oropharyngeal surgery where it will continue to provide a clear airway and protect the respiratory tract. It is more sensible in this situation for patients to be recovered in the lateral position to allow the continual drainage of blood and secretions. They should be moved into the lateral position while still deeply anesthetized. The LMA may be removed with the cuff fully inflated provided care is taken to avoid damaging the cuff on sharp teeth. Rarely it may be difficult to remove the device inflated due to the cuff becoming caught under the base of the tongue.

Training

Delegating responsibility for removal of the LMA is controversial and should only be undertaken after consideration of the operating room layout, nursing expertise and the immediate availability of an anesthesiologist[219]. The LMA requires a fresh approach to postoperative care and the unique aspects of caring for patients with the LMA in situ make it essential that some form of training and certification is undertaken. Brimacombe et al have suggested a training program which involves acquiring both theoretical and practical knowledge about the LMA[238]. Trainees are expected to firstly view the laryngeal mask instruction video, read specified material relevant to its use in PACU and observe a trained nurse or anesthesiologist managing five patients with the LMA in situ. Certification requires the successful completion of a questionnaire, which includes identification of complications and knowledge of their management. Finally trainees must demonstrate they are competent at LMA removal at least 10 times depending on prior experience. Oral questioning is undertaken at this time. This training program has been safely implemented and no major problems have arisen over a 3 year period.

Miscellaneous

The LMA has been used during recovery for the management of laryngeal spasm[239], inadequate reversal[240] and for ventilatory assistance in a post thoracotomy patient with reactive airways disease. This cannot be justified where an adequate seal is obtained with a face mask since the LMA may occasionally trigger laryngeal spasm. In some instances its use has continued into the intensive care unit (ICU)[241]. Runcie et al have shown when comparing propofol 3 mg kg^{-1} with thiopentone 5 mg kg^{-1} using a spontaneous ventilation anesthetic via the LMA in children that recovery is quicker with propofol[242].

Postoperative aspects

General

Once the LMA is removed and the patient has recovered from the immediate effects of anesthesia any minor morbidity may become apparent. Sore throat occurs in approximately 10% of adult patients and is usually mild[182,236,243–247] (see Chapter 9, *Pharyngolaryngeal morbidity: Minor morbidity*). The advantages of the LMA in terms of sore throat have not been adequately demonstrated in children[248,249]. Other minor complications potentially related to the LMA are hoarseness[250,251], dry mouth[251,252], dysphagia[253] and a feeling of 'fullness'[254]. Not all postoperative airway complications are related to the LMA. Nair and Thompsett reported a case of late postoperative stridor in a 3-year-old following tonsillectomy with the LMA which turned out to be undiagnosed subglottic stenosis[255]. A potential benefit in the postoperative period is a reduction in analgesic requirements[236]. It has been speculated that this may be related to a central pre-emptive analgesic effect. Japanese workers have shown that the LMA does not reduce the incidence of postoperative nausea and vomiting after major gynecological surgery under balanced regional anesthesia[256]. Stanley et al compared postoperative laryngeal competence between the LMA and tracheal tube by asking 40 patients to swallow barium dye upon discharge to the ward followed by an immediate X-ray. Only one case of silent aspiration occurred and this was in a patient who was intubated[257].

PACU Hints

1. Always recover in the operating room if there are no staff in the PACU trained in recovery techniques with the LMA
2. Recovery in the PACU has become standard practice in many centers in the UK where PACU personnel have considerable experience with the LMA. However, it has been suggested that PACU staff should receive training in recovering patients with the LMA[238].
3. Pain from the wound commonly provokes an increase in muscle tone as anesthetic agents are eliminated. The pharyngeal constrictor muscles will thus increase intracuff pressure. The blue pilot balloon will be seen to expand, a useful sign of returning consciousness.
4. Lifting the patient from the operating table may consititute a strong stimulus. If the pilot balloon is already distending (indicating returning awareness) remove enough air to restore normal cuff pressure before moving the patient. This reduces patient discomfort and so prolongs the period during which the LMA can be tolerated.
5. Try to keep cuff pressure around 60 cm H_2O to avoid stimulating the patient.
6. After removing or adding air to the cuff, always check for airway patency.
7. Always ensure a bite block is in place before patients are transferred to a recovery area with the LMA in place.
8. **Do not** remove all the air before the patient is completely awake – this allows secretions to enter the larynx which may cause spasm.
9. **Do not** remove the bite block before the LMA is removed.
10. **Do not** allow patients to recover in areas where there are no personnel trained in LMA use.

11. **Do not** allow PACU personnel to stimulate patients with the LMA in place as a means of hastening recovery.
12. Apart from patients in whom operations have been carried out in the oropharynx, there is no need to suction the oropharyngeal cavity while the mask is in place or after it is removed, since the airway is protected by the mask from oral secretions. However, suction may be necessary if the mask is removed before the patient is able to swallow effectively.
13. **Do not** allow PACU personnel to routinely suction the pharynx with the LMA in place. The patient should be able to perform their own pharyngeal toilet by swallowing secretions as the device is removed, provided removal is timed to coincide with return of full effective reflexes.

References

1 McLure HA. Dental damage to the laryngeal mask. *Anaesthesia* 1996;**51**:1078–1079.

2 Martlew RA, Meakin G, Wadsworth R, Sharples A, Baker RD. Dose of propofol for laryngeal mask insertion in children: effect of premedication with midazolam. *Br J Anaesth* 1996;**76**:308–309.

3 Withington DE, Wrigley SF, Jones HE, Johnston DF, Robb PF. The laryngeal mask airway in paediatric anaesthesia. *Anaesthesia* 1991;**46**:321–322.

4 Mason DG, Bingham RM. The laryngeal mask airway in children. *Anaesthesia* 1990;**45**:760–763.

5 St Claire Logan A, Morris P. Complications following use of the laryngeal mask airway in children. *Paed Anaesth* 1993;**3**:297–300.

6 Williams PJ, Bailey PM. The reinforced laryngeal mask airway in paediatric radiotherapy. *Br J Anaesth* 1993;**71**:172.

7 Rolly G, Versichelen L, Huyghe L, Mungroop H. Effect of speed of injection on induction of anaesthesia using propofol. *Br J Anaesth* 1985;**57**:743–746.

8 Kinirons B, Hubbard K, Cunningham AJ. Laryngeal mask airway – optimum time for insertion? *Br J Anaesth* 1995;**75**:664–665 (Abstract).

9 Blake DW, Dawson P, Donnan G, Bjorksten A. Propofol induction for laryngeal mask airway insertion: dose requirements and cardiorespiratory effects. *Anaesth Intens Care* 1992;**20**:479–483.

10 Leslie K, Crankshaw DP. Potency of propofol for loss of consciousness after a single dose. *Br J Anaesth* 1990;**64**:734–736.

11 Brimacombe J, Berry A, Yaddanapudi LN, Kashyap L. Neuromuscular blockade and insertion of the laryngeal mask airway. *Br J Anaesth* 1993;**71**:166–167.

12 Uchiyama M, Yoshino A, Kato S, Hashimoto Y, Hirashima J. Effectiveness of low dose suxamethonium for laryngeal mask insertion. *11th World Congress of Anesthesiology, Sydney, 14–20 April 1996, Abstract Handbook* p.423 (Abstract).

13 Brodrick PM, Webster NR, Nunn JF. The laryngeal mask airway. A study of 100 patients during spontaneous breathing. *Anaesthesia* 1989;**44**:238–241.

14 Brimacombe J, Berry A. Insertion of LMA – an indication for propofol? *Anaesth Intens Care* 1992;**20**:394–395.

15 Hollande J. Diprivan et ventilation: le masque larynge. *Ann Fr Anesth Reanim* 1994;**13**:613–616.

16 Brain AIJ. The development of the laryngeal mask – a brief history of the invention, early clinical studies and experimental work from which the laryngeal mask evolved. *Eur J Anaesthesiol* 1991;**4**:5–17.

17 Brown GW, Patel N, Ellis FR. Comparison of propofol and thiopentone for laryngeal mask insertion. *Anaesthesia* 1991;**46**:771–772.

★ 18 Scanlon P, Carey M, Power M, Kirby F. Patient response to laryngeal mask insertion after induction of anaesthesia with propofol or thiopentone. *Can J Anaesth* 1993;**40**:816–818.
Prospective study of 72 patients comparing propofol 2.5 mg kg^{-1} with thiopentone 5 mg kg^{-1} for LMA insertion. Showed that conditions for placement were better with propofol.

19 Glausch-Wild M, Perras J, Buttner. Laryngeal mask anaesthesia, induction with propofol versus thiopentone. *11th World Congress of Anesthesiology, Sydney, 14–20 April 1996, Abstract Handbook* p.369 (Abstract).

20 Stoneham MD, Bree SE, Sneyd JR. Facilitation of laryngeal mask insertion. Effects of lignocaine given intravenously before induction with propofol. *Anaesthesia* 1995;**50**:464–466.

21 Driver IK, Mills P, Howard-Griffin R. Induction end point and laryngeal mask placement. *Anaesthesia* 1995;**50**:921.

22 Driver I, Wiltshire S, Mills P, Howard-Griffin R. Midazolam before induction improves conditions for laryngeal mask insertion. *Br J Anaesth* 1995;75:664 (Abstract).

23 Driver IK, Wiltshire S, Mills P, Lillywhite N, Howard-Griffin R. Midazolam co-induction and laryngeal mask insertion. *Anaesthesia* 1996;**51**:782–784.

24 Chan MSH, Mui KS, Kan AF. Insertion of LMA: Thiopentone with topical lignocaine. *Anaesth Intens Care* 1993;**21**:130.

25 Seavell CR, Cook TM, Cox CM. Topical lignocaine and thiopentone for the insertion of the laryngeal mask airway. *Anaesthesia* 1996;**51**:699–701.

26 Cook TM, Seavell CR, Cox CM. Lignocaine to aid the insertion of the laryngeal mask airway with thiopentone. A comparison between topical and intravenous administration. *Anaesthesia* 1996;**51**:787–790.

27 Bapat P, Joshi RN, Young E, Jago RH. Comparison of propofol versus thiopentone with midazolam or lidocaine to facilitate laryngeal mask insertion. *Can J Anaesth* 1996;**43**:564–568.

28 Mecklem D. Metoclopramide reduces propofol induction dose. *Anaesth Intens Care* 1996;**24**:110 (Abstract).

29 Taguchi M, Watanabe S, Asakura N, Inomata S. End-tidal sevoflurane concentrations for laryngeal mask airway insertion and for tracheal intubation in children. *Anesthesiology* 1994;**81**:628–631.

30 Holden R, Morsman CD, Butler J, Clark GS, Hughes DS, Bacon PJ. Intra-ocular pressure changes using the laryngeal mask airway and tracheal tube. *Anaesthesia* 1991;**46**:922–924.

31 Teles ASS, Gerez MC, Fortuna A. Alteracoes cardiovasculares na colocacao da mascara laringea (ML): inducao com etomidato e alfentanyl. *Rev Brasil Anestesiol* 1992;**42**:CBA 011.

32 Lauretti GR, Azevedo VMS, Reis MP. Etomidato associado ao alfentanyl ou sufentanyl para a insercao da mascara laringea. *Rev Brasil Anestesiol* 1995;**45**:CBA 256 (Abstract).

33 Lauretti GR, Silva RI. Estudo comparativo entre propofol, etomidate e tiopental com ou lidocaina para a insercao da mascara laringea. *Rev Brasil Anestesiol* 1995;**45**:CBA 253 (Abstract).

34 Prasiko D, Shrestha BM. Laryngeal mask airway in pediatric burn contractures in Nepal. *11th World Congress of Anesthesiology, Sydney, 14–20 April 1996, Abstract Handbook* p.119 (Abstract).

35 Mizikov V, Variuschina T, Esakov I. The laryngeal mask in paediatric anaesthesia: the first experience in Russia. *11th World Congress of Anesthesiology, Sydney, 14–20 April 1996, Abstract Handbook* p.465 (Abstract).

36 Dasey N, Mansour N. Coughing and laryngospasm with the laryngeal mask. *Anaesthesia* 1989;**44**:865.

37 Dingley J, Asai T. Insertion methods of the laryngeal mask airway. A survey of current practice in Wales. *Anaesthesia* 1996;**51**:596–599.

38 Magill IW. Technique in endotracheal anaesthesia. *Br Med J* 1930;**ii**:817–820.

★ 39 Ishimura H, Minami K, Sata T, Shigematsu A, Kadoya T. Impossible insertion of the laryngeal mask airway and oropharyngeal axes. *Anesthesiology* 1995;**83**:867–869.
Case report describing failed insertion of the LMA in a patient with a fixed flexion deformity. Includes laboratory work illustrating why insertion is difficult if the oropharyngeal axis is less than 90 degrees.

40 Morikawa S, Safar P, DeCarlo J. Influence of the head–jaw position upon upper airway patency. *Anesthesiology* 1996;**22**:265–279.

41 Boidin MP. Airway patency in the unconscious patient. *Br J Anaesth* 1985;**57**:306–310.

42 Pennant JH, Pace NA, Gajraj NM. Role of the laryngeal mask airway in the immobile cervical spine. *J Clin Anesth* 1993;**5**:226–230.

43 Brimacombe J, Berry A. Laryngeal mask airway insertion. A comparison of the standard verses neutral position in normal patients with a view to its use in cervical spine instability. *Anaesthesia* 1993;**48**:670–671.

44 Logan A. Use of the laryngeal mask in a patient with an unstable fracture of the cervical spine. *Anaesthesia* 1991;**46**:987.

45 Lee JJ, Yau K, Barcroft J. LMA and respiratory arrest after anterior cervical fusion. *Can J Anaesth* 1993;**40**:395–396.

46 Milligan KA. Laryngeal mask in the prone position. *Anaesthesia* 1994;**49**:449.

47 Chen CH, Lin CC, Tan PP. [Clinical experience of laryngeal mask airway in lateral position during anesthesia]. *Acta Anaesthesiol Sin* 1995;**33**:31–34.

48 Fukutome T. Correct positioning of the epiglottis for application of the Brain laryngeal mask airway. *Anaesthesia* 1995;**50**:818–819.

49 Brain AIJ. The laryngeal mask – a new concept in airway management. *Br J Anaesth* 1983;**55**:801–805.

50 Brain AI, McGhee TD, McAteer EJ, Thomas A, Abu Saad MA, Bushman JA. The laryngeal mask airway. Development and preliminary trials of a new type of airway. *Anaesthesia* 1985;**40**:356–361.

51 Storey AT. A functional analysis of sensory units innervating epiglottis and larynx. *Exp Neurol* 1968;**20**:366–383.

52 Sant'Ambrogio G, Mathew OP, Fisher JT, Sant'Ambrogio FB. Laryngeal receptors responding to transmural pressure, airflow and local muscle activity. *Resp Physiol* 1983;**54**:317–330.

53 Nishino T. Swallowing as a protective reflex for the upper respiratory tract. *Anesthesiology* 1993;**79**:588–601.

54 Brain AIJ. Modification of laryngeal mask insertion technique in children. *Anesth Analg* 1995;**81**:212.

55 Wilkins CJ, Cramp PG, Staples J, Stevens WC. Comparison of the anesthetic requirement for tolerance of laryngeal mask airway and endotracheal tube. *Anesth Analg* 1992;**75**:794–797.

★ 56 Brimacombe J, Berry A. Insertion of the laryngeal mask airway – a prospective study of four techniques. *Anaesth Intens Care* 1993;**21**:89–92.
The first randomized prospective trial comparing four different insertion techniques. Showed that the standard technique was superior and that insertion with the cuff deflated was better than with the cuff inflated.

★ 57 Lopez-Gil M, Brimacombe J, Cebrian J, Arranz J. The laryngeal mask airway in pediatric practice – a prospective study of skill acquisition by resident anesthesiologists. *Anesthesiology* 1996;**84**:807–811.
A prospective study of eight anesthesiology trainees to detemine the rate of skill acquisition with the LMA in pediatric practice. Showed that there was a dramatic reduction in the number of complications in all phases of anesthesia over the first 75 uses. Suggests that problem rates greater than 10% might represent suboptimal usage.

58 Brimacombe J, Berry A. Laryngeal mask airway insertion – which way is best and what should we teach? *Anaesth Intens Care* 1993;**21**:897–898.

★ 59 Brimacombe J. Analysis of 1500 laryngeal mask uses by one anaesthetist in adults undergoing routine anaesthesia. *Anaesthesia* 1996;**51**:76–80.
Large series by a single LMA user utilizing the standard insertion technique. High success rate, low problem rate and no correlation with Mallampati score. Also provides evidence for long-term learning curve.

★ 60 Verghese C, Brimacombe J. Survey of laryngeal mask usage in 11 910 patients – safety and efficacy for conventional and nonconventional usage. *Anesth Analg* 1996;**82**:129–133.
This survey of 11 910 LMA anaesthetics demonstrates that the technique has a high success rate for both spontaneous and controlled ventilation (99.81%), and with a low critical incident rate (0.37%). One patient aspirated, but did not require intensive care management. There were 3 cases of failed tracheal intubation in which the airway was secured with the LMA. The LMA was used for 1469 laparoscopic procedures and 644 laparotomies, including 404 abdominal hysterectomies. It was also used on 304 occasions for procedures > 3 hr. The frequency of problems was similar to that for more routine uses.

61 Van Damme E. Die Kehlopfmaske in der ambulanten Anasthesie – Eine Auswertung von 5000 ambulanten Narkosen. *Anaesthesiol Intensivmed Notfalmed Schmerzther* 1994;**29**:284–286.

62 Rose DK, Cohen MM. The airway: problems and predictions in 18 500 patients. *Can J Anaesth* 1994;**41**:372–383.

63 Maltby JR, Loken RG, Beriault MT, Archer DP. Laryngeal mask airway with mouth opening less than 20 mm. *Can J Anaesth* 1995;**42**:1140–1142.

64 van Heerden PV, Kirrage D. Large tonsils and the laryngeal mask airway. *Anaesthesia* 1989;**44**:703.

65 Collier C. A hazard with the laryngeal mask airway. *Anaesth Intens Care* 1991;**19**:301.

66 Brimacombe J, Berry A, Brain AIJ. Optimal cuff pressures with the laryngeal mask. *Br J Anaesth* 1996;**77**:295–296.

67 Morris GN, Marjot R. Laryngeal mask airway performance: effect of cuff deflation during anaesthesia. *Br J Anaesth* 1996;**76**:456–458.

68 Marjot RM, Morris G. Optimal intracuff pressures with the laryngeal mask. *Br J Anaesth* 1996;**77**:296.

69 Brimacombe J, Berry A. Size selection and the sixth LMA. *J Clin Anesth* 1995;**7**:265–266.

70 Ahmad NS, Yentis SM. Laryngeal mask airway and lingual nerve injury. *Anaesthesia* 1996;**51**:707–708.

71 Brimacombe J. Laryngoscopy through the LMA – a useful skill to acquire. *Anaesth Intens Care* 1992;**20**:535.

72 Wee MYK. The oesophageal detector device. Assessment of a new method to distinguish oesophageal from tracheal intubation. *Anaesthesia* 1988;**43**:27–29.

73 Ainsworth QP, Calder I. The oesophageal detector device and the laryngeal mask. *Anaesthesia* 1990;**45**:794.

74 Wafai Y, Salem MR, Tartaglione A, Joseph NJ. Facilitation of positioning of the laryngeal mask airway by the self-inflating bulb. *Anesthesiology* 1994;**81**:A628 (Abstract).

75 Asai T. The oesophageal detector device is not useful for the laryngeal mask. *Anaesthesia* 1995;**50**:175.

76 Haynes SR, Morton NS. The laryngeal mask airway: a review of its use in paediatric anaesthesia. *Paediatr Anaesth* 1993;**3**:65–73.

77 Kondo Y, Suzuki Y, Miyasaka K. Use of laryngeal mask airway (LMA) in routine paediatric anaesthesia. *Paediatr Anaesth* 1993;**3**:318.

78 Haynes SR, McGinn G, Morton NS. Use of laryngeal mask airway (LMA) in routine paediatric anaesthesia (reply). *Paediatr Anaesth* 1993;**3**:318–319.

79 Alexander CA, Leach AB, Thompson AR, Lister JB. Use your Brain! *Anaesthesia* 1988;**43**:893–894.

80 Lee JJ, Brain AIJ. Laryngeal mask and trauma to uvula. *Anaesthesia* 1989;**44**:1014–1015.

81 Coyne BJ. The use of the laryngeal mask airway in day case and short stay surgery. *Ir J Med Sci* 1990;**159**:185–186.

82 Jenkins J. The laryngoscope and the laryngeal mask airway. *Anaesthesia* 1993;**48**:735.

83 Brimacombe J, Berry A. The laryngoscope and the laryngeal mask airway. *Anaesthesia* 1994;**49**:82.

84 Jewell WE, Frerk C. The laryngeal mask airway – a useful tip. *Anaesthesia* 1994;**49**:543.

85 Wright E. The laryngeal mask airway. *Today's Anaesthetist* 1990;**5**:223.

86 Brain AIJ, Nunn JF. The laryngeal mask airway – insertion technique. *Today's Anaesthetist* 1991;**6**:18.

87 Cino PJ, Webster AC. Laryngeal mask insertion – a useful tip. *Anaesthesia* 1993;**48**:1012.

88 Brimacombe J, Berry A. Laryngeal mask insertion – a useful tip? *Anaesthesia* 1994;**49**:358.
89 Newman PTF. Insertion of a partially inflated laryngeal mask airway. *Anaesthesia* 1991;**46**:235.
90 O'Neill B, Templeton JJ, Caramico L, Schreiner MS. The laryngeal mask airway in pediatric patients: factors affecting ease of use during insertion and emergence. *Anesth Analg* 1994;**78**:659–662.
91 Young TM. The laryngeal mask in dental anaesthesia. *Eur J Anaesthesiol* 1991;**4**:53–59.
92 Cass L. Inserting the laryngeal mask. *Anaesth Intens Care* 1991;**19**:615.
93 Leader GL. Facilitation of the insertion of the laryngeal mask. *Anaesthesia* 1991;**46**:987.
94 Chow BF, Lewis M, Jones SE. Laryngeal mask airway in children: insertion technique. *Anaesthesia* 1991;**46**:590–591.
95 Garcia-Pedrajas F, Monedero P, Carrascosa F. Modification of Brain's technique for insertion of laryngeal mask airway. *Anesth Analg* 1994;**79**:1024–1025.
96 McNicol LR. Insertion of the laryngeal mask airway in children. *Anaesthesia* 1991;**46**:330.
97 Sing G. The laryngeal mask airway and the Guedel airway. *Anaesthesia* 1994;**49**:171.
98 Brimacombe J. The Guedel airway and the laryngeal mask airway? *Anaesthesia* 1994;**49**:643.
99 Rabenstein K. Alternative techniques for laryngeal mask insertion. *Anaesthesia* 1994;**49**:80–81.
100 Harding JB. A 'skid' for easier insertion of the laryngeal mask airway. *Anaesthesia* 1993;**48**:80.
101 Brimacombe J, Berry A. Alternative techniques for laryngeal mask airway insertion. *Anaesthesia* 1993;**48**:638.
102 Amos M, Navaratnam S, Biswas TK. Insertion of laryngeal mask airway (LMA) by non-anaesthetic personnel. *Anaesth Intens Care* 1994;**22**:97 (Abstract).
103 Navaratnam S, Tayler S. The laryngeal mask – another insertion technique. *Anaesth Intens Care* 1993;**21**:250.
104 Philpott B, Renwick M. An introducer for the flexible laryngeal mask airway. *Anaesthesia* 1993;**48**:174.
105 Asai T, Stacey M, Barclay K. Stylet for reinforced laryngeal mask airway. *Anaesthesia* 1993;**48**:636.
106 Moylan SL, Luce MA. The reinforced laryngeal mask airway in paediatric radiotherapy. *Br J Anaesth* 1993;**71**:172.
107 Hunter AR. Problems of anaesthesia in artificial pneumothorax. *Proc Roy Soc Med* 1955;**48**:765.
108 Palmer JHM. Introducing the reinforced laryngeal mask airway. *Anaesthesia* 1994;**49**:1098.
109 Dingley J, Whitehead MJ. A comparative study of sore throat with the laryngeal mask airway. *Anaesthesia* 1994;**49**:251–254.
110 Brimacombe J, Berry A. Active swallowing to aid LMA insertion in awake patients. *Anesth Analg* 1994;**78**:1029.
111 Omi A, Fukuhara T, Isshiki A, Arakawa K, Goto H. Effectiveness of the J-shaped LMA-holding forceps (J-forceps) for LMA insertion. *Anesthesiology* 1994;**81**:A627 (Abstract).
112 Costa e Silva L, Brimacombe J. The laryngeal mask airway for stereotactic implantation of fetal hypophysis. *Anesth Analg* 1996;**82**:430–431.
113 Matta BF, Marsh DS, Nevin M. Laryngeal mask airway: a more successful method of insertion. *J Clin Anesth* 1995;**7**:132–135.
114 James Kao Y. Spoons to assist the insertion of the laryngeal mask airway. *Anesthesiology* 1995;**83**:1381.
115 Beahan PG. An aid to placing the laryngeal mask airway. *Anaesth Intens Care* 1996;**24**:511.
116 Adejumo SWA, Davies MW. The laryngeal mask airway – another trick. *Anaesthesia* 1996;**51**:604.
117 Kumar SK. A modified technique of introducing laryngeal mask airway (a comparative study). *Indian J Anaesth* 1995;**43**:379–384.
118 Brimacombe J. Laryngeal mask airway: a more successful method for insertion? *J Clin Anesth* 1996;**8**:82–83.
119 Pennant JH, Walker MB. Comparison of the endotracheal tube and laryngeal mask in airway management by paramedical personnel. *Anesth Analg* 1992;**74**:531–534.
120 Tighe SQ, Davies PR, Greenslade GL, Evans GH. Laryngeal mask airway. *Lancet* 1991;**337**:375–376.
121 Martin PD, Cyna AM, Hunter WAH, Henry J, Pamayya GP. Training nursing staff in airway management for resuscitation – a clinical comparison of the facemask and laryngeal mask. *Anaesthesia* 1993;**48**:33–37.
122 Stone BJ, Leach AB, Alexander CA, et al. The use of the laryngeal mask airway by nurses during cardiopulmonary resuscitation – results of a multicentre trial. *Anaesthesia* 1994;**49**:3–7.
123 Aoyama K, Takenaka I, Sata T, Shigematsu A. The triple airway manoeuvre for insertion of the laryngeal mask airway in paralysed patients. *Can J Anaesth* 1996;**42**:1010–1016.
124 Elwood T, Cox RG. Laryngeal mask insertion with a laryngoscope in paediatric patients. *Can J Anaesth* 1996;**43**:435–437.
125 Brimacombe J. Jaw thrust and laryngeal mask insertion – a warning. *Anaesthesia* 1996;**51**:203.
126 Charters P. Digital exploration and the laryngeal mask. *Anaesthesia* 1996;**51**:990.
127 Elwood T, Cox RG. Laryngeal mask insertion in pediatric patients is facilitated with a laryngoscope. *Anesth Analg* 1995;**80**:S114 (Abstract).
128 Prosperi M, Heinen M, Fantini G. La maschera laringea nell'anestesia ambulatoriale pediatrica. *Minerva Anestesiol* 1995;**61**:53–55.
129 Welsh BE. Use of a modified Magill's forceps to place a flexible laryngeal mask. *Anaesthesia* 1995;**50**:1002–1003.
130 Welsh BE. A modified placement stilette. *Today's Anaesthetist* 1995;129.
131 Brimacombe J. Gastroesophageal reflux with the laryngeal mask. *Anesth Analg* 1996;**82**:215.

132 Rowbottom SJ, Simpson DL, Grubb D. The laryngeal mask airway in children. A fibreoptic assessment of positioning. *Anaesthesia* 1991;**46**:489–491.

133 Brain AIJ. *The role of the reinforced tube laryngeal mask*. London: Intavent, 1992.

134 Ravalia D, Kumar N. Rotation of reinforced laryngeal mask airway. *Anaesthesia* 1994;**49**:541–542.

135 Brain AIJ. Rotation of reinforced laryngeal mask airway. *Anaesthesia* 1994;**49**:542.

136 Brimacombe J, Berry A. Use of an introducer for the reinforced laryngeal mask airway. *Anaesthesia* 1993;**48**:637.

137 Webster AC, Morley-Forster PK, Dain S, et al. Anaesthesia for adenotonsillectomy: a comparison between tracheal intubation and the armoured laryngeal mask airway. *Can J Anaesth* 1993;**40**:1171–1177.

138 Brimacombe J, Dunbar-Reid K. The effect of introducing fibreoptic bronchoscopes on gas flow in laryngeal masks and tracheal tubes. *Anaesthesia* 1996;**51**:923–928.

139 Squires SJ, Woods K. Fragmented laryngeal mask airway. *Anaesthesia* 1992;**47**:274.

140 Kramer-Kilper OT. Removal of laryngeal mask airway during light anaesthesia. *Anaesthesia* 1992;**47**:816.

141 O'Connor B. Rotation of the laryngeal mask airway. *Anaesthesia* 1994;**49**:169.

142 Paterson SJ, Byrne PJ, Molesky MG, Seal RF, Finucane BT. Neonatal resuscitation using the laryngeal mask airway. *Anesthesiology* 1994;**80**:1248–1253.

143 Bignell S, Brimacombe J. LMA stability and fixation. *Anaesth Intens Care* 1994;**22**:745.

144 Baum J, Sachs G. The laryngeal mask airway – fixation, gags and stability. *Anaesthesiol Intensivmed Notfalmed Schmerzther* 1995;**30**:130.

145 Worsley MH, Howie CC. Fixation of the laryngeal mask airway. *Anaesthesia* 1990;**45**:1001.

146 Nott MR. A tie for the laryngeal mask airway. *Anaesthesia* 1993;**48**:1013.

147 Conacher ID. A method of fixing of laryngeal mask airways. *Anaesthesia* 1993;**48**:638.

148 Brimacombe J, Berry A. Laryngeal mask airway cuff pressure and position: the effect of adding nitrous oxide to the cuff. *Anesthesiology* 1994;**80**:957–958.

149 Brimacombe J, Berry A. Laryngeal mask airway cuff pressure and position during anaesthesia lasting 1–2 hours. *Can J Anaesth* 1994;**41**:589–593.

150 Brimacombe J. The laryngeal mask airway – fixation, gags and stability. *Anaesthesiol Intensivmed Notfalmed Schmerzther* 1995;**30**:129.

151 Heath ML, Sinnathamby SW. The reinforced laryngeal mask airway for adenotonsillectomy. *Br J Anaesth* 1994;**72**:728–729.

152 Williams PJ, Bailey PM. The reinforced laryngeal mask airway for adenotonsillectomy. *Br J Anaesth* 1994;**72**:729.

153 Molloy AR. Unexpected position of the laryngeal mask airway. *Anaesthesia* 1991;**46**:592.

154 Nandi PR, Nunn JF, Charlesworth CH, Taylor SJ. Radiological study of the laryngeal mask. *Eur J Anaesthesiol* 1991;**4**:33–39.

155 Ball AJ. Laryngeal mask misplacement – a nonproblem. *Anesth Analg* 1995;**81**:204.

156 Yanagimoto M, Mizogami M, Fujibayashi T, Harada J, Goto Y. Effect of position of the epiglottis on volume–pressure curve during use of the LM. *J Jpn Soc Clin Anesth (Nihon rinsho-masui Gakkai Shi)* 1992;**12**:738–741.

157 Fiani N, Scandella C, Giolitto N, Prudhomme G, Leon A. Comparison of reinforced laryngeal mask vs endotracheal tube in tonsillectomy. *Anesthesiology* 1994;**81**:A491 (Abstract).

158 Lumb AB, Wrigley MW. The effect of nitrous oxide on laryngeal mask cuff pressure. In vitro and in vivo studies. *Anaesthesia* 1992;**47**:320–323.

159 Marjot R. Pressure exerted by the laryngeal mask airway cuff upon the pharyngeal mucosa. *Br J Anaesth* 1993;**70**:25–29.

160 O'Kelly SW, Heath KL, Lawes EG. A study of laryngeal mask inflation. Pressures exerted on the pharynx. *Anaesthesia* 1993;**48**:1075–1078.

161 Gursoy F, Algren JT, Skjonsby BS. The effect of nitrous oxide (N_2O) on laryngeal mask airway (LMA) volume and pressure in children. *Anesthesiology* 1994;**81**:A1319 (Abstract).

162 Ri J, Iwasaki H, Yamakage M, Yamasaki Y, Kirita A, Namiki A. Intracuff pressure of the laryngeal mask during anaesthesia. *J Clin Anesth (Rinsho-Masui)* 1991;**15**:1424–1426.

163 Marjot R. Laryngeal mask cuff pressures. *Anaesthesia* 1994;**49**:447.

164 Brimacombe J, Berry A. Laryngeal mask cuff pressures. *Anaesthesia* 1994;**49**:447–448.

165 Asai T, Morris S. Inflation of the cuff of the laryngeal mask. *Anaesthesia* 1994;**49**:1098–1099.

166 Sarma VJ. The use of a laryngeal mask airway in spontaneously breathing patients. *Acta Anaesthesiol Scand* 1990;**34**:669–672.

167 Goodwin APL, Rowe WL, Ogg TW. Day case laparoscopy – a comparison of two anaesthetic techniques using the laryngeal mask during spontaneous breathing. *Anaesthesia* 1992;**47**:892–895.

168 Rungreungvanich M, Sriswasdi S, Soranastaporn C. Comparison of halothane and isoflurane for laryngeal mask insertion in pediatric patients. *11th World Congress of Anesthesiology, Sydney, 14–20 April 1996, Abstract Handbook* p.395 (Abstract).

169 Fujibayashi T, Goto Y. Use of the LM and sevoflurane for a patient with a history of asthmal attack. *J Clin Anesth (Rinsho-Masui)* 1990;**14**:1509.

170 Hamakawa T, Nakamura S, Kawasaki Y. Intracuff pressure of the LM and pressure on the pharynx. *J Clin Anesth (Rinsho-Masui)* 1993;**17**:1165–1167.

171 Smith I, White PF. Use of the laryngeal mask airway as an alternative to a face mask during outpatient arthroscopy. *Anesthesiology* 1992;**77**:850–855.

172 Van Damme E. Die Brauchbarkeit der Larynxmaske in der ambulanten Anasthesie: Eine Auswertung von 200 ambulanten Narkosen. *Anaesthetist* 1992;**41**:542.

173 Goodwin A, Ogg TW, Lamb W, Adlam D. The reinforced laryngeal mask airway in dental day surgery. *Ambulatory Surg* 1993;**1**:31–35.

174 Dyer RA, Llewellyn RL, James MFM. Total i.v. anaesthesia with propofol and the laryngeal mask for orthopaedic surgery. *Br J Anaesth* 1995;**74**:123–128.

175 Palomba R, Sica G, Scibelli G, Bardari G, Llardo A. L'impiego della maschera laringea (LMA) in chirurgia generale. *Minerva Anestesiol* 1995;**61**:45–50.

176 Phillips J, Brimacombe J, Simpson D. Anaesthetic induction with isoflurane or halothane. Oxygen saturation during induction with isoflurane or halothane in unpremedicated children. *Anaesthesia* 1988;**43**:927–929.

177 Verghese C, Smith TGC, Young E. Prospective survey of the use of the laryngeal mask airway in 2359 patients. *Anaesthesia* 1993;**48**:58–60.

178 Recio A, Jacobson K, Gronert B, Motoyama E. The use of the LMA in children under halothane anesthesia: is spontaneous ventilation acceptable? *Anesthesiology* 1995;**83**:A1153 (Abstract).

179 Brimacombe J, Shorney N. The laryngeal mask airway and prolonged balanced anaesthesia. *Can J Anaesth* 1993;**40**:360–364.

180 Brimacombe J, Archdeacon J. The laryngeal mask airway for unplanned prolonged procedures. *Can J Anaesth* 1995;**42**:1176.

181 Brimacombe J, Berry A. IPPV and the laryngeal mask airway – what are the risks? *Today's Anaesthetist* 1995;**10**:5.

182 Denny NM, Gadelrab R. Complications following general anaesthesia for cataract surgery: a comparison of the laryngeal mask airway with tracheal intubation. *J Roy Soc Med* 1993;**86**:521–522.

183 Wainwright AC. Positive pressure ventilation and the laryngeal mask airway in ophthalmic anaesthesia. *Br J Anaesth* 1995;**75**:249–250.

★ **184** Devitt JH, Wenstone R, Noel AG, O'Donnell RRT. The laryngeal mask airway and positive-pressure ventilation. *Anesthesiology* 1994;**80**:550–555.
Study of 48 patients comparing leak pressures for the LMA and tracheal tube. Showed that leak was less likely with the tracheal tube, but that the LMA provided adequate ventilation in all patients.

185 Berry A, Verghese C. Changes in pulmonary mechanics during IPPV with the laryngeal mask airway compared to the tracheal tube. *Anesth Analg* 1994;**78**:S38 (Abstract).

186 Graziotti PJ. Intermittent positive pressure ventilation through a laryngeal mask airway – is a nasogastric tube useful? *Anaesthesia* 1992;**47**:1088–1089.

187 Epstein RH. Maintenance of airway sealing pressures of the laryngeal mask airway in children. *Anesthesiology* 1994;**81**:A1322 (Abstract).

188 Heinrichs W, Weiler N, Latorre F, Eberie B. Respiratory mechanics, gastric insufflation pressure and air leakage of the laryngeal mask airway. *Anesthesiology* 1995;**83**:A1227 (Abstract).

189 Epstein RH, Ferouz F, Jenkins MA. Airway sealing pressures of the laryngeal mask airway in pediatric patients. *J Clin Anesth* 1996;**8**:93–98.

190 Brimacombe J, Berry A. Preliminary experience with the Size 5 laryngeal mask airway. *Anaesth Intens Care* 1993;**21**:888–889.

191 Van Damme E. Die Larynxmaske Grosse 5 – Erste Erfahrungen. *Anaesthesiol Intensivmed Notfalmed Schmerzther* 1994;**29**:293.

★ **192** Brimacombe J. Positive pressure ventilation with the size 5 LMA. *J Clin Anesth* (in press).
Study of 179 patients undergoing PPV with the size 5 LMA. Showed that gastric insufflation pressure was 31 (23–45 cm H_2O) and oropharyngeal leak was 33 (8–44 cm H_2O). At tidal volumes of 8 ml kg^{-1} no patient had gastric insufflation and one patient had an oropharyngeal leak. The device performed equally well in the obese and nonobese patient.

193 Haden RM, Pinnock CA, Campbell RL. The laryngeal mask for intraocular surgery. *Br J Anaesth* 1993;**71**:772.

194 Brimacombe J, Berry A. The incidence of aspiration associated with the laryngeal mask airway – a meta-analysis of published literature. *J Clin Anesth* 1995;**7**:297–305.

195 Isserles SA, Rozenberg B. LMA – reduction of gas leak. *Can J Anaesth* 1995;**41**:449.

196 Brimacombe J, Berry A. Leak reduction with the laryngeal mask airway – the application of external neck pressure. *Can J Anaesth* 1996;**43**:537.

197 Valentine J, Stakes AF, Bellamy MC. Reflux during positive pressure ventilation through the laryngeal mask. *Br J Anaesth* 1994;**74**:543–545.

198 Brain AIJ, Brimacombe J, Berry A, Verghese C. Reflux during positive pressure ventilation through the laryngeal mask airway? *Br J Anaesth* 1995;**74**:489–490.

199 Wang W, Tovar JA, Eizaguirre I, Aldazabal P. Airway obstruction and gastroesophageal reflux: an experimental study on the pathogenesis of this association. *J Pediatr Surg* 1993;**28**:995–998.

200 O'Mullane EJ. Vomiting and regurgitation during anaesthesia. *Lancet* 1954;**i**:1209–1212.

201 Lang SA, Duncan PC, Shephard DA, Ha HC. Pulmonary oedema associated with airway obstruction. *Can J Anaesth* 1990;**37**:210–218.

202 Arosio EM, Conci F. Use of the laryngeal mask airway for respiratory distress in the intensive care unit. *Anaesthesia* 1995;**50**:635–636.

203 Smith I, Joshi G. The laryngeal mask airway for outpatient anesthesia. *J Clin Anesth* 1993;**5**:22S-28S.

204 Groudine SB, Lumb PD, Sandison MR. Pressure support ventilation with the laryngeal mask airway: a method to manage severe reactive airway disease postoperatively. *Can J Anaesth* 1995;**42**:341–343.

205 Capdevila X, Biboulet P, Vallee M, Drissi S, D'Athis F. Pressure support ventilation with a laryngeal mask during general anesthesia. *Anesthesiology* 1995;**83**:A1226 (Abstract).

206 Groudine SB, Lumb PD. Noninvasive ventilatory support with the laryngeal mask airway. *Am J Anesthesiol* 1996;124–128.

207 Smirnova V, Lickvantsev V, Sitnikov V, Vinogradov V. Low flow anaesthesia with laryngeal mask. *11th World Congress of Anesthesiology, Sydney, 14–20 April 1996, Abstract Handbook* p.406 (Abstract).

208 Husum B. Mutagenicity of inhalational anaesthetics studied by the sister chromatid exchange test in lymphocytes of patients. *Dan Med Bull* 1987;**34**:159–170.

209 Guirguiss SS, Pelmear PL, Roy ML, Wong L. Health effects associated with exposure to anaesthetic gases in Ontario hospital personnel. *Br J Ind Med* 1990;**47**:490–497.

210 National Institute for Occupational Safety and Health Criteria for a recommended standard – occupational exposure to waste anesthetic gases and vapours. *National Institute for Occupational Safety and Health*, 1977:77–140.

211 Reinhart DJ, Hansen K, Odesseus K. The laryngeal mask airway and trace gases in the operating room. *Anesthesiology* 1994;**81**:A555 (Abstract).

★ 212 Hoerauf KH, Koller C, Jakob W, Taeger K, Hobbhahn J. Isoflurane waste gas exposure during general anaesthesia: the laryngeal mask compared with tracheal intubation. *Br J Anaesth* 1996;**77**:189–193.
Study determining the level of isoflurane pollution during PPV with the LMA and tracheal tube. Shows that levels were slightly higher with the LMA but that both devices met the safety requirements.

213 Mollhoff T, Burgard G, Prien T. Low-flow and minimal flow anesthesia and the laryngeal mask airway. *Anesthesiology* 1995;**83**:A499 (Abstract).

214 Stacey MRW, Shambrook A. Laryngeal mask airway and low flow anaesthesia. *Anaesthesia* 1992;**47**:1108.

215 Berry A, Brimacombe J. The laryngeal mask airway and recovery room pollution. *Anaesthesia* 1993;**48**:541–542.

216 Erskine RJ, Rabey PG. The laryngeal mask airway in recovery. *Anaesthesia* 1992;**47**:354.

217 Edwards ND. Lignocaine gel and the laryngeal mask airway. *Anaesthesia* 1995;**50**:746–747.

218 Brain AIJ. The laryngeal mask and the oesophagus. *Anaesthesia* 1991;**46**:701–702.

219 Brimacombe J. The laryngeal mask airway: tool for airway management. *J Post Anaes Nurs* 1993;**8**:88–95.

220 Gataure PS, Latto IP, Rust S. Complications associated with removal of the laryngeal mask airway: a comparison of removal in deeply anaesthetised versus awake patients. *Can J Anaesth* 1995;**42**:1113–1116.

221 Sorba F, Courreges P, Lecoutre D, Bayard-Gary R. Evaulation du Masque Larynge. *Cahiers d'Anesthesiol* 1994;**42**:567–570.

222 Chan ST, Med M, Tham CS. The effects of 2% lignocaine gel on incidence of retching with the use of the laryngeal mask airway. *Anaesthesia* 1995;**50**:257–258.

223 Millett SV, Allman KG. Lignocaine gel and the laryngeal mask airway. *Anaesthesia* 1995;**50**:747.

224 Brain AIJ. Studies on the laryngeal mask: first, learn the art. *Anaesthesia* 1991;**46**:417–427.

225 Brain AIJ. *The Intavent laryngeal mask – instruction manual.* London: Intavent, 1991;1–58.

226 Koehli N. Aspiration and the laryngeal mask airway. *Anaesthesia* 1991;**46**:419.

227 Lewis RP, Porter M. Supplementary oxygen and the laryngeal mask airway. *Anaesthesia* 1991;**46**:70.

228 Broadway PJ, Royle P. Supplementary oxygen and the laryngeal mask airway. *Anaesthesia* 1990;**45**:792–793.

229 Goodwin APL. Postoperative oxygen via the laryngeal mask airway. *Anaesthesia* 1991;**46**:700.

230 Kennedy R, Meyer M, Joyce C. Supplemental oxygen using an LMA. *Anaesth Intens Care* 1992;**20**:118.

231 Brimacombe J, Washbourne D, Hill D, Mousa A, Lai M. Anterior neck stethoscopy and capnography for monitoring respiratory function with the laryngeal mask airway in the PACU. *J Post Anaes Nurs* (in press).

232 Brimacombe J, Berry A. A simple method of ventilation via the laryngeal mask during transportation and recovery from anaesthesia. *Acta Anaesthesiol Scand* (in press).

233 Brimacombe J, Berry A. Barotrauma and the laryngeal mask airway. *Anaesthesia* 1994;**49**:1009.

234 John RE, Hill S, Hughes TJ. Airway protection by the laryngeal mask – a barrier to dye placed in the pharynx. *Anaesthesia* 1991;**46**:366–367.

235 Cork RC, Kaul B, Frink EJ, Jr, Standen JR, Depa R. Comparison of laryngeal mask with endotracheal tube for airway control. *Anesthesiology* 1992;**75**:A1112 (Abstract).

236 Cork RC, Depa RM, Standen JR. Prospective comparison of use of the laryngeal mask and endotracheal tube for ambulatory surgery. *Anesth Analg* 1994;**79**:719–727.

237 Langenstein H, Moller F, Krause R, Kluge R, Vogelsang H. Die Handhabung der Larynxmaske bei Augenoperationen. *Congress on Anaesthesia in Eye Surgery, Congress-Centrum Stadtpark, Hannover, 10–11 May 1996* (Abstract).

238 Brimacombe J, Berry A, Fletcher D. A training program for laryngeal mask airway removal in the PACU. *J Post Anaes Nurs* 1993;**8**:236–237.

239 Michel MZ, Stubbing JF. Laryngeal mask airway and laryngeal spasm. *Anaesthesia* 1991;**46**:71.

240 Kumar CM. Laryngeal mask airway for inadequate reversal. *Anaesthesia* 1990;**45**:792.

241 Aoyagi M. Application of the laryngeal mask airway in ICU. *40th Meeting of the Japanese Society of Anesthesiology, Iwate Prefectual Hall, Japan, 22 April 1993,* pp.6–7 (Abstract).

242 Runcie CJ, Mackenzie SJ, Arthur DS, Morton NS. Comparison of recovery from anaesthesia induced in children with either propofol or thiopentone. *Br J Anaesth* 1993;**70**:192–195.

243 Braude N, Clements EA, Hodges UM, Andrews BP. The pressor response and laryngeal mask insertion. A comparison with tracheal intubation. *Anaesthesia* 1989;**44**:551–554.

244 Akhtar TM, McMurray P, Kerr WJ, Kenny GNC. A comparison of laryngeal mask airway with tracheal tube for intra-ocular ophthalmic surgery. *Anaesthesia* 1992;**47**:668–671.

245 Harris TM, Johnston DF, Collins SRC, Heath ML. A new general anaesthetic technique for use in singers: the Brain laryngeal mask airway verses endotracheal intubation. *J Voice* 1990;**4**:81–85.

246 Swann DG, Spens H, Edwards SA, Chestnut RJ. Anaesthesia for gynaecological laparoscopy – a comparison between the laryngeal mask airway and tracheal intubation. *Anaesthesia* 1993;**48**:431–434.

247 Reinhart DJ. Comparison of effects of placement of the laryngeal mask airway (LMA) vs endotracheal tube (ETT) on the cardiovascular response. *Anesthesiology* 1993;**79**:A1052 (Abstract).

248 Johnston DF, Wrigley SR, Robb PJ, Jones HE. The laryngeal mask airway in paediatric anaesthesia. *Anaesthesia* 1990;**45**:924–927.

249 Splinter WM, Smallman B, Rhine EJ, Komocar L. Postoperative sore throat in children and the laryngeal mask airway. *Can J Anaesth* 1994;**41**:1081–1083.

250 Fujii Y, Tanaka H, Toyooka H. [Effects of laryngeal mask airway on circulation and on incidence of postoperative sore throat and hoarseness]. *Masui* 1993;**42**:1559–1562.

251 O'Neill BL, Foley EP, Chang A. Effects of humidification of inspired gases with the laryngeal mask airway. *Anesthesiology* 1994;**81**:A52 (Abstract).

252 Alexander CA, Leach AB. Incidence of sore throats with the laryngeal mask. *Anaesthesia* 1989;**44**:791.

253 Ferrut O, Toulouse C, Lancon JP, Douvier S, Fayolle JL. The laryngeal mask for elective gynecologic surgery: a very attractive oral airway dispositive. *Anesth Analg* 1994;**78**:S110 (Abstract).

254 Daum REO, Downes RN, Vardy S. Day-stay cataract surgery under general anaesthesia. *Today's Anaesthetist* 1992;**7**:24–28.

255 Nair I, Thompsett C. Laryngeal mask airway and late postoperative stridor. *Anaesthesia* 1994;**49**:449–450.

256 Kumagai A, Iwasaki H, Kawana S, Namiki A. Laryngeal mask airway does not reduce the incidence of post-operative nausea and vomiting after gynaecological surgery. *Anesth Analg* 1996;**81**:S255 (Abstract).

257 Stanley GD, Bastianpillai BA, Mulcahy K, Langton JA. Postoperative laryngeal competence. The laryngeal mask airway and tracheal tube compared. *Anaesthesia* 1995;**50**:985–986.

7 Advantages and disadvantages

Compared with the face mask

Advantages

The advantages over the face mask include provision of a clearer airway while freeing the anesthesiologist's hands for other important tasks such as administration of drugs and record keeping. The hands of the anesthesiologist often get tired when holding a face mask[1], particularly if they are arthritic[2], and in effect the LMA allows more effective airway management for longer periods. Remote anesthesia is also possible[3–5]. An effective airtight seal is more easily obtained, making ventilation and monitoring of tidal gases and low flow anesthesia easier[6]. The quality of airway is generally unaffected by anatomical factors which make the application of a face mask difficult, e.g. the edentulous[7–9], bearded[10], oriental[11] and neonatal[12] patient. It may be useful where application of the face mask may worsen facial pathology[13,14] or cannot be applied[15]. Less skill is required to successfully use the LMA than the face mask for trainees/inexperienced personnel[16]. Comparative studies with the face mask suggest that hypoxia is less likely to occur with the LMA[1,17–19]. Furthermore the LMA provides direct access to the glottis without loss of airway control, facilitating visualization and instrumentation of the vocal cords and large airways. Compression of the eyeballs, facial and infraorbital nerves is avoided[20]. Procedures to the head and neck are more feasible, particularly with the FLMA, since surgical access is greatly improved. The relative lack of need for manipulation of the head and neck may be advantageous with an unstable cervical spine[21]. Operating room and PACU pollution is also less likely with the LMA[22–24].

Disadvantages

The main disadvantage of the LMA compared with the face mask is that reflux is considered to be more likely. However, this theory remains controversial (see Chapter 3, *Gastrointestinal system: The esophagus*) and data from large audit or epidemiology studies suggests the incidence of aspiration is similar to that for the tracheal tube and face mask during elective surgery[25,26].

Compared with the tracheal tube

Advantages

The advantages over the tracheal tube include avoidance of laryngoscopy, less invasion of the respiratory tract, avoidance of the risks of endobronchial or esophageal intubation, avoidance of muscle relaxing drugs and less trauma to local tissues. There have been no reports of damage to teeth associated with use of the LMA and the incidence of sore throat (in adults)[27] and bacteremia[28] is less. In addition, placement is easy to learn[29–31] and generally unaffected by factors which make tracheal intubation difficult[32]. Adverse airway events such as difficult placement and laryngeal spasm probably occur less frequently with the LMA than with the tracheal tube[33,34]. Patients tolerate the LMA at lighter levels of anesthesia than they do the tracheal tube[35–37] and are usually awake before objecting to its presence. The incidence of coughing, straining and breathholding is reduced during emergence[38,39]. Insertion and removal have minimal effect on cardiovascular response[40–45], intraocular pressure[38,46,47] and possibly intracranial pressure (D. Ferson, personal communication, 1996). The potential advantages in terms of respiratory function have been outlined[48]. Barotrauma is less likely with the LMA[49]. Emergence times may be shorter with the LMA compared with the tracheal tube[50]. The approximate ratio of adverse events for tracheal intubation compared with the LMA are given in Table 7.1[51].

Table 7.1 The approximate ratio of adverse events for tracheal intubation and the LMA. The references provided are representative of the consensus of data from independent tracheal tube (TT) or LMA studies (referenced separately), or studies directly comparing the tracheal tube and LMA (referenced with the adverse event)

Adverse event	*TT (%)*	*LMA (%)*	*Ratio TT:LMA*
Clinically significant problems[33]	3.4	0.9	3.8
Laryngeal spasm[33]	0.38	0.12	3.2
Aspiration	0.017[56]	0.02[25]	0.85
Sore throat[27,57]	50	10	5
Laryngeal trauma	6.2[58]	–	–
BP/HR increase on insertion[40,57]	25	5	5
IOP increase on insertion[38,46,47]	25	10	2.5
Coughing during recovery[59]	60	2	30

Data derived from a meta-analysis of published literature[25].

Key: BP = blood pressure; HR = heart rate; IOP = intraocular pressure.
Reproduced with permission from reference 51, *Today's Anaesthetist*.

Disadvantages

The main disadvantage of the LMA compared with the tracheal tube is that it does not protect against aspiration[25]. Also, leak and gastric insufflation are more likely[24,36,52–54]. The extent to which this occurs depends on the airway pressure generated and probably also on the precise position of the LMA. Also, the LMA does not secure the airway as effectively as a tracheal tube and airway obstruction at the glottic and subglottic level cannot be prevented. The LMA is probably unsuitable for patients with collapsible airways[55]. Fixation of the LMA requires more spatial orientation than the tracheal tube and dislodgment is therefore more likely.

Compared with the esophageal tracheal combitube

As yet there are no published studies directly comparing the esophageal tracheal combitube (ETC)[60] with the LMA. Potential advantages over the ETC are ease of insertion, simplicity of use, minimal trauma and the facility for use in both children and adults. The ETC is unsuitable for use during general anesthesia other than as an emergency airway device, and is currently only available in one size. Anesthesiologists are unlikely to have much experience with the ETC. The main advantage of the ETC is that it protects the airway and facilitates high airway pressure ventilation when placed correctly[61,62].

Meta-analysis

Brimacombe performed a meta-analysis on randomized prospective trials from peer review journals comparing the LMA with other forms of airway management to determine if the LMA offered any significant advantages over the tracheal tube or face mask[63]. Of the 858 LMA publications identified to December 1994, 52 met the criteria for the analysis. Thirty-two different issues were tested using Fisher's method for combining the *P* values. The LMA had 13 significant advantages over the tracheal tube and four over the face mask. The LMA had two significant disadvantages over the tracheal tube and one over the face mask. There were 12 issues where neither device had a significant advantage. These data were derived from 37 papers[1,16,17,19,29,30,35,37–42,46,47,52,53,59,64–82] and 15 abstracts[24,36,54,57,83–93]. Advantages over the tracheal tube included: increased speed and ease of placement by inexperienced personnel; increased speed of placement by anesthesiologists; improved hemodynamic stability at induction and during emergence; minimal rise in intraocular pressure following insertion; reduced anesthetic requirements for airway tolerance; lower frequency of coughing during emergence; improved oxygen saturation during emergence; and lower incidence of sore throat in adults. Advantages over the face mask included: easier placement by inexperienced personnel; improved oxygen saturation; less hand fatigue; and improved operating conditions during minor pediatric otological surgery. Disadvantages over the tracheal tube were lower seal pressures and a higher frequency of gastric insufflation. The only disadvantage compared with the face mask was that esophageal reflux was more likely. It was not possible to assess the significance of these findings in terms of patient outcome and the data were not considered to be sufficiently homogeneous to make meaningful estimates of the size of the difference between the airway devices. It is important to recognize that some of the benefits of the LMA cannot be measured in randomized controlled studies, particularly in situations where the LMA complements other forms of airway management or when it is used in unique situations such as airway rescue or as an aid to intubation. Also, where one form of airway management is contraindicated, comparisons between airway devices cannot be made. The results are summarized in Tables 7.2 and 7.3.

Table 7.2 Advantages/disadvantages of the LMA over the tracheal tube demonstrated by prospective randomized studies

Advantages/disadvantages	*Reference number*
Advantages	
• placement easier for nonanesthesiologists	29,30,72,75
• placement quicker for nonanesthesiologists	29,30,72,75
• placement quicker for anesthesiologists	40,47,79,90
• pulse rate changes less during insertion	40,41,46,47,57,72,74,76
• blood pressure changes less during insertion	40,41,46,47,57,72,74,76
• pulse rate changes less during emergence	46,72,87
• blood pressure changes less during emergence	46,72,87
• intraocular pressure rise less during placement	38,39,46,47,74
• frequency of cough less during emergence	38,39,59,64,72,78
• oxygen saturation higher during emergence	36,71,72,85,91
• sore throat is less in adults	39,40,57,59,64,71,78
• airways better tolerated	35–37
• voice analysis is less impaired	64,65
Disadvantages	
• gastric insufflation more likely	52,53
• air leak more likely	24,36,53,54

Adapted from reference 63 with permission from the Canadian Society of Anesthesiologists.

Table 7.3 Advantages/disadvantages of the LMA over the face mask demonstrated by prospective randomized studies

Advantages/disadvantages	*Reference number*
Advantages	
• placement easier for nonanesthesiologists	1,68,70
• oxygen saturation higher	1,17,19,69
• surgical conditions superior for minor otological surgery in children	17,19
• hand fatigue is less	1,90
Disadvantages	
• frequency of esophageal reflux is higher	66,67,83,84

Adapted from reference 63 with permission from the Canadian Society of Anesthesiologists.

Potential patient benefits

There are several areas where the LMA has the potential to benefit patients compared with the tracheal tube. The increased speed and reliability of placement by inexperienced personnel suggests a potential role in resuscitation. The hemodynamic stability at induction and during emergence may be of benefit to patients with cardiovascular disease[94]. The minimal changes in intraocular pressure may be of benefit to patients with glaucoma[74]. The low frequency of coughing during emergence may be beneficial to patients following open eye or ENT surgery where excessive straining is potentially harmful. Postoperatively, the low incidence of sore throat and voice alteration may have advantages for professional voice users and reduce overall morbidity. Patients in whom muscle relaxants are relatively contraindicated (suxamethonium apnea, myasthenia gravis) or in whom spontaneous ventilation is desirable (e.g. mediastinal mass, pneumothorax, some patients with right to left shunts) might benefit from the LMA.

References

1 Smith I, White PF. Use of the laryngeal mask airway as an alternative to a face mask during outpatient arthroscopy. *Anesthesiology* 1992;**77**:850–855.

2 Alexander CA, Leach AB. The laryngeal mask – experience of its use in a District General Hospital. *Today's Anaesthetist* 1989;**4**:200–205.

3 Moylan SL, Luce MA. The reinforced laryngeal mask airway in paediatric radiotherapy. *Br J Anaesth* 1993;**71**:172.

4 Van Obbergh LJ, Muller G, Zeippen B, Dooms G. Propofol (P) infusion (I) and laryngeal mask (LMA) for magnetic resonance imaging (MRI) in children. *Anesthesiology* 1992;**77**:A1177 (Abstract).

5 Stevens JE, Burden G. Reinforced laryngeal mask airway and magnetic resonance imaging. *Anaesthesia* 1994;**49**:79–80.

6 Mollhoff T, Burgard G, Prien T. Low-flow and minimal flow anesthesia and the laryngeal mask airway. *Anesthesiology* 1995;**83**:A499 (Abstract).

7 Bremner WGM. Fixing the laryngeal mask airway during eye surgery. *Anaesthesia* 1993;**48**:542.

8 Baraka A. Laryngeal mask airway for edentulous patients. *Can J Anaesth* 1994;**41**:78–79.

9 O'Connor B. Rotation of the laryngeal mask airway. *Anaesthesia* 1994;**49**:169.

10 Pothmann W, Fullekrug B, Schulte am Esch J. [Fiberoptic determination of the position of the laryngeal mask]. *Anaesthesist* 1992;**41**:779–784.

11 Miyasaka K, Suzuki Y, Kondo Y, Nakagawa S, Asahara S. The use of the laryngeal mask airway in paediatric anaesthesia. *J Anaesth* 1991;**5**:160–165.

12 Paterson SJ, Byrne PJ, Molesky MG, Seal RF, Finucane BT. Neonatal resuscitation using the laryngeal mask airway. *Anesthesiology* 1994;**80**:1248–1253.

13 Russell R, Judkins KC. The laryngeal mask airway and facial burns. *Anaesthesia* 1990;**45**:894.

14 Alexander R. The laryngeal mask airway and ocular surgery. *Can J Anaesth* 1993;**40**:901–902.

15 Judkins KC. When the chips are down – the laryngeal mask in anger. *Anaesthesia* 1993;**48**:353.

16 Martin PD, Cyna AM, Hunter WAH, Henry J, Pamayya GP. Training nursing staff in airway management for resuscitation – a clinical comparison of the facemask and laryngeal mask. *Anaesthesia* 1993;**48**:33–37.

17 Johnston DF, Wrigley SR, Robb PJ, Jones HE. The laryngeal mask airway in paediatric anaesthesia. *Anaesthesia* 1990;**45**:924–927.

18 Watcha MF, Garner FT, White PF. Perioperative conditions with face mask – oral airway or laryngeal mask airway during bilateral myringotomy in children. *Anesth Analg* 1993;**76**:S456 (Abstract).

19 Watcha MF, Garner FT, White PF, Lusk R. Laryngeal mask airway vs face mask and Guedel airway during pediatric myringotomy. *Arch Otolaryngol Head Neck Surg* 1994;**120**:877–880.

20 Maltby JR, Loken RG, Watson NC. The laryngeal mask airway: clinical appraisal in 250 patients. *Can J Anaesth* 1990;**37**:509–513.

21 Brimacombe J, Berry A. Laryngeal mask airway insertion. A comparison of the standard verses neutral position in normal patients with a view to its use in cervical spine instability. *Anaesthesia* 1993;**48**:670–671.

22 Lamber-Jensen P, Christensen NE, Brynnum J. Laryngeal mask and anaesthetic waste gas exposure. *Anaesthesia* 1992;**47**:697–700.

23 Sarma VJ, Leman J. Laryngeal mask and anaesthetic waste gas concentrations. *Anaesthesia* 1990;**45**:791–792.

24 Reinhart DJ, Hansen K, Odesseus K. The laryngeal mask airway and trace gases in the operating room. *Anesthesiology* 1994;**81**:A555 (Abstract).

25 Brimacombe J, Berry A. The incidence of aspiration associated with the laryngeal mask airway – a meta-analysis of published literature. *J Clin Anesth* 1995;**7**:297–305.

26 Haden RM, Pinnock CA, Scott PV. Incidence of aspiration with the laryngeal mask airway. *Br J Anaesth* 1994;**72**:496.

27 Alexander CA, Leach AB. Incidence of sore throats with the laryngeal mask. *Anaesthesia* 1989;**44**:791.

28 Stone JM, Karalliedde LD, Carter ML, Cumerland NS. Bacteraemia and insertion of laryngeal mask airways. *Anaesthesia* 1992;**47**:77.

29 Pennant JH, Walker MB. Comparison of the endotracheal tube and laryngeal mask in airway management by paramedical personnel. *Anesth Analg* 1992;**74**:531–534.

30 Davies PRF, Tighe SQ, Greenslade GL, Evans GH. Laryngeal mask airway and tracheal tube insertion by unskilled personnel. *Lancet* 1990;**336**:977–979.

31 Reinhart DJ. Laryngeal mask airway (LMA) vs endotracheal tube (ETT) placement by paramedics, respiratory therapists and registered nurses. *Anesthesiology* 1993;**79**:A1058 (Abstract).

32 Mahiou P, Narchi P, Veyrac P, Germond M, Gory G, Bazin G. Is laryngeal mask easy to use in case of difficult intubation? *Anesthesiology* 1992;**77**:A1228 (Abstract).

33 Haden RM, Pinnock CA, Campbell RL. The laryngeal mask for intraocular surgery. *Br J Anaesth* 1993;**71**:772.

34 Sher M, Brimacombe J, Laing D. Anaesthesia for laser pharyngoplasty – a comparison of the tracheal tube verses reinforced laryngeal mask airway. *Anaesth Intens Care* 1995;**23**:149–154.

35 Taguchi M, Watanabe S, Asakura N, Inomata S. End-tidal sevoflurane concentrations for laryngeal mask airway insertion and for tracheal intubation in children. *Anesthesiology* 1994;**81**:628–631.

36 Fiani N, Scandella C, Giolitto N, Prudhomme G, Leon A. Comparison of reinforced laryngeal mask vs endotracheal tube in tonsillectomy. *Anesthesiology* 1994;**81**:A491 (Abstract).

37 Wilkins CJ, Cramp PG, Staples J, Stevens WC. Comparison of the anesthetic requirement for tolerance of laryngeal mask airway and endotracheal tube. *Anesth Analg* 1992;**75**:794–797.

38 Holden R, Morsman CD, Butler J, Clark GS, Hughes DS, Bacon PJ. Intra-ocular pressure changes using the laryngeal mask airway and tracheal tube. *Anaesthesia* 1991;**46**:922–924.

39 Akhtar TM, McMurray P, Kerr WJ, Kenny GNC. A comparison of laryngeal mask airway with tracheal tube for intra-ocular ophthalmic surgery. *Anaesthesia* 1992;**47**:668–671.

40 Braude N, Clements EA, Hodges UM, Andrews BP. The pressor response and laryngeal mask insertion. A comparison with tracheal intubation. *Anaesthesia* 1989;**44**:551–554.

41 Wilson IG, Fell D, Robinson SL, Smith G. Cardiovascular responses to insertion of the laryngeal mask. *Anaesthesia* 1992;**47**:300–302.

42 Hickey S, Cameron AE, Asbury AJ. Cardiovascular response to insertion of Brain's laryngeal mask. *Anaesthesia* 1990;**45**:629–633.

43 Wood MLB, Forrest ETS. Haemodynamic response to insertion of laryngeal mask. *Anaesthesia* 1989;**44**:1001.

44 Smigovec E, Sakic K, Tripkovic B. [The laryngeal mask – news in orthopedic anesthesia]. *Lijec Vjesn* 1993;**115**:166–169.

45 Fujii Y, Tanaka H, Toyooka H. [Effects of laryngeal mask airway on circulation and on incidence of postoperative sore throat and hoarseness]. *Masui* 1993;**42**:1559–1562.

46 Lamb K, James MFM, Janicki PK. The laryngeal mask airway for intraocular surgery: effects on intraocular pressure and stress responses. *Br J Anaesth* 1992;**69**:143–147.

47 Watcha MF, White PF, Tychsen L, Steven JL. Comparative effects of laryngeal mask airway and endotracheal tube insertion on intraocular pressure in children. *Anesth Analg* 1992;**75**:355–360.

48 Ferrari L, Goudsouzian N. Comparison of the laryngeal mask with the endotracheal tube in children with bronchopulmonary dysplasia. *Anesth Analg* 1995;**80**:S122 (Abstract).

49 Brimacombe J, Berry A. Barotrauma and the laryngeal mask airway. *Anaesthesia* 1994;**49**:1009.

50 Fung ST, Cheung HK, Jawan B, Tsai PS, Chen CC, Lee JH. Use of the laryngeal mask in off-floor anesthesia for hepatic angiography in pediatric liver transplant candidates. *Transplant Proc* 1996;**28**:1723–1724.

51 Brimacombe J, Berry A. IPPV and the laryngeal mask airway – what are the risks? *Today's Anaesthetist* 1995;**10**:5.

52 Graziotti PJ. Intermittent positive pressure ventilation through a laryngeal mask airway – is a nasogastric tube useful? *Anaesthesia* 1992;**47**:1088–1089.

53 Devitt JH, Wenstone R, Noel AG, O'Donnell RRT. The laryngeal mask airway and positive-pressure ventilation. *Anesthesiology* 1994;**80**:550–555.

54 Barnett R, Gallant B, Fossey S, Finegan B. Nitrous oxide environmental pollution. A comparison between face mask, laryngeal mask airway and endotracheal tube. *Can J Anaesth* 1992;**39**:A151 (Abstract).

55 Asai T, Morris S. The laryngeal mask and patients with 'collapsible' airways. *Anaesthesia* 1994;**49**:169–170.

56 Kallar SK. Aspiration pneumonitis: fact or fiction? *Probl Anesth* 1988;**2**:29–36.

57 Reinhart DJ. Comparison of effects of placement of the laryngeal mask airway (LMA) vs endotracheal tube (ETT) on the cardiovascular response. *Anesthesiology* 1993;**79**:A1052 (Abstract).

58 Harmer M. Complications of tracheal intubation. In: Latto IP, Rosen M, eds. *Difficulties in tracheal intubation.* London: Baillière Tindall, 1987;36–48.

59 Denny NM, Gadelrab R. Complications following general anaesthesia for cataract surgery: a comparison of the laryngeal mask airway with tracheal intubation. *J Roy Soc Med* 1993;**86**:521–522.

60 Frass M, Frezner R, Zdrahal F, Hoflehner G, Porges P, Lackner F. The esophageal tracheal combitube: preliminary results with a new airway for cardiopulmonary resuscitation. *Ann Emerg Med* 1987;**16**:768–772.

61 Wissler RN. The esophageal-tracheal combitube. *Anaesth Rev* 1993;**20**:147–152.

62 Pepe PE, Zachariah BS, Chandra NC. Invasive airway techniques in resuscitation. *Ann Emerg Med* 1993;**22**:393–403.

★ 63 Brimacombe J. The advantages of the LMA over the tracheal tube or facemask: a meta-analysis. *Can J Anaesth* 1995;**42**:1017–1023.

A meta-analysis of randomized prospective trials comparing the LMA with other forms of airway management to determine if it offered any significant advantages over the tracheal tube or face mask. The LMA had 13 significant advantages over the tracheal tube and four over the face mask. The LMA had two significant disadvantages over the tracheal tube and one over the face mask. There were 12 issues where neither device had a significant advantage.

64 Harris TM, Johnston DF, Collins SRC, Heath ML. A new general anaesthetic technique for use in singers: the Brain laryngeal mask airway versus endotracheal intubation. *J Voice* 1990;**4**:81–85.

65 Lee SK, Hong KH, Choe H, Song HS. Comparison of the effects of the laryngeal mask airway and endotracheal intubation on vocal function. *Br J Anaesth* 1993;**71**:648–650.

66 Barker P, Langton JA, Murphy PJ, Rowbotham DJ. Regurgitation of gastric contents during general anaesthesia using the laryngeal mask airway. *Br J Anaesth* 1992;**69**:314–315.

67 Rabey PG, Murphy PJ, Langton JA, Barker P, Rowbotham DJ. Effect of the laryngeal mask airway on lower oesophageal sphincter pressure in patients during general anaesthesia. *Br J Anaesth* 1992;**69**:346–348.

68 Tolley PM, Watts DJ, Hickman JA. Comparison of the use of the laryngeal mask and face mask by inexperienced personnel. *Br J Anaesth* 1992;**69**:320–321.

69 Williams PJ, Bailey PM. Comparison of the reinforced laryngeal mask airway and tracheal intubation for adenotonsillectomy. *Br J Anaesth* 1993;**70**:30–33.

70 Alexander R, Hodgson P, Lomax D, Bullen C. A comparison of the laryngeal mask airway and Guedel airway, bag and facemask for manual ventilation following formal training. *Anaesthesia* 1993;**48**:231–234.

71 Swann DG, Spens H, Edwards SA, Chestnut RJ. Anaesthesia for gynaecological laparoscopy – a comparison between the laryngeal mask airway and tracheal intubation. *Anaesthesia* 1993;**48**:431–434.

72 Webster AC, Morley-Forster PK, Dain S, et al. Anaesthesia for adenotonsillectomy: a comparison between tracheal intubation and the armoured laryngeal mask airway. *Can J Anaesth* 1993;**40**:1171–1177.

73 Epstein RH, Halmi BH. Oxygen leakage around the laryngeal mask airway during laser treatment of port-wine stains in children. *Anesth Analg* 1994;**78**:486–489.

74 Barclay K, Wall T, Wareham K, Asai T. Intra-ocular pressure changes in patients with glaucoma – comparison between the laryngeal mask airway and tracheal tube. *Anaesthesia* 1994;**49**:159–162.

75 Reinhart DJ, Simmons G. Comparison of placement of the laryngeal mask airway with endotracheal tube by paramedics and respiratory therapists. *Ann Emerg Med* 1994;**24**:260–263.

76 Hollande J, Riou B, Guerrero M, Landault C, Viars P. Comparison des effets hemodynamiques du masque larynge et du tube orotracheal. *Ann Fr Anesth Reanim* 1994;**12**:372–375.

77 Valentine J, Stakes AF, Bellamy MC. Reflux during positive pressure ventilation through the laryngeal mask. *Br J Anaesth* 1994;**74**:543–545.

78 Cork RC, Depa RM, Standen JR. Prospective comparison of use of the laryngeal mask and endotracheal tube for ambulatory surgery. *Anesth Analg* 1994;**79**:719–727.

79 Pace NA, Gajraj NM, Pennant JH, Victory RA, Johnson ER, White PF. Use of the laryngeal mask airway after oesophageal intubation. *Br J Anaesth* 1994;**73**:688–689.

80 Boisson-Bertrand D, Hannhart B, Rousselot JM, Duvivier C, Quilici N, Peslin R. Comparative effects of laryngeal mask and tracheal tube on total respiratory resistance in anaesthetised patients. *Anaesthesia* 1994;**49**:846–849.

81 Pennant JH, Pace NA, Gajraj NM. Role of the laryngeal mask airway in the immobile cervical spine. *J Clin Anesth* 1993;**5**:226–230.

82 Splinter WM, Smallman B, Rhine EJ, Komocar L. Postoperative sore throat in children and the laryngeal mask airway. *Can J Anaesth* 1994;**41**:1081–1083.

83 El Mikatti N, Luthra AD, Healy TEJ, Mortimer AJ. Gastric regurgitation during general anaesthesia in the supine position with the laryngeal and face mask airways. *Br J Anaesth* 1992;**68**:529P–530P. (Abstract).

84 Owens T, Robertson P, Twomey K, Doyle M, McShane AJ. Incidence of gastroesophageal reflux with the laryngeal mask. *Anesthesiology* 1993;79:A1053 (Abstract).

85 Cros AM, Boudey C, Esteben D, Milacic M, Dardel E. Intubation vs laryngeal mask. Incidence of desaturations and spasms during adenoidectomy. *Anesthesiology* 1993;**79**:A1155 (Abstract).

86 Phan Thi H, Ivens D, Khayat Y. Evolution of the gradient $Pa\text{CO}_2$-ETCO$_2$ during anesthesia on spontaneous ventilation with face mask verses laryngeal mask. *Anesthesiology* 1993;**79**:A37 (Abstract).

87 Joshi GP, Morrison SG, Gajraj NM, Okonkwo N, White PF. Hemodynamic changes during emergence from anesthesia: use of the laryngeal mask airway vs endotracheal tube. *Anesth Analg* 1994;**78**:S185 (Abstract).

88 Berry A, Verghese C. Changes in pulmonary mechanics during IPPV with the laryngeal mask airway compared to the tracheal tube. *Anesth Analg* 1994;**78**:S38 (Abstract).

89 Joshi GP, Morrison SG, Miciotto CJ, White PF. Evaluation of work of breathing during anesthesia: use of laryngeal mask airway versus tracheal tube. *Anesthesiology* 1994;**81**:A1449 (Abstract).

90 Watcha MF, Tan TSH, Safavi F, Payne CT, Teufel AE. Comparison of outcome with the use of the laryngeal mask, face mask–oral airway and endotracheal tube in children. *Anesth Analg* 1994;**78**:S471 (Abstract).

91 Cros AM, Boudey C, Esteben D, Milacic M, Dardel E. Intubation versus masque larynge – incidence des spasmes et des desaturations en per et postoperatoire. *Ann Fr Anesth Reanim* 1994;**12**:R87 (Abstract).

92 Green D, Ward B, Hughes N. Absence of pressor response following early insertion of laryngeal mask airway after induction with fentanyl and propofol. *Br J Anaesth* 1994;**72**:A54.

93 Joshi GP, Morrison SG, Okonkwo N, Gajraj NM, Pennant JH, White PF. Continuous hypopharyngeal pH monitoring: use of laryngeal mask airway versus tracheal tube. *Anesthesiology* 1994;**81**:A1281 (Abstract).

94 Fujii Y, Tanaka H, Toyooka H. Circulatory responses to laryngeal mask airway insertion or tracheal intubation in normotensive and hypertensive patients. *Can J Anaesth* 1995;**42**:32–36.

8 Indications and contraindications

Indications

The precise indications for use of the LMA have not been fully established and in many specialized areas its use is only supported by case reports and uncontrolled studies. The relative indications will vary according to patient and user factors and the perceived advantages and disadvantages over the face mask and tracheal tube. As a broad generalization the LMA is indicated where use of a face mask would be appropriate, but not when a tracheal tube is advisable[1]. This is not an absolute rule and is highly dependent on what is considered advisable. The indications for tracheal intubation can be broadly classified into four surgical categories: mandatory, preferable, optional and not justified[1]. Maltby suggested that some anesthesiologists consider the LMA should only be used when the tracheal tube is not justified[1], a viewpoint supported by a survey of consultant opinion on LMA practice in the UK[2]. However, the LMA has been used where tracheal intubation would be considered mandatory, preferable and optional. In some situations, such as for adenotonsillectomy, laser pharyngoplasty and open eye surgery, some advantages have been demonstrated over tracheal intubation, although outcome studies have yet to be performed. It may be more logical to consider the indications for tracheal intubation in terms of purpose rather than surgical category. Classically, indications for elective tracheal intubation would be reliable and secure maintenance of a clear airway, use of PPV, noninterference with the surgical field, protection against aspiration from the oropharynx, protection against aspiration from the stomach[1]. When the LMA is correctly placed the first four requirements are fulfilled to a reasonable and safe degree, but the fifth is not. In practice the extent of use depends on the clinician's level of experience and training with the LMA, patient factors, and the requirements of the surgeon.

Contraindications

The LMA is contraindicated in patients at risk of aspiration due to the presence of a full stomach, hiatus hernia, morbid obesity[3-5], intestinal obstruction, delayed gastric emptying, in patients unable to give accurate histories and who are not definitely within fasting guidelines[6,7]. The LMA should be avoided in injured patients, especially those who have eaten within 6 h of injury since, despite long periods of fasting and particularly where opioids have been administered, an empty stomach cannot be guaranteed and aspiration may still occur[8,9]. The LMA is also contraindicated in patients with low lung/chest compliance or high airway resistance (e.g. acute bronchospasm[10,11], pulmonary edema or fibrosis, thoracic trauma, morbid obesity). The LMA is relatively contraindicated in patients with glottic or subglottic airway obstruction, collapsible airways, limited mouth opening, pharyngeal pathology (abscess, hematoma, tissue disruption), one lung ventilation, some situations of difficult access to the airway and in some situations where the airway is difficult. It is also relatively contraindicated in the presence of bleeding diatheses[12–14] (Table 8.1). It has been suggested that placement is only relatively contraindicated in patients with a bleeding diathesis since the LMA can be inserted gently and under continual fiberoptic control[14].

Table 8.1 Contraindications

Patient factors increasing risk of pulmonary aspiration • not fasted • upper gastrointestinal pathology • morbid obesity • >14 weeks pregnant • trauma • severe pain • poor historian • gastrointestinal obstruction • autonomic neuropathy • opiate-delayed gastric emptying
Operative factors increasing risk of pulmonary aspiration • upper abdominal surgery • peritoneal traction • increased intra-abdominal pressure • steep Trendelenburg tilt
Patient factors with high inflation pressure • low compliance of lungs or chest wall • high airway resistance • glottic pathology (especially radiation to the larynx/pharynx)
Operative factors with need for high inflation pressure • intrathoracic surgery • intra-abdominal procedures leading to diaphragmatic splinting
Some diseases of the mouth and pharynx (including previous radiotherapy)
Bleeding diathesis (relative)

References

★ 1 Maltby JR. The laryngeal mask airway in anaesthesia. *Can J Anaesth* 1994;**41**:888–893.
Editorial discussing the indications and contraindication to LMA usage.

2 Akhtar TM, Shankar RK, Street MK. Is Guedel's airway and facemask dead? *Today's Anaesthetist* 1994;**9**:56–58.

3 Hill SA. Obese patient with coexisting anaesthetic problems. *Br J Hosp Med* 1993;**50**:205.

4 Hood DD, Dewan DM. Anesthetic and obstetric outcome in morbidly obese parturients. *Anesthesiology* 1993;**79**:1210–1218.

5 Fisher A, Waterhouse TD, Adams AP. Obesity: its relation to anaesthesia. *Anaesthesia* 1975;**30**:633–647.

6 Goresky GV, Maltby JR. Fasting guidelines for elective surgical patients. *Can J Anaesth* 1990;**37**:493–495.

7 Kallar SK, Everett LL. Potential risks and preventive measures for pulmonary aspiration: new concepts in preoperative fasting guidelines. *Anesth Analg* 1993;**77**:171–182.

8 Nanji GM, Maltby JR. Vomiting and aspiration pneumonitis with the laryngeal mask airway. *Can J Anaesth* 1992;**39**:69–70.

9 Wilkinson PA, Cyna AM, MacLeod DM, Campbell JR, Criswell J, John R. The laryngeal mask: cautionary tales. *Anaesthesia* 1990;**45**:167–168.

10 Cook T. Bronchospasm and the laryngeal mask airway. *Anaesthesia* 1994;**49**:82.

11 Brain AIJ. Bronchospasm and the laryngeal mask airway. *Anaesthesia* 1994;**49**:542–543.

12 Thompsett C, Cundy JM. Use of the laryngeal mask airway in the presence of a bleeding diathesis. *Anaesthesia* 1992;**47**:530–531.

13 Brain AIJ. Laryngeal mask misplacement – causes, consequences and solutions. *Anaesthesia* 1992;**47**:531–532.

14 Brimacombe J. Laryngeal mask and bleeding diathesis. *Anaesthesia* 1992;**47**:1004–1005.

9 Problems and complications

Problem overview

The LMA confers many advantages for the patient, anesthesiologist and surgeon (see Chapter 7). In most patients the technique is easily performed and relatively free from problems/complications. Nevertheless, both minor and very occasionally major problems/complications have been documented, many of which are associated with misuse and misplacement of the device (Table 9.1). The incidence of problems/ complications, as with all procedures, is related to the experience and expertise of the clinician[1]. Minor problems (e.g. coughing, sore throat, difficulty in placement) are relatively common, but major problems (e.g. aspiration, hypoxia, gross trauma) are uncommon and a number of very rare/unique complications (e.g. vocal cord paralysis, tongue cyanosis) have been reported. After 6 years of widespread use, there have been no deaths recorded in the scientific literature as directly attributable to LMA usage[2]. A number of device problems have been documented.

The frequency of problems/complications will vary according to user skill, patient factors, the type of anesthetic, the phase of anesthesia and the criteria by which the

Table 9.1 Classification of problems and complications with the LMA

Problem/complication	*Problem/complication*
Failed use[6] • insertion failure • excessive oropharyngeal leak Aspiration[11] Regurgitation[11] Vomiting[11] Leak[6,14,15] • oropharyngeal (inadequate ventilation) • esophagus (gastric insufflation) Breathholding[4,18] Pharyngolaryngeal reflexes • bronchospasm[4] • coughing[20] • gagging[22,23] • hiccup[4] • laryngeal spasm[26,27] • retching[22,23] • transient glottic closure[4,31] Trauma • arytenoid dislocation[10] • minor abrasions[4,31,36] • epiglottis[38] • larynx[40] • posterior pharyngeal wall[42] • tonsils[43] • uvula[45] Neurovascular • tongue cyanosis[47] • lingual nerve paralysis[49,50] • hypoglossal nerve paralysis[52] • vocal cord paralysis[53–56] • parotid gland swelling[57]	Postoperative • dry mouth[7,8] • dysarthria[9,10] • dysphagia[12] • dysphonia[12] • feeling of fullness[13] • hoarseness[7,16] • sore throat[17] • stridor[10] • mouth ulcer[19] • pharyngeal ulcer (L. Costa e Silva, personal communication, 1996) Device problems • cuff herniation[21] • pilot tube occlusion[24] • fractured LMA tube[25] • fragmentation of tube[28,29] • separation tube from bowl[30] • kinking[32–34] • damaged aperture bars[35] Miscellaneous • foreign body in tube[37] • wrong cleaning solution[39] • cuff damage by rotten tooth[41] Coincidental • pulmonary edema[44] • laryngeal hematoma[40] • infection transmission[46] • stridor[48] • head and neck edema[51] Nonairway • myocardial ischemia[6] • dysrhythmias[6]

problems are defined[3]. There is a significant reduction in the number of problems as experience is gained[1,4]. Problems are more likely to occur during induction or emergence from anesthesia[1]. Lopez-Gil et al have shown that there is a short-term learning curve with LMA usage in pediatric anesthetic practice and the average problem rate per patient can be reduced from 62 to 2% within 75 uses[1]. The overall incidence of problems is approximately 10% in both adults[4] and children[5], but is entirely dependent on problem definitions. The severity of problems may be quantified according to the minimum oxygen saturation. In a study of 1500 adult patients, problems occurred in 6.27%, but oxygen saturation fell below 90% on only 10 occasions and below 80% on one occasion[4]. The percentage of problems fell significantly from 8.7% during the first 750 uses to 3.9% during the last 750 uses. The first time insertion rate was 95.5% with an overall failure rate after three attempts of 0.4%. In a study of 1400 pediatric patients the overall problem rate was 11.5%, but oxygen saturation briefly fell below 90% on 23 occasions[5]. Placement was successful in 90% at the first attempt, 8% at the second attempt and 2% required an alternative technique. In a survey of 11 910 patients there were a total of 18 critical incidents related to the airway: regurgitation occurred in four patients; vomiting in two patients and aspiration occurred once; laryngeal spasm and bronchospasm occurred in eight and three patients, respectively[6]. There was only one actual adverse outcome related to airway management: a 68-year-old ASA 1 female who aspirated, but did not require ICU management.

Pulmonary aspiration, regurgitation and vomiting

Aspiration

The single most limiting feature of the LMA is the potential for aspiration. The anatomical and physiological reasons why aspiration may occur with the LMA have already been outlined (see Chapters 2 and 3). Large pre-LMA epidemiological studies have documented low incidences of perioperative pulmonary aspiration in both adults and children[58,59]. The overall incidence of aspiration related to general anesthesia has been variably reported as 1.4–6.5 per 10 000 with an associated mortality of approximately 5%[59–63]. A recent large prospective trial of 215 488 non-LMA general anesthetics, in which rigid criteria were used to define aspiration, estimated that aspiration occurred in 11 per 10 000 patients undergoing emergency surgery and 2.6 per 10 000 undergoing elective surgery[64]. The overall mortality, which was confined to patients ASA 3–5, was 0.14 per 10 000. A large survey of 529 150 outpatient anesthetics showed an aspiration rate of 1.7 per 10 000, with no significant difference between the face mask and tracheal tube[63].

A meta-analysis of published literature on the LMA to September 1993 (547 publications) suggested that the overall incidence of pulmonary aspiration was in the region of 2 per 10 000 (5 : 24 562)[11]. This comprised 3 : 6562 from papers where there were no problems or aspiration was specifically excluded; 2 : 8500 from Brain's personal series[45,65]; 0 : 7000 from Leach and Alexander[66]; and 0 : 2500 from Moylan and Luce (pediatric)[67]. There have been no published reports of long-term morbidity or mortality associated with the LMA secondary to aspiration. More recent studies have confirmed these figures. Haden et al reported a figure of 1 : 3500[68], Van Damme 0 : 5000 (controlled ventilation)[69], Braun and Fritz 1 : 3000 (pediatric)[70], Lopez-Gil et al 0 : 2000 (pediatric)[1,5], Brimacombe 0 : 1500[4] and Wainwright 0 : 1877[71]. Verghese and Brimacombe reported only one aspiration from a survey of 11 910 patients (44% controlled ventilation)[6]. Critical anesthetic events are consistently under-reported[72,73], but the fact that there were no admissions to the intensive care unit (ICU) from critical airway incidents in this latter study supports the concept that clinically significant aspiration is rare. Brain reported that only four cases of aspiration had been detected in 35 000 LMA anaesthetics at the Conquest Hospital, UK, and none had a serious outcome[2]. In three out of four cases use of the device was subsequently found to have been contraindicated. There appears to be no increased risk of aspiration with controlled versus spontaneous ventilation or in the pediatric population[74].

There had only been 18 cases of suspected pulmonary aspiration of gastric contents documented in the literature to September 1993[11]. Comprehensive details were lacking in many of these cases and in only 10 could pulmonary aspiration be confirmed (Table 9.2). The age range was 8–74 years and the male to female ratio was 6 : 5 and included two children. ASA grade was 1–3. In four cases aspiration occurred at or shortly after induction, in two cases during the procedure, in two cases at the end of the procedure, and in two cases timing was unspecified. Most cases had one or more predisposing factors including emergency anesthesia[75,76], obesity[65], dementia[76,77], previous gastric surgery[76,77], elective upper abdominal surgery[65,78], Trendelenburg position with intra-

Table 9.2 Analysis of cases of pulmonary aspiration

Reference	*Age*	*Sex*	*ASA*	*Diagnostic criteria met*	*Timing*	*Predisposing conditions*	*Outcome*
75	50	F	n/a	Yes	1.5 h after induction	Multitrauma. Fasting 26 h. Opioids ++	n/a
75	29	F	1	Yes	Just before end of procedure		n/a
78	26	F	1	Yes	After surgery during epidural insertion	Patient movement. Cholecystectomy. Cuff deflated early	ICU for 24 h. No PPV. Good recovery
79	51	M	2	Yes	Immediately after insertion	Hiccup following insertion	ICU. PPV 20 h. Good recovery
76	74	M	?3	Yes	Following displacement of femoral head	Fractured neck of femur. Dementia. PMH peptic ulcer and esophageal dilatation. Opioids	ICU. PPV for 4 days. Discharged to ward day 5
65	n/a	n/a	n/a	Yes	During anesthesia	n/a	No sequelae
65	n/a	F	n/a	Yes	At induction	Obesity. Cholecystectomy	No sequelae
80	8	F	?2	Yes	Following transfer and positioning in lithotomy	Movement. Procedure abandoned	Full recovery
82	55	M	1–2	Yes	During procedure	Bronchospasm. LMA removed. Aspiration during PPV with FM	No sequelae
81	15	n/a	1–2	n/a	After 2 h	Inadequate anesthetic depth	ICU. No PPV. Rapid recovery
77*	75	M	3	Yes	During anesthesia	Lithotomy position, dementia, hiatus hernia	PPV for 1 week. Survived

* Survey of Australian Intensive Care Units. A total of eight alleged cases. Lack of detail.

Key: n/a = not available, PMH = past medical history.
Reproduced with permission from reference 11, *Journal of Clinical Anesthesia*.

abdominal insufflation[75], inadequate anesthetic depth[78–81] and airway difficulties[82]. There was no correlation with ventilatory mode. Significant pulmonary complications occurred in three patients who then required PPV postoperatively for between 20 and 168 h[77–79]. All patients subsequently recovered fully with no long-term disability. A small number of similar cases have been reported since September 1993[6,83–85]. The case reports of aspiration must represent the tip of the iceberg. If the LMA has been used in 30 million patients and the incidence of aspiration is 2 per 10 000 there should have been at least 6000 cases of aspiration associated with its use worldwide. Less than 0.5% of this hypothetical subgroup of patients have been documented in the LMA literature. Detailed reports from all of this hypothetical group could provide invaluable information for evaluating risk factors and determining the benefits of therapeutic regimens. A suggested strategy for managing aspiration with the LMA is given in Table 9.3. Meticulous attention to selection of low risk patients[86,87] and appropriate operative procedures, and avoidance of light anesthesia, should reduce the incidence even further (Table 9.4).

Table 9.3 Management of regurgitation/aspiration

If regurgitation/aspiration occurs during anesthesia, the following steps should be taken:

1. Tilt the patient head down
2. Leave LMA in situ, disconnect the circuit temporarily to allow free fluid drainage
3. Deepen the anesthetic using propofol
4. Control ventilation manually, using low flows and small tidal volumes to avoid forcing any fluids present in the trachea into the bronchial tree
5. Give 100% oxygen
6. Suck out the LMA tube if necessary
7. Suck out the bronchial tree preferably using a fiberscope
8. Standard appropriate treatment should be instigated without delay if aspiration is confirmed bronchoscopically

Table 9.4 Guidelines to minimize risk of aspiration

1. Meticulous selection of patients
2. Avoid inadequate anesthesia during surgery
3. Meticulous selection of surgical procedure
4. Only insert the LMA when anesthetic depth is adequate
5. Avoid lubrication of anterior surface or excessive lubrication or use of lidocaine gel or gels containing nonaqueous solvents or silicones
6. Ensure adequate neuromuscular reversal prior to termination of general anesthesia
7. Avoid airway obstruction by ensuring adequate placement
8. Avoid gastric dilatation (minimize peak airway pressures, avoid inadequate paralysis and routinely place a gastric tube when anesthetizing small infants)
9. Routine use of device performance tests
10. Avoid disturbance of the patient during emergence (including stimulation from an overinflated cuff or turning the patient into the lateral position)
11. Keep the cuff inflated until the patient is awake.
12. Avoid use for prolonged procedures (> 2 h)*

* Controversial.

Finally, a large, randomized prospective trial comparing the incidences of regurgitation and aspiration between the LMA, the face mask and oral airway, and the tracheal tube in 'low risk' patients would be valuable. Such studies, however, are probably unrealistic given the large sample size required (>500 000 patients)[11,88,89]. Furthermore, because aspiration is such a rare event, it would also be difficult to study the impact of any management regimen on outcome.

Regurgitation

The incidence of regurgitation of small amounts of gastric contents is estimated at between 4 and 26% in general anesthesia[90–92], and subsequent aspiration into the tracheobronchial tree ranges from 10 to 20%[90,91,93]. This is of uncertain significance, although it has been suggested as one of the causes of postoperative pulmonary complications[94]. Blitt et al demonstrated that regurgitation occurs in 4.5% of patients undergoing general anesthesia with a face mask and 12.5% with a tracheal tube, and of these 17% and 7% respectively go on to aspirate[93]. The incidence of gastroesophageal reflux in children is approximately 2.5% and does not correlate with adverse respiratory events[95]. The incidence of clinically detectable regurgitation with the LMA varies between 0 and 150 per 10 000 patients with an average of 8.9 per 10 000. These data were derived from the following publications: 5 : 8500[45,65], 8 : 546[75], 5 : 2359[96], 4 : 11 910[6], 0 : 1500[4]. The higher figures come from earlier trials where experience with the device was limited. Regurgitation has been noted on two occasions in non-fasted patients[97,98], in a patient with a small hiatus hernia[99], and in a 45-year-old man undergoing routine myringoplasty with no predisposing condition[100]. The presence of fluid in the tube of the LMA indicates that regurgitation has occurred and that aspiration is about to occur or is already occurring[101]. Regurgitation of a large tablet into the LMA was described by Cairo[37], although it is equally possible that the tablet was never swallowed in the first place. This patient had dementia and diabetes – known risk factors for regurgitation/swallowing difficulties[102].

Vomiting

Physiologically, vomiting differs from regurgitation, the glottis being closed, and aspiration is less likely. The incidence of vomiting is variably reported at between 2 and 500 per 10 000[4–6,18,82,103,104] and tends to occur either at induction or, more commonly, during the recovery phase following LMA removal. The incidence of postoperative nausea and vomiting with the LMA is similar to the tracheal tube following gynecological surgery[105].

Aspiration from above the cuff

Although the LMA cuff does not isolate the respiratory tract from the gastrointestinal tract, it forms a reliable seal across the oropharyngeal inlet[39,106,107]. If the mask is correctly positioned and the leak pressure >10 cm H_2O the device should protect the trachea even if the mouth is flooded with fluid. If the cuff is dislodged, however, aspiration is possible and this has been reported in a patient with chronic purulent sinusitis[108]. Movement of the head and neck may make the LMA less effective in protecting against oropharyngeal soiling. Methylene blue dye was found within the bowl in 3/50 patients following prolonged surgery (mean 152 min) in which the head and neck was deliberately rotated, flexed and extended[109]. Samarkandi et al found that dye staining was present inside the mask in 5/50 pediatric patients, but no mention was made of leak pressures and suboptimal placement may have occurred[110]. The management of aspiration from above the cuff will involve oropharyngeal suction followed by removal of aspirated material, either through the LMA or a tracheal tube.

Oropharyngeal leak, gastric distension and barotrauma

As airway pressure increases during PPV, gas leaks occur into the oropharynx and, more importantly, the esophagus. Malposition increases the risk of leaks and overpressure (>25 cm H_2O) may lift the LMA tip from its correct position in the hypopharynx, elevate the distal cuff from the larynx and expose the esophageal inlet[111]. If the leak is sufficiently large or prolonged, gastric distension may occur[18,112–115], ventilation may be inadequate and there will be increased operating room pollution. Gastric distension may lead to impaired respiratory function and increase the risk of regurgitation, but even in children this may not be associated with any clinical problem[116]. The passage of small quantities of air into the stomach can be detected by auscultation of the epigastrium during PPV and this should be performed in all patients undergoing PPV. Although the reliability of this method has not been demonstrated with the LMA, Lawes et al have suggested that volumes as low as 5 ml passing from the esophagus to the stomach can be detected by epigastric auscultation during face mask ventilation[117]. Gastric distension may also occur in spontaneously breathing patients due to recurrent swallowing when anesthesia is too light[118].

One of the advantages of a low pressure seal with the larynx is that it protects the patient from barotrauma[66,119]. The supported normal lung requires pressures of 80–140 cm H_2O before rupture occurs and the maximum safe intrapulmonary pressure is considered to be about 70 cm H_2O[120]. Such high airway pressures could only be generated with the LMA if very high flow rates were used, or if the LMA cuff was forced more tightly onto the glottic perimeter such as might occur during coughing. There has only been one report of barotrauma associated with the LMA[121]. This occurred in a neonate during resuscitation and may have arisen spontaneously. Barotrauma is more likely to occur with future designs of the LMA which faciliate higher seal pressures (see Chapter 17, *Future designs*).

Pharyngolaryngeal reflexes

Laryngeal spasm[26,27], coughing[20], gagging, retching, bronchospasm[22,23,82] and breath-holding[18] may be associated with LMA usage, particularly if anesthesia is inadequate, or the device is malpositioned or inserted incorrectly. Activation of these reflexes is more likely to occur during placement and emergence, but can occur during maintenance[1,5]. For adults, in the hands of highly experienced LMA users (>750 uses) and using a fentanyl/propofol/O_2/N_2O/isoflurane technique, the incidence of perioperative pharyngolaryngeal reflex activation was: bronchospasm, 0.13%; glottic closure (either transient glottic closure or laryngeal spasm), 0.8%; hiccup, 1.1%; and coughing/gagging/retching, 0.8%[4]. For children, in the hands of moderately experienced LMA users, the incidence of upper airway reflex activation was 3%[5]. Severe bronchospasm requiring intubation would appear to be rare with one case reported (associated with inadequate anesthesia and minor aspiration) in 7239 patients taken from six large prospective surveys[67,82,96,122,123]. It is generally considered that complications occur more frequently in children, particularly during emergence, but this is unproven[124–126]. Impaction of the LMA tip with the glottis might precipitate bronchospasm, although this particular malposition is perhaps more likely to cause laryngeal spasm, stridor or mechanical airway obstruction. To distinguish bronchospasm from obstruction from a misplaced mask tip, the authors recommend anterolateral auscultation of the neck in addition to peripheral lung field auscultation.

Pharyngolaryngeal morbidity

Minor morbidity

The incidence of sore throat is approximately 10%, but varies between 0 and 70%[7,8,12,13,16,31,97,103,115,122,123,127–136]. This is usually mild, may not be directly related to the LMA, and is generally less than that reported for the tracheal tube (>30%)[137,138] and similar to that for the face mask (15–22%)[17]. Pharyngeal erythema and dry throat may occur more frequently with the LMA than with the face mask in children[139]. Two trials have failed to demonstrate a difference in sore throat compared with the tracheal tube[140,141]. Minor pharyngeal abrasions have been reported on the soft palate in 2% of patients[142]. The incidence of macroscopic blood on the LMA varies between 1 and 22% depending on insertion technique[4,31,36]. It is not clear why the reported incidence of sore throat is so varied, but many factors may potentially affect the incidence including insertion skill and technique, type of lubricant, cuff pressure, duration of operation, the presence of a throat pack[39] and use of the wrong cleaning solution. The only factor which has been clearly shown to reduce the incidence of sore throat is cuff pressure control. In a study of 200 patients Burgard et al demonstrated that reducing cuff pressure to the minimum required for an adequate seal produced a significant reduction in sore throat[134]. This has been confirmed by Lacroix et al, who also showed that the incidence of sore throat was 70% if the cuff pressure had increased by more than 50% compared with only 23% if the increase was less than 50%[135]. In a small study, O'Neill et al demonstrated a higher incidence of sore throat if gases were humidified, but a larger study is required before conclusions can be drawn[7]. Harada and Namiki compared the incidence of sore throat with the LMA versus the tracheal tube in 188 patients undergoing mastectomy and lower abdominal surgery and found the incidence to be similar[136]. Other minor complications potentially related to the LMA are hoarseness (4–47%)[7,12,16,140], dry mouth[7,8], dysphagia (4–24%)[12,140], and a feeling of 'fullness' (25%)[13]. It is likely that there is a distinct pattern of pharyngolaryngeal morbidity with the LMA compared with the tracheal tube[140].

Major morbidity

Lumb and Wrigley suggested that damage might occur by compression of parts of the pharynx against surrounding tissues such as the hyoid bone or cervical vertebrae[143]. This is more likely if the cuff is overinflated, as commonly occurs when attempting to produce an adequate seal with too small a mask. In this situation the surface of the cuff becomes stiff and local high pressure points may develop. Nonetheless, there is no evidence that the LMA significantly damages the pharynx over periods of 1–2 h[144]. Operations of up to 8 h duration have resulted in no adverse pharyngeal sequelae[118,145–147]. The LMA has been used in the ICU to provide respiratory support for 10–24 h[148,149]. There is anecdotal evidence that transient hypoglossal nerve paralysis[52], lingual nerve palsy[49,50] and tongue cyanosis[47] may occur with the LMA, although this probably represents a malposition of the cuff or tube[49] and/or cuff overinflation[150]. Laxton and Kipling reported a case of lingual nerve palsy which took 4 months to resolve[50]. Trauma to the uvula[45], tonsils[43], posterior pharyngeal wall[42], epiglottis[38] and larynx[40] have been reported, but are rare. McKinney and Grigg reported a case of epiglottitis requiring tracheal intubation which developed 12 h following an LMA anesthetic[151]. Major pharyngeal morbidity has been reported on one occasion in a child with Down's syndrome who received 14 LMA anesthetics within 1 month[42]. Costa e Silva has reported the development of a small area of pharyngeal necrosis when the LMA was left in situ for 8 days in the ICU (Costa e Silva, personal communication, 1996). Transient swelling of the parotid glands has also been reported and may be related to stimulation of salivary glands and mechanical compression of the parotid duct[57]. This latter complication occurs in approximately 0.2% of tracheal tube anesthetics[152]. There has been one case where an adult patient developed severe mouth ulcers 6 days after a 75 min LMA anesthetic[19]. It has been postulated that lingual nerve injury may occur where the nerve distal to its gingival branch is compressed by the LMA tubing against the side of the tongue (a malposition)[49].

Vocal cord function

Tracheal intubation causes transient changes in vocal function in the majority of patients[153]. These are thought to be multifactorial in origin relating to laryngeal and extralaryngeal factors. Although the LMA tip may occasionally impact with the larynx, correct LMA placement involves no laryngeal penetration. It has been shown that over the first 4–24 h postoperatively the LMA is associated with a much reduced incidence of postoperative laryngeal damage compared with the tracheal tube as determined by indirect stroboscopic laryngoscopy, electroglottography, vocal profile analysis[154] and acoustic waveform analysis[155]. The later study, however, could demonstrate no differences after 24 h[155]. Satoh et al conducted a phonetic evaluation of patients receiving balanced regional anesthesia with the LMA and found a tendency for the pitch perturbation quotient and amplitude perturbation quotient to increase 2 h posteratively, returning to normal at 24 h[156].

Transient dysarthria may occur if the cuff is overinflated during prolonged procedures[9]. Transient vocal cord paralysis has been reported on four occasions[53–56]: following a 1.5 h LMA anesthetic which took 14 days to resolve[53]; following a routine total abdominal hysterectomy which lasted less than 1 h[54]; and following a 35 min minor procedure in a 72 kg male[55,157]. Fawcett et al reported two cases of unilateral vocal cord paralysis following use of the LMA which resolved over 6–12 weeks[56,158]. Severe dysphonia lasting several months has been reported in two patients: in a 19-year-old male undergoing a 90 min inguinal hernia repair and in a 54-year-old female undergoing a D&C[10]. Several mechanisms of injury have been proposed: (1) misplacement of the LMA tip between the false cords might cause pressure on the vocal cords and lead to paresis[55]; (2) hyperextension of the neck could result in stretching of the vagus nerve[54]; (3) local diffusion of the viscous lidocaine jelly applied to the LMA cuff[54]; (4) a reaction to products used for cleaning[54]; or (5) pressure neuropraxia from an overinflated cuff due to N_2O diffusion[54,56,116]. It is generally considered that the likely mechanism is a pressure neuropraxia by the cuff of the LMA in the cricoid region at the lower part of the pyriform fossa (see Chapter 2, *Mouth: Neurovascular considerations*)[10,54,56,116], but this is unproven. Cros and Pitti reported a case of severe dysphonia secondary to arytenoid cartilage dislocation after LMA anesthesia[10]. The authors considered that the injury was either due to (1) direct trauma, (2) cuff inflation with the tip in the laryngeal inlet, or (3) swallowing against a malpositioned LMA during emergence. Brain[159] and Cros and Pitti[10] consider that limiting cuff pressures to 60 cm H_2O and using the standard insertion technique may help reduce the risk of these problems[159]. There is circumstantial evidence that granuloma of the larynx occurs in 1 : 10 000 following tracheal intubation[160], but there have been no reports of this complication in over 30 million LMA anesthetics. No major pharyngolaryngeal morbidity was reported from a prospective series of 11 910 patients[6]. Although it is reasonable to presume that major vocal complications might be reduced with the LMA compared with the tracheal tube, this has not been proven.

Coincidental and non-airway complications

Coincidental complications

Ezri et al reported two cases of pulmonary edema associated with use of the LMA[44]. This was considered to have occurred secondary to airway obstruction, a well-known cause of pulmonary edema in adults[161] and children[162]. Several authors commented that this complication was not a fault of the device itself, but rather of the way in which it was used[163–166]. On a number of occasions complications initially attributed to the LMA were due to unrecognized coincidental pathology. Marked head and neck edema and airway obstruction has occurred following removal of the LMA, but was probably related to metastatic breast disease[51]. A case of stridor occurring 1 day after adenotonsillectomy with the LMA was caused by recognized subglottic stenosis secondary to laryngotracheitis[48].

Thompsett and Cundy reported its use in a patient with a low platelet count for insertion of a right subclavian line for chemotherapy for a severe myelodysplastic syndrome. The patient subsequently developed a right laryngeal hematoma and required intubation[40]. Because of his bleeding tendency and his laryngeal hematoma, chemotherapy was never instituted and his condition deteriorated; he died 4 days later. Placement of the subclavian central line insertion was a likely cause of the hematoma[167,168]. This is the only patient in whom death has been tentatively linked to LMA usage in the literature.

Non-airway complications

In a survey of 11 910 patients undergoing LMA anesthesia there were 26 critical cardiovascular incidents which were not related to airway management[6]. This is fewer than reported prior to the availability of the LMA. In a cross-sectional study of complications of inhalational anesthesia in 16 995 patients conducted before the release of the LMA, the incidence of arrhythmia was 2.2% and myocardial ischemia 0.2%[23]. This compares with 0.09% and 0% for the LMA survey[6]. The extent to which this reflects patient selection, under-reporting, inadequate monitoring, use of different anesthetic drugs or the cardiovascular stability of the LMA[107] could not be determined from these data. The incidence of cardiac arrest in this series was 0.06% and would be considered relatively high, but the overall mortality rate was low (0.009%). Four out of the seven arrests were brief asystolic events which were directly related to surgical stimulation. One was secondary to massive hemorrhage and the other two occurred in elderly patients.

Infection transmission

Provided correct cleaning and sterilization procedures are adhered to, there is no direct risk of patient cross-contamination from the LMA. A controversial paper published in Australia suggested that hepatitis C transmission was possible via contaminated anesthetic breathing systems and indicated that by providing a clear airway the LMA facilitated passage of contaminants into the anesthetic breathing system when compared with the face mask[46]. It was suggested that organisms could enter the patient via small abrasions to the upper airway. These are reported to occur in approximately 2% of patients[142] (see this chapter, *Pharyngolaryngeal morbidity: Minor morbidity*). It is likely that circuit contamination may be promoted equally by either the LMA or the tracheal tube. By providing a superior airway to the face mask, both the LMA and the tracheal tube increase the risk of material reaching the anesthetic circuit and flowing back into a subsequent patient. It is imperative that a bacterial filter is inserted between the LMA and the circuit; alternatively the circuit should be changed between cases. It is recommended that gloves be worn at all times when handling the LMA. After LMA insertion, the inserting gloves should be discarded to prevent contamination of the trolley or other equipment by patient secretions.

Device problems/complications

A number of device complications have been documented in the literature. Herniation of the cuff may be caused by overinflation or overuse and may lead to airway obstruction[21,169–172]. Failure to inflate the cuff has been caused by the patient biting down on the pilot tube[24], or the pilot tube becoming looped around the mask aperture bars[173]. To avoid this it has been suggested that the pilot tube should be included in the lumen of the LMA tube[24,173]. However, if the airway tube is accidentally bitten into, it is likely that the pilot tube, if incorporated in its wall, would be severed, resulting in complete loss of seal. Thus the manufacturer has kept the pilot tube separate from the main tube in the interests of patient safety. On several occasions the LMA has broken apart in situ[25,28–30]. On one occasion the LMA tube separated from the cuff during removal[30] and on another the tube fractured mid-shaft[25]. More seriously the LMA has fragmented in situ[28,29]. These problems are probably related either to overuse, tube damage from biting, severe heat aging or a failure to follow the correct sterilization procedures. It is also possible that incorrect postcuring at the manufacturing stage may have been to blame[28]. If the LMA does break in situ, it should be remembered that the patient can still be ventilated by the application of a face mask since damage to the tube will not automatically result in cuff deflation[174,175]. A further mechanical problem which was noted in an early production model was kinking of the size 2 LMA[32–34]. This has since been rectified by the manufacturer[176]. A solution offered by Wilson and Eastley was to pass a reinforced tracheal tube down the shaft of the LMA to provide additional strength[177]. Where surgery makes kinking a concern, the FLMA should be used. Kinking may occur if the FLMA tube has been previously damaged (usually by biting following failure to place a bite block)[178,179]. Careful preoperative testing of the LMA and FLMA should prevent these problems (see Chapter 5, *Pre-use tests*).

References

★ 1 Lopez-Gil M, Brimacombe J, Cebrian J, Arranz J. The laryngeal mask airway in pediatric practice – a prospective study of skill acquisition by resident anesthesiologists. *Anesthesiology* 1996;**84**:807–811.
A prospective study of eight anesthesiology trainees to detemine the rate of skill acquisition with the LMA in pediatric practice. Presents data about the incidence of problems in 600 pediatric patients undergoing total intravenous or volatile anesthesia.

2 Brain AIJ. Use of the laryngeal mask airway (LMA) in general anaesthesia. *Minerva Anestesiol* 1996;**61**:9–11.

3 Down MP. Success rate of laryngeal mask passage. *Anaesthesia* 1996;**51**:795.

★ 4 Brimacombe J. Analysis of 1500 laryngeal mask uses by one anaesthetist in adults undergoing routine anaesthesia. *Anaesthesia* 1996;**51**:76–80.
Large series by a single LMA user utilizing the standard insertion technique. Presents data about the incidence of complications in 1500 adults following a standardized anesthetic.

★ 5 Lopez-Gil M, Brimacombe J, Alvarez M. Safety and efficacy of the laryngeal mask airway – a prospective survey of 1400 paediatric patients. *Anaesthesia* 1996;**51**:969–972.
Prospective survey of 1400 LMA uses in pediatrics. Presents data about the frequency of problems during induction, maintenance and emergence. The overall problem rate was 11.5% and the oxygen saturation fell briefly below 90% in 1.7%.

★ 6 Verghese C, Brimacombe J. Survey of laryngeal mask usage in 11 910 patients – safety and efficacy for conventional and nonconventional usage. *Anesth Analg* 1996;**82**:129–133.
This survey of 11 910 LMA anesthetics demonstrates that the technique has a high success rate for both spontaneous and controlled ventilation (99.81%). Presents data about critical incidents for conventional and nonconventional use.

7 O'Neill BL, Foley EP, Chang A. Effects of humidification of inspired gases with the laryngeal mask airway. *Anesthesiology* 1994;**81**:A52 (Abstract).
8 Alexander CA, Leach AB. Incidence of sore throats with the laryngeal mask. *Anaesthesia* 1989;**44**:791.
9 Brain AIJ. *The Intavent laryngeal mask – instruction manual.* London: Intavent, 1991;1–58.
10 Cros AM, Pitti R. Severe dysphonia following use of a laryngeal mask airway. *Anesthesiology* (in press).
★ 11 Brimacombe J, Berry A. The incidence of aspiration associated with the laryngeal mask airway – a meta-analysis of published literature. *J Clin Anesth* 1995;7:297–305.
Meta-analysis of publications to September 1993 determining the incidence of aspiration with the LMA. Suggests that the incidence is 2 : 10 000 and similar to that for the tracheal tube and face mask for outpatient anesthesia.
12 Ferrut O, Toulouse C, Lancon JP, Douvier S, Fayolle JL. The laryngeal mask for elective gynecologic surgery: a very attractive oral airway dispositive. *Anesth Analg* 1994;**78**:S110 (Abstract).
13 Daum REO, Downes RN, Vardy S. Day-stay cataract surgery under general anaesthesia. *Today's Anaesthetist* 1992;7:24–28.
14 Devitt JH, Wenstone R, Noel AG, O'Donnell RRT. The laryngeal mask airway and positive-pressure ventilation. *Anesthesiology* 1994;**80**:550–555.
15 Brimacombe J. Positive pressure ventilation with the size 5 LMA. *J Clin Anesth* (in press).
16 Fujii Y, Tanaka H, Toyooka H. [Effects of laryngeal mask airway on circulation and on incidence of postoperative sore throat and hoarseness]. *Masui* 1993;**42**:1559–1562.
17 Latto IP. The cuff. In: Latto IP, Rosen M, eds. *Difficulties in tracheal intubation.* London: Baillière Tindall, 1984;48–74.
18 Mason DG, Bingham RM. The laryngeal mask airway in children. *Anaesthesia* 1990;**45**:760–763.
19 Van Dongen VCPC, Langemeijer JJM. An unusual complication of the laryngeal mask airway. *Anaesthesia* 1994;**49**:1097–1098.
20 Thomson KD. The effect of the laryngeal mask airway on coughing after eye surgery under general anaesthetic. *Ophthalmic Surg* 1992;**23**:630–631.
21 Welsh BE, Martin DW. Will we ever learn? *Anaesthesia* 1990;**45**:892.
22 Shnider SM, Papper EM. Anesthesia for the asthmatic patient. *Anesthesiology* 1961;**22**:886.
23 Lew JKL, Spence AA, Elton RA. Cross-sectional study of complications of inhalational anaesthesia in 16 995 patients. *Anaesthesia* 1991;**46**:810–815.
24 George A. Failed cuff inflation of a laryngeal mask. *Anaesthesia* 1994;**49**:80.
25 Vickers R, Springer A, Hindmarsh J. Problem with the laryngeal mask airway. *Anaesthesia* 1992;**47**:639.
26 Haden RM, Pinnock CA, Campbell RL. The laryngeal mask for intraocular surgery. *Br J Anaesth* 1993;**71**:772.
27 Runcie CJ, Mackenzie SJ, Arthur DS, Morton NS. Comparison of recovery from anaesthesia induced in children with either propofol or thiopentone. *Br J Anaesth* 1993;**70**:192–195.
28 Squires SJ, Woods K. Fragmented laryngeal mask airway. *Anaesthesia* 1992;**47**:274.
29 Crawford M, Davidson G, Woods K. A problem with a laryngeal mask airway. *Anaesthesia* 1992;**47**:76.
30 Khoo ST. The laryngeal mask airway – an unusual complication. *Anaesth Intens Care* 1993;**21**:249–250.
31 Brimacombe J, Berry A. Insertion of the laryngeal mask airway – a prospective study of four techniques. *Anaesth Intens Care* 1993;**21**:89–92.
32 Rowbottom SJ, Simpson DL. Partial obstruction of the laryngeal mask airway. *Anaesthesia* 1990;**45**:892.
33 Goldberg PL, Evans PF, Filshie J. Kinking of the laryngeal mask airway in two children. *Anaesthesia* 1990;**45**:487–488.
34 Herrick MJ, Kennedy DJ. Airway obstruction and the laryngeal mask airway in paediatric radiotherapy. *Anaesthesia* 1992;**47**:910.
35 Wat LI, Templin PA, Lynch ME, Hammamura RK, White PF. Use of the laryngeal mask airway for ambulatory anesthesia: utilization, longevity and cost. *American Society of Anesthesiologist's Annual General Meeting, New Orleans, October 1996* (Abstract).
36 Dingley J, Whitehead MJ. A comparative study of sore throat with the laryngeal mask airway. *Anaesthesia* 1994;**49**:251–254.
37 Cairo SA. An unusual result of using a laryngeal mask airway. *Anaesth Intens Care* 1994;**22**:231–237.
38 Miller AC, Bickler P. The laryngeal mask airway. An unusual complication. *Anaesthesia* 1991;**46**:659–660.
39 Quinn AC, Samaan A, McAteer EM, Moss E, Vucevic M. The reinforced laryngeal mask airway for dento-alveolar surgery. *Br J Anaesth* 1996;**77**:185–188.
40 Thompsett C, Cundy JM. Use of the laryngeal mask airway in the presence of a bleeding diathesis. *Anaesthesia* 1992;**47**:530–531.
41 McLure HA. Dental damage to the laryngeal mask. *Anaesthesia* 1996;**51**:1078–1079.
42 Marjot R. Trauma to the posterior pharyngeal wall caused by a laryngeal mask airway. *Anaesthesia* 1991;**46**:589–590.
43 van Heerden PV, Kirrage D. Large tonsils and the laryngeal mask airway. *Anaesthesia* 1989;**44**:703.
44 Ezri T, Priscu V, Szmuk P, Soroker D. Laryngeal mask and pulmonary edema. *Anesthesiology* 1993;**78**:219.

45 Lee JJ, Brain AIJ. Laryngeal mask and trauma to uvula. *Anaesthesia* 1989;**44**:1014–1015.

46 Chant K, Kociuba K, Munro R, et al. Investigation of possible patient-to-patient transmission of hepatitis C in a hospital. *New South Wales Hlth Bull* 1994;**5**:47–51.

47 Wynn JM, Jones KL. Tongue cyanosis after laryngeal mask insertion. *Anesthesiology* 1994;**80**:1403–1404.

48 Nair I, Thompsett C. Laryngeal mask airway and late postoperative stridor. *Anaesthesia* 1994;**49**:449–450.

49 Ahmad NS, Yentis SM. Laryngeal mask airway and lingual nerve injury. *Anaesthesia* 1996;**51**:707–708.

50 Laxton CH, Kipling R. Lingual nerve paralysis following the use of the laryngeal mask airway. *Anaesthesia* 1996;**51**:869–870.

51 Kawaguchi M. Upper airway obstruction after removal of the LM. *J Clin Anesth (Rinsho-Masui)* 1993;**17**:97–98.

52 Nagai K, Sakuramoto C, Goto F. Unilateral hypoglossal nerve paralysis following the use of the laryngeal mask airway. *Anaesthesia* 1994;**49**:603–604.

53 Morikawa M. Vocal cord paralysis after use of the LM. *J Clin Anesth (Rinsho-Masui)* 1992;**16**:1194.

54 Inomata S, Nishikawa T, Suga A, Yamashita S. Transient bilateral vocal cord paralysis after insertion of a laryngeal mask airway. *Anesthesiology* 1995;**82**:787–788.

55 Lloyd Jones FR, Hegab A. Recurrent laryngeal nerve palsy after laryngeal mask airway insertion. *Anaesthesia* 1996;**51**:171–172.

56 Daya H, Fawcett W, Weir N. Vocal cord palsy after use of the laryngeal mask airway. *J Laryngol Otol* 1996;**110**:383–384.

57 Harada M. Transient swelling of the parotid glands following laryngeal mask airway. *Can J Anaesth* 1992;**39**:745–746.

58 Tiret L, Nivoche Y, Hatton F, Desmonts JM, Vourc'h G. Complications related to anaesthesia in infants and children. A prospective survey of 40 240 anaesthetics. *Br J Anaesth* 1988;**61**:263–269.

59 Olsson GL, Hallen B, Hambraeus Jonzon K. Aspiration during anaesthesia: a computer-aided study of 185 358 anaesthetics. *Acta Anaesthesiol Scand* 1986;**30**:84–92.

60 Cohen MM, Duncan PG, Pope WDB, Wolkenstein C. A survey of 112 000 anaesthetics at one teaching hospital. *Can Anaesth Soc J* 1986;**33**:22–31.

61 Tiret L, Desmonts JM, Hatton F, Vourc'h G. Complications associated with anaesthesia: a prospective survey in France. *Can Anaesth Soc J* 1986;**33**:336–344.

62 Leigh JM, Tytler JA. Admissions to the intensive care unit after complications of anaesthetic techniques over 10 years. *Anaesthesia* 1990;**45**:814–820.

63 Kallar SK. Aspiration pneumonitis: fact or fiction? *Probl Anesth* 1988;**2**:29–36.

64 Warner MA, Warner WE, Webber JG. Clinical significance of pulmonary aspiration during the perioperative period. *Anesthesiology* 1993;**78**:56–62.

65 Brain AIJ. The laryngeal mask and the oesophagus. *Anaesthesia* 1991;**46**:701–702.

66 Leach AB, Alexander CA. The laryngeal mask – an overview. *Eur J Anaesthesiol* 1991;**4**:19–31.

67 Moylan SL, Luce MA. The reinforced laryngeal mask airway in paediatric radiotherapy. *Br J Anaesth* 1993;**71**:172.

68 Haden RM, Pinnock CA, Scott PV. Incidence of aspiration with the laryngeal mask airway. *Br J Anaesth* 1994;**72**:496.

69 Van Damme E. Die Kehlopfmaske in der ambulanten Anasthesie – Eine Auswertung von 5000 ambulanten Narkosen. *Anaesthesiol Intensivmed Notfalmed Schmerzther* 1994;**29**:284–286.

70 Braun U, Fritz U. Die Kehlopfmaske in der Kinderanasthesie. *Anaesthesiol Intensivmed Notfalmed Schmerzther* 1994;**29**:286–288.

71 Wainwright AC. Positive pressure ventilation and the laryngeal mask airway in ophthalmic anaesthesia. *Br J Anaesth* 1995;**75**:249–250.

72 Cooper JB, Newbower RS, Kitz RJ. An analysis of major errors and equipment failures in anaesthesia management: considerations for prevention and detection. *Anesthesiology* 1984;**60**:34–42.

73 Cooper JB, Newbower RS, Long CD, McPeek B. Preventable anesthesia mishaps: a study of human factors. *Anesthesiology* 1978;**49**:399–406.

74 Brimacombe J, Berry A. LMA-related aspiration in children. *Anaesth Intens Care* 1994;**22**:313–314.

75 Wilkinson PA, Cyna AM, MacLeod DM, Campbell JR, Criswell J, John R. The laryngeal mask: cautionary tales. *Anaesthesia* 1990;**45**:167–168.

76 Nanji GM, Maltby JR. Vomiting and aspiration pneumonitis with the laryngeal mask airway. *Can J Anaesth* 1992;**39**:69–70.

77 Brimacombe J, Berry A. Aspiration and the laryngeal mask airway – a survey of Australian intensive care units. *Anaesth Intens Care* 1992;**20**:534–535.

78 Griffin RM, Hatcher IS. Aspiration pneumonia and the laryngeal mask airway. *Anaesthesia* 1990;**45**:1039–1040.

79 Koehli N. Aspiration and the laryngeal mask airway. *Anaesthesia* 1991;**46**:419.

80 Alexander R, Arrowsmith JE, Frossard RJ. The laryngeal mask airway: safe in the X ray department. *Anaesthesia* 1993;**48**:734.

81 Maroof M, Khan RM, Siddique MS. Intraoperative aspiration pneumonitis and the laryngeal mask airway. *Anesth Analg* 1993;77:409–410.

82 Langer A, Hempel V, Ahlhelm T, Heipertz W. Die Kehlkopfmaske bei > 1900 Allgemeinanasthesien – Erfahrungsbericht. *Anaesthesiol Intensivmed Notfalmed Schmerzther* 1993;**28**:156–160.

83 Cortes J, Franco A, Bouzada M, Cortinas J, Pedraza I, Alvarez J. La mascarilla laringea. *Actual Anesthesiol Reanim* 1995;5:21–28.

84 Lopez-Gil MT, Verghese C. La mascarilla laringea. *Actual Anesthesiol Reanim* 1995;**5**:181.

85 Ismail-Zade IA, Vanner RG. Regurgitation and aspiration of gastric contents in a child during general anaesthesia using the laryngeal mask airway. *Paed Anaesth* 1996;**6**:325–328.

86 Ball DR. LMA masks and children. *Can J Anaesth* 1994;**41**:1235.

87 Tham LCH. LMA masks and children – reply. *Can J Anaesth* 1994;**41**:1235.

88 Koller JP, Hackmann T. Laryngeal mask and aspiration of gastric contents. *Anesth Analg* 1996;**83**:441.

89 Joshi GP, White PF. Laryngeal mask and aspiration of gastric contents. *Anesth Analg* 1996;**83**:441–442.

90 Berson W, Adriani J. 'Silent' regurgitation and aspiration during anesthesia. *Anesthesiology* 1954;**15**:644.

91 Weiss WA. Regurgitation and aspiration of gastric contents during inhalational anesthesia. *Anesthesiology* 1950;**11**:102.

92 Carlsson C, Islander G. Silent gastropharyngeal regurgitation and aspiration during anesthesia. *Anesth Analg* 1981;**60**:655.

93 Blitt CD, Gutman HL, Cohen DD, Weisman H, Dillon JB. 'Silent' regurgitation and aspiration during general anaesthesia. *Anesth Analg* 1970;**49**:707–713.

94 Cameron JL, Zuidema GD. Aspiration pneumonia. Magnitude and frequency of the problem. *J Am Med Assoc* 1972;**219**:1194.

95 Milross JG, Negus BH, Street NE, Gaskin KJ. Gastro-oesophageal reflux and adverse respiratory events in children under anaesthesia. *Anaesth Intens Care* 1995;**23**:587–590.

96 Verghese C, Smith TGC, Young E. Prospective survey of the use of the laryngeal mask airway in 2359 patients. *Anaesthesia* 1993;**48**:58–60.

97 Brain AIJ. The development of the laryngeal mask – a brief history of the invention, early clinical studies and experimental work from which the laryngeal mask evolved. *Eur J Anaesthesiol* 1991;**4**:5–17.

98 Bonner SM. A fasted patient? *Anaesthesia* 1992;**47**:916.

99 Cook TM. Aspiration, the LMA and day case surgery. *Today's Anaesthetist* 1993;**8,2**:32.

100 Lack A. Regurgitation using a laryngeal mask. *Anaesthesia* 1993;**48**:734.

101 Brain AIJ. Regurgitation through a laryngeal mask. *Can J Anaesth* 1993;**40**:797.

102 Brimacombe J. An unusual complication in an unsuitable patient. *Anaesth Intens Care* 1994;**22**:504.

103 Reddy SVG, Win N. Brain laryngeal mask – study in 50 spontaneously breathing patients. *Sing Med J* 1990;**31**:338–340.

104 Young TM. The laryngeal mask in dental anaesthesia. *Eur J Anaesthesiol* 1991;**4**:53–59.

105 Kumagai A, Iwasaki H, Kawana S, Namiki A. Laryngeal mask airway does not reduce the incidence of post-operative nausea and vomiting after gynaecological surgery. *Anesth Analg* 1996;**81**:S255 (Abstract).

106 John RE, Hill S, Hughes TJ. Airway protection by the laryngeal mask – a barrier to dye placed in the pharynx. *Anaesthesia* 1991;**46**:366–367.

★ 107 Cork RC, Depa RM, Standen JR. Prospective comparison of use of the laryngeal mask and endotracheal tube for ambulatory surgery. *Anesth Analg* 1994;**79**:719–727.
Complex paper investigating several aspects of LMA usage including efficacy for PPV, fiberoptic position, efficacy as a throat pack and differing trends in PPV compared with the tracheal tube. Also suggests that patients managed with the LMA may require less analgesia postoperatively.

108 Terada H, Ootaka H, Ohta S, Suzuki MI. Airway obstruction due to pus from sinusitis during the use of the LM. *J Clin Anesth (Rinsho-Masui)* 1993;**17**:673–674.

109 Fujii T, Watanabe S, Taguchi N, Takeshima R. Airway protection by the laryngeal mask during various neck positions and during protracted surgeries: sealing to dye placed in the pharynx. *Anesth Analg* 1996;**82**:S118 (Abstract).

110 Samarkandi AH, Ali MS, Elgammal M, Bakhamees HS. Airway protection by the laryngeal mask airway in children. *Middle East J Anesthesiol* 1995;**13**:107–113.

111 Pothmann W, Fullekrug B, Schulte am Esch J. [Fiberoptic determination of the position of the laryngeal mask]. *Anaesthesist* 1992;**41**:779–784.

112 Miyasaka K, Suzuki Y, Nakagawa S, Asahara S. The use of the laryngeal mask in pediatric anesthesia. *8th Asian–Australian Congress of Anaesthesiologists* 1990;**1, S 5–6**:158 (Abstract).

113 Wittmann PH, Wittmann FW. Laryngeal mask and gastric dilatation. *Anaesthesia* 1991;**46**:1083.

114 Hammond JE. Controlled ventilation and the laryngeal mask airway. *Anaesthesia* 1989;**44**:616–617.

115 Jeong J, Yang H, Cho H. Clinical investigation of laryngeal mask airway. *J Kor Soc Anesthesiol* 1993;**25**:708–718.

116 Gursoy F, Algren JT, Skjonsby BS. Positive pressure ventilation with the laryngeal mask airway in children. *Anesth Analg* 1996;**82**:33–38.

117 Lawes EG, Campbell I, Mercer D. Inflation pressure, gastric insufflation and rapid sequence induction. *Br J Anaesth* 1987;**59**:315–318.

118 Brimacombe J. Laryngeal mask anaesthesia and recurrent swallowing. *Anaesth Intens Care* 1991;**19**:275–276.

119 Brimacombe J, Berry A. Barotrauma and the laryngeal mask airway. *Anaesthesia* 1994;**49**:1009.

120 Mushin WW, Rendell-Baker L, Thompson PW, Mapleson WW, eds. Physiological aspects. In *Automatic ventilation of the lungs*. Oxford: Blackwell Scientific Publications, 1980;1–32.

121 Paterson SJ, Byrne PJ, Molesky MG, Seal RF, Finucane BT. Neonatal resuscitation using the laryngeal mask airway. *Anesthesiology* 1994;**80**:1248–1253.

122 McCrirrick A, Ramage DT, Pracilio JA, Hickman JA. Experience with the laryngeal mask airway in two hundred patients. *Anaesth Intens Care* 1991;**19**:256–260.

123 Maltby JR, Loken RG, Watson NC. The laryngeal mask airway: clinical appraisal in 250 patients. *Can J Anaesth* 1990;**37**:509–513.

124 Haynes SR, Morton NS. The laryngeal mask airway: a review of its use in paediatric anaesthesia. *Paed Anaesth* 1993;**3**:65–73.

125 St Claire Logan A, Morris P. Complications following use of the laryngeal mask airway in children. *Paed Anaesth* 1993;**3**:297–300.

126 Wilson IG. The laryngeal mask airway in paediatric practice. *Br J Anaesth* 1993;**70**:124–125.

127 Miranda AF, Reddy SVG. Controlled ventilation with Brain laryngeal mask. *Med J Malaysia* 1991;**45**:65–69.

128 Slappendel R, Harbers JBM, ten Have FTM, Moll JE. Eerste ervaringen met het larynxmasker. *Nederlands Tijdschrift voor Anaesthesie* May 1991:16–20.

129 Morley AP. Hoarseness and the use of the laryngeal mask. *Anaesthesia* 1992;**47**:713.

130 Sarma VJ. The use of a laryngeal mask airway in spontaneously breathing patients. *Acta Anaesthesiol Scand* 1990;**34**:669–672.

131 Coyne BJ. The use of the laryngeal mask airway in day case and short stay surgery. *Ir J Med Sci* 1990;**159**:185–186.

132 Santamaria LB, Badessa P, Practico C, Fedale V, Monanini S. Anaesthesia with propofol and laryngeal mask airway is useful and safe in dental surgery. *10th World Congress of Anaesthesiologists, Den Haag, 1992*, A815 (Abstract).

133 Splinter WM, Smallman B, Rhine EJ, Komocar L. The effect of the laryngeal mask airway on postoperative sore throat in children. *Anesth Analg* 1994;**78**:S414 (Abstract).

★ **134** Burgard G, Mollhoff T, Prien T. The effect of laryngeal mask cuff pressure on postoperative sore throat incidence. *J Clin Anesth* 1996;**8**:198–201.
Prospective study of 200 gynecological patients showing that limiting cuff pressure to 'just seal' pressure reduces the incidence of sore throat.

135 Lacroix O, Billard V, Bourgain JL, Debaene B. Prevention of postoperative sore throat during use of the laryngeal mask airway. *European Society of Anaesthesiologists Annual Congress, London, 1–5 June 1996*, A51 (Abstract).

136 Harada Y, Namiki A. Incidence of sore throat after endotracheal intubation is not different from that after use of the laryngeal mask airway. *11th World Congress of Anesthesiology, Sydney, 14–20 April 1996, Abstract Handbook*, p.511 (Abstract).

137 Brindle GF, Soliman MG. Anaesthetic complications in surgical outpatients in surgical outpatients. *Can Anaesth Soc J* 1975;**22**:613–619.

138 Jones MW, Catling S, Evans E, Green DH, Green JR. Hoarseness after tracheal intubation. *Anaesthesia* 1992;**47**:213–216.

139 Johnston DF, Wrigley SR, Robb PJ, Jones HE. The laryngeal mask airway in paediatric anaesthesia. *Anaesthesia* 1990;**45**:924–927.

140 Rieger A, Brunne B, Has I, et al. Laryngo-pharyngeal complaints following laryngeal mask airway and endotracheal intubation. *J Clin Anesth* (in press).

141 Splinter WM, Smallman B, Rhine EJ, Komocar L. Postoperative sore throat in children and the laryngeal mask airway. *Can J Anaesth* 1994;**41**:1081–1083.

142 Shrestha BM, Basnyat NB. Experience with the laryngeal mask airway in Nepal. *Today's Anaesthetist* 1993;**8**:133–134.

143 Lumb AB, Wrigley MW. The effect of nitrous oxide on laryngeal mask cuff pressure. In vitro and in vivo studies. *Anaesthesia* 1992;**47**:320–323.

144 Brimacombe J, Berry A. Laryngeal mask airway cuff pressure and position during anaesthesia lasting 1–2 hours. *Can J Anaesth* 1994;**41**:589–593.

145 Brain AIJ. *The laryngeal mask – instruction manual*. London: Intavent, 1990;1–38.

146 Brimacombe J, Shorney N. The laryngeal mask airway and prolonged balanced anaesthesia. *Can J Anaesth* 1993;**40**:360–364.

147 Brimacombe J, Archdeacon J. The laryngeal mask airway for unplanned prolonged procedures. *Can J Anaesth* 1995;**42**:1176.

148 Aoyagi M. Application of the laryngeal mask airway in ICU. *40th Meeting of the Japanese Society of Anesthesiology, Iwate Prefectual Hall, Japan, 22 April 1993,* pp.6–7 (Abstract).
149 Arosio EM, Conci F. Use of the laryngeal mask airway for respiratory distress in the intensive care unit. *Anaesthesia* 1995;**50**:635–636.
150 Brain AIJ. Course of the hypoglossal nerve in relation to the position of the laryngeal mask airway. *Anaesthesia* 1995;**50**:82–83.
151 McKinney B, Grigg R. Epiglottitis after anaesthesia with a laryngeal mask. *Anaesth Intens Care* 1995;**23**:618–619.
152 Reilly DJ. Benign transient swelling of the parotid glands following general anesthesia: 'Anesthesia Mumps'. *Anesth Analg* 1970;**49**:560–563.
153 Beckford NS, Mayo R, Wilkinson A, Tierney M. Effects of short-term endotracheal intubation on vocal function. *Laryngoscope* 1990;**100**:331–336.
★ **154** Harris TM, Johnston DF, Collins SRC, Heath ML. A new general anaesthetic technique for use in singers: the Brain laryngeal mask airway verses endotracheal intubation. *J Voice* 1990;**4**:81–85.
Double blind study comparing vocal function following LMA or tracheal tube anesthesia. Showed using vocal profile analysis, indirect stroboscopic laryngoscopy and electroglottography that the LMA interfered with vocal function less than the tracheal tube.
155 Lee SK, Hong KH, Choe H, Song HS. Comparison of the effects of the laryngeal mask airway and endotracheal intubation on vocal function. *Br J Anaesth* 1993;**71**:648–650.
156 Satoh M, Shigematsu T, Yoruzo T, Miyazwa N. Phonetic evaluation of the patient after using the laryngeal mask airway. *11th World Congress of Anesthesiology, Sydney, 14–20 April 1996, Abstract Handbook,* p.611 (Abstract).
157 Inomata S, Nishikawa T. Vocal cord paralysis and a laryngeal mask airway. *Anaesthesia* 1996;**51**:1079.
158 Fawcett WJ, Daya H, Weir N. Recurrent laryngeal nerve palsy and the laryngeal mask airway. *Anaesthesia* 1996;**51**:708.
159 Brain AIJ. Pressure in laryngeal mask airway cuffs. *Anaesthesia* 1996;**51**:603.
160 Snow JC, Harano M, Balogy K. Postintubation granuloma of the larynx. *Anesth Analg* 1966;**45**:425.
161 Price SL, Hacker BR. Pulmonary oedema following airway obstruction in a patient with Hodgkin's disease. *Br J Anaesth* 1987;**59**:518–521.
162 Lee KWT, Downes JJ. Pulmonary edema secondary to laryngospasm in children. *Anesthesiology* 1983;**59**:347–349.
163 Brimacombe J, Berry A. Laryngeal mask airway and pulmonary edema: III. *Anesthesiology* 1993;**79**:185.
164 Gajraj NM, Pennant JH, Joshi GP. Laryngeal mask airway and pulmonary edema: I. *Anesthesiology* 1993;**79**:184.
165 Stiff G, Old S, Bapat P, Verghese C. Laryngeal mask airway and pulmonary edema: II. *Anesthesiology* 1993;**79**:184–185.
166 Ezri T, Szmuk P, Soroker D. Laryngeal mask airway and pulmonary edema (reply). *Anesthesiology* 1993;**79**:186.
167 Brain AIJ. Laryngeal mask misplacement – causes, consequences and solutions. *Anaesthesia* 1992;**47**:531–532.
168 Brimacombe J. Laryngeal mask and bleeding diathesis. *Anaesthesia* 1992;**47**:1004–1005.
169 Newnam PFT. Discarding used laryngeal mask airways – can there still be life after 40? *Anaesthesia* 1994;**49**:81.
170 Boge E, Brandis K. Testing the laryngeal mask. *Anaesth Intens Care* 1995;**23**:751–752.
171 Sleth JC, Sidawy P. Hernie peroperatoire du coussinet d'un masque larynge. *Ann Fr Anesth Reanim* 1995;**14**:240–241.
172 Leonetti MA. Hernie peroperatoire du coussinet d'un masque larynge. *Ann Fr Anesth Reanim* 1995;**14**:241.
173 Richards JT. Pilot tube of the laryngeal mask airway. *Anaesthesia* 1994;**49**:450.
174 Woods K. Pilot tube of the laryngeal mask airway. *Anaesthesia* 1994;**49**:450–451.
175 Woods K. Failed cuff inflation of a laryngeal mask. *Anaesthesia* 1994;**49**:80.
176 Martin DW. Kinking of the laryngeal mask airway in two children. *Anaesthesia* 1990;**45**:488.
177 Wilson IG, Eastley R. A modification of the laryngeal mask airway. *Anesthesiology* 1991;**74**:1157 (Abstract).
178 Dempsey GA, Barrett PJ. Hazard with the reinforced laryngeal mask airway. *Anaesthesia* 1995;**50**:660–661.
179 Woods KD. Hazard with the reinforced laryngeal mask airway. *Anaesthesia* 1995;**50**:661.

10 Training and basic uses

Training

Although insertion and ventilation can be readily achieved with minimal training, as illustrated by controlled studies of nonanesthesiologists[1-3], optimal use in anesthesia requires the acquisition of a wide range of new skills. The inventor has suggested that skill in using the LMA increases appreciably with time[4] and there is some data supporting this concept[5-9] including both a short (75 uses)[10] (Figure 10.1) and long-term learning curve (750 uses)[9]. Training programs should be standardized to ensure complete coverage of LMA usage, and should include formal lectures, adherence to guidelines in the instruction manual and video and experience in LMA insertion in an intubating mannequin prior to practical experience in the operating room[11]. One to one training with an experienced LMA user is recommended and training centers have been established in the UK and USA. Some form of certification and continued training

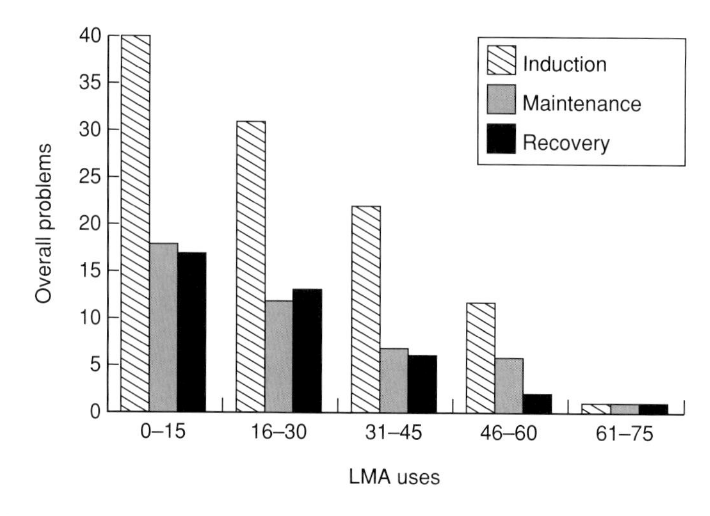

Figure 10.1 Problems with LMA[10]. Reproduced with permission, International Anesthesia Research Society.

would also be desirable[11]. An LMA compatible mannequin is now available from Ambu (Demark).

Some authors have expressed concern that face mask and tracheal intubation skills are being jeopardized by trainees over-reliant on the LMA[12-15]. It has been suggested that trainees should not be allowed to use the LMA until skills with the face mask and tracheal tube have been acquired[13]. It would seem more logical if skills with all three airway management techniques were acquired synchronously, particularly since the LMA might be required for airway rescue at any stage during training[16].

Basic uses

Whilst gaining initial experience with the LMA its use should be confined to short, simple procedures (<1 h) in ASA 1–2 patients in whom spontaneous ventilation is an acceptable modality. Patient position should preferably be confined to the supine position or lithotomy (without Trendelenburg tilt) for brief procedures (<30 min). Such procedures would include anesthesia for operations to the extremities, minor urological and gynecological procedures and surface operations on the trunk. In some of these areas the advantages of the LMA have been demonstrated in controlled trials[17-20].

Monitored anesthesia care (MAC)

The advantages of using a propofol/LMA/isoflurane or LMA/propofol infusion technique over pure sedation/variable flow oxygen mask are: the airway is more reliably maintained and manually assisted ventilation may be given if respiration becomes depressed – airway obstruction may be avoided; concentration of oxygen delivered can be increased to 100%; end-tidal carbon dioxide may be accurately monitored; the risk of awareness and patient distress is reduced as light anesthesia is avoided; excessive sedation and therefore prolonged patient recovery times are avoided should the surgical procedure take a long time. The LMA is frequently used in combination with regional anesthesia. However, the level of anesthesia required is that which is sufficient to tolerate the LMA, i.e. somewhat deeper than MAC anesthesia. The cost of the LMA and using deeper anesthesia may be offset by using low flow systems and faster patient discharge times.

Day surgery

The use of the LMA for day surgery has been reviewed by McGoldrick[21] and Smith and Joshi[22]. The criteria for use would include the majority of day surgery patients[23,24]. Usage rates for day surgery exceed 70% in some institutions. Day surgery units in the USA have recently reported LMA usage rates of 28%, with usage rates for the tracheal tube of 52% and the face mask of 20%[25]. The safety and efficacy of the LMA for day surgery has been demonstrated by Van Damme in a series of 5000 patients[26]. The technique was successful in over 99.9% of patients and in only 1.5% was the oxygen saturation less than 90%. There were no episodes of regurgitation or aspiration. Prosperi et al reported its use for day surgery in 100 children aged 1–3 years[27]. Not all uses of the LMA in day surgery can be considered basic uses. Advanced day case uses include dental surgery[7,28,29], bronchoscopy[30], open eye surgery[31], most head, neck and ENT procedures and gynecological laparoscopy[32].

Advanced uses

Once basic skills have been acquired, the practitioner may consider using the LMA for so-called 'advanced' clinical situations, techniques and surgical procedures (Chapters 11–13). The point at which the practitioner could embark on advanced uses will vary according to the rate of practitioner skill acquisition and the specific clinical situation. Advice should be sought from more experienced LMA users before attempting many advanced uses. It would be sensible to avoid advanced uses until reasonable levels of skill have been achieved. It has been suggested that reasonable levels of skill could be defined as: (1) problem rates less than 10% in children[10]; (2) first time insertion rates greater than 90% in adults [9]; (3) overall success rates greater than 95% in adults[9]; and (4) median fiberoptic scoring greater than 3.0 in adults[9].

References

1 Pennant JH, Walker MB. Comparison of the endotracheal tube and laryngeal mask in airway management by paramedical personnel. *Anesth Analg* 1992;**74**:531–534.

2 Tighe SQ, Davies PR, Greenslade GL, Evans GH. Laryngeal mask airway. *Lancet* 1991;**337**:375–376.

3 Martin PD, Cyna AM, Hunter WAH, Henry J, Pamayya GP. Training nursing staff in airway management for resuscitation – a clinical comparison of the facemask and laryngeal mask. *Anaesthesia* 1993;**48**:33–37.

4 Brain AIJ. Laryngeal mask airway. *Anesthesiology* 1992;**76**:1061.

5 McCrirrick A, Ramage DT, Pracilio JA, Hickman JA. Experience with the laryngeal mask airway in two hundred patients. *Anaesth Intens Care* 1991;**19**:256–260.

6 Brodrick PM, Webster NR, Nunn JF. The laryngeal mask airway. A study of 100 patients during spontaneous breathing. *Anaesthesia* 1989;**44**:238–241.

7 Young TM. The laryngeal mask in dental anaesthesia. *Eur J Anaesthesiol* 1991;**4**:53–59.

8 Webster AC, Morley-Forster PK, Dain S, et al. Anaesthesia for adenotonsillectomy: a comparison between tracheal intubation and the armoured laryngeal mask airway. *Can J Anaesth* 1993;**40**:1171–1177.

★ 9 Brimacombe J. Analysis of 1500 laryngeal mask uses by one anaesthetist in adults undergoing routine anaesthesia. *Anaesthesia* 1996;**51**:76–80.
Large series by a single LMA user utilizing the standard insertion technique. Provides evidence for a long-term learning curve over the first 1500 uses.

★ 10 Lopez-Gil M, Brimacombe J, Cebrian J, Arranz J. The laryngeal mask airway in pediatric practice – a prospective study of skill acquisition by resident anesthesiologists. *Anesthesiology* 1996;**84**:807–811.
A prospective study of eight anesthesiology trainees to detemine the rate of skill acquisition with the LMA in pediatric practice. Showed that there was a dramatic reduction in the number of complications over the first 75 uses from 60% to less than 2% when comparing the first with the last 15 use epoch.

11 Brimacombe J, Berry A, Fletcher D. A training program for laryngeal mask airway removal in the PACU. *J Post Anaes Nurs* 1993;**8**:236–237.

12 Pennant JH, White PF. The laryngeal mask airway. Its uses in anesthesiology. *Anesthesiology* 1993;**79**:144–163.

13 Tuckey J. Does the use of the laryngeal mask airway result in loss of airway management skills? *Anaesthesia* 1994;**49**:824.

14 Akhtar TM, Shankar RK, Street MK. Is Guedel's airway and facemask dead? *Today's Anaesthetist* 1994;**9**:56–58.

15 Asai T, Morris S. The laryngeal mask airway: its features, effects and role. *Can J Anaesth* 1994;**41**:930–960.
16 Koppel JN, Reed AP. Formal instruction in difficult airway management. A survey of anesthesiology residency programs. *Anesthesiology* 1995;**83**:1343–1346.
17 Johnston DF, Wrigley SR, Robb PJ, Jones HE. The laryngeal mask airway in paediatric anaesthesia. *Anaesthesia* 1990;**45**:924–927.
18 Watcha MF, Garner FT, White PF, Lusk R. Laryngeal mask airway vs face mask and Guedel airway during pediatric myringotomy. *Arch Otolaryngol Head Neck Surg* 1994;**120**:877–880.
19 Smith I, White PF. Use of the laryngeal mask airway as an alternative to a face mask during outpatient arthroscopy. *Anesthesiology* 1992;**77**:850–855.
20 Cork RC, Depa RM, Standen JR. Prospective comparison of use of the laryngeal mask and endotracheal tube for ambulatory surgery. *Anesth Analg* 1994;**79**:719–727.
21 McGoldrick KE. The laryngeal mask airway. *Day Surg Patient* 1993;**2**:1–5.
22 Smith I, Joshi G. The laryngeal mask airway for outpatient anesthesia. *J Clin Anesth* 1993;**5**:22S–28S.
23 Coyne BJ. The use of the laryngeal mask airway in day case and short stay surgery. *Ir J Med Sci* 1990;**159**:185–186.
24 Stillman PC. Introduction of the laryngeal mask airway in a community outpatient surgical centre. *Anesthesiology* 1993;**79**:A559 (Abstract).
25 Wat LI, Templin PA, Lynch ME, Hammamura RK, White PF. Use of the laryngeal mask airway for ambulatory anesthesia: utilization, longevity and cost. *American Society of Anesthesiologist's Annual General Meeting, New Orleans, October 1996* (Abstract).
★ 26 Van Damme E. Die Kehlopfmaske in der ambulanten Anasthesie – Eine Auswertung von 5000 ambulanten Narkosen. *Anaesthesiol Intensivmed Notfalmed Schmerzther* 1994;**29**:284–286.
Prospective survey of 5000 day case patients showing a low incidence of problems and desaturation events. Assessed leak pressures in 4866 patients and showed that a leak pressure of < 15 cm H_2O occurred in only 2.7%.
27 Prosperi M, Heinen M, Fantini G. La maschera laringea nell'anestesia ambulatoriale pediatrica. *Minerva Anestesiol* 1995;**61**:53–55.
28 Noble H, Wooller DJ. Laryngeal masks and chair dental anaesthesia. *Anaesthesia* 1991;**46**:591.
29 Goodwin A, Ogg TW, Lamb W, Adlam D. The reinforced laryngeal mask airway in dental day surgery. *Ambulatory Surg* 1993;**1**:31–35.
30 Du Plessis MC, Marshall Barr A, Verghese C, Lyall JRW. Fibreoptic bronchoscopy under general anaesthesia using the laryngeal mask airway. *Eur J Anaesthesiol* 1993;**10**:363–365.
31 Daum REO, Downes RN, Vardy S. Day-stay cataract surgery under general anaesthesia. *Today's Anaesthetist* 1992;**7**:24–28.
32 Brimacombe J. The laryngeal mask airway for outpatient anaesthesia. *J Clin Anesth* 1994;**6**:452–453.

11 Advanced uses: clinical situations

Obesity

Management of anesthesia in the obese patient is influenced by unfavorable alterations in anatomical and physiological function[1]. Those alterations relevent to airway management include a restrictive ventilatory defect, arterial hypoxemia, increased gastric acidity/risk of reflux and difficult airway management. These risks generally increase with increasing body mass index, but will vary considerably and risk assessment based on body mass index alone is probably unreliable.

Apart from the above considerations, the obese patient may present problems with face mask anesthesia since the abundant soft tissue makes upper airway obstruction common. Tracheal intubation is frequently more difficult in the obese patient and hypoxia occurs more rapidly[2]. Some authors consider awake intubation to be mandatory in this population, but preference for this technique must be balanced by the realization that most episodes of gastroesophageal reflux occur from and during bucking[3,4]. The LMA has been used as an aid to awake intubation in a morbidly obese patient requiring an urgent cesarean section[5].

The LMA is not recommended for use in the morbidly obese patient[6] because of the associated increased incidence of reflux, but it can be appropriate in some obese patients provided the patient has no symptoms of reflux and the anesthesiologist is experienced with the LMA, and takes care to avoid inadequate anesthesia. There is some evidence supporting the use of the LMA in these circumstances. Verghese et al did not detect any increase in problem rate in patients who were moderately obese[7]. Brimacombe reported use of the size 5 LMA in 52 obese patients (body mass index 30–50) and the incidence of problems was similar to acceptible weight and overweight patients (body mass index 25–30)[8].

In practice, a size 4 or 5 LMA will usually be appropriate irrespective of gender. It is wise to ensure a further dose of the induction agent used is available immediately and short acting relaxants and facilities for tracheal intubation should be at hand. Unless surgery demands neuromuscular blockade, the length of operation may dictate whether spontaneous or controlled ventilation is used. It is often useful, even in short procedures, to assist ventilation by gentle squeezing of the reservoir bag when using the LMA in moderately obese patients. This reduces the tendency to atelectasis and the risk of reflux associated with increased negative intrathoracic pressures which may develop if there is any degree of upper respiratory obstruction.

Respiratory disease

The physiological advantages of the LMA for the tracheobronchial tree have already been discussed (see Chapter 3, *Respiratory system*). Despite some initial concerns expressed by Gunawardene, who encountered difficulties with 15 patients with chronic obstructive pulmonary disease (COPD)[9], the LMA is a suitable device for patients with respiratory disease who do not require high airway pressure ventilation provided patients are managed appropriately[10]. Brain has emphasized that it is important to ensure that anesthetic depth is sufficient to prevent triggering of upper airway reflexes[10], which may be more active in these patients[11]. Its use in patients with pulmonary pathology has been widely documented including patients with COPD[9], vocal cord[12], tracheal[13], carinal[14], bronchial[15–17], mediastinal tumors[18] and Hodgkin's lymphoma[19], pulmonary infection[15–17,19,20], pneumothorax[21], postoperative respiratory failure[22,23], asthma[24], bronchopulmonary dysplasia[25,26], inhaled foreign body[20], tracheal stenosis[27,28], lung transplantation[19] and neonatal respiratory distress syndrome[29].

Langenstein et al reported use of the LMA in 100 patients with severe asthma undergoing eye surgery and suggested that the device produces less bronchial activity than the tracheal tube[30]. Buzzetti et al showed that patients with respiratory failure returned to their previous respiratory condition within 1 h of fiberoptic bronchoscopy via the LMA[19]. The LMA has also been used in the management of two patients, one with a preoperative pneumothorax from a central line undergoing total abdominal hysterectomy (lasting over 5 h) and the other at risk of a pneumothorax from a large bulla undergoing repair of clavicle[21]. Both cases were managed with a balanced regional technique with the patients breathing spontaneously and thus thoracentesis was avoided. There is some evidence from children with bronchopulmonary dysplasia that the LMA may be superior to the tracheal tube in terms of recovery characteristics[26]. The LMA is not suitable in patients with acute asthma although it has been used to facilitate weaning of an asthmatic in the ICU[24] (see Chapter 15, *Intensive care*).

Oropharyngeal pathology

The LMA is relatively contraindicated in patients with oropharyngeal pathology and should only be used after careful consideration of the extent of the pathology and the relative risk/benefit compared with other airway options. Any pathology lying along the path followed by the LMA might impede placement or be exacerbated during the attempt. Insertion may be difficult in patients with limited mouth opening since the finger cannot be placed on the hard palate, making adherence to the standard technique impossible. However, provided the mask is pushed through the gap tilted cranially it will be forced up against the hard palate and successful placement may be possible even with mouth opening of <1 cm. Successful insertion in a patient with mouth opening of 12 mm has been reported[31]. In this respect an 'underslung jaw' actually favors correct placement. In patients with restricted incisal opening, an alternative method is to pass the LMA as far as possible between the teeth and then slide it laterally until it can be passed behind the molar teeth into the pharynx. Once the mask is within the mouth, the tube can be slid back into the midline and the device fed into place by pushing the tube cranially. Pathology of the palate or oropharynx, such as tonsillar hypertrophy[32] or a high arched palate[33], will similarly interfere with placement, as can laryngopharyngeal pathology. Because the LMA follows a posterior path, tongue lesions tend not to interfere with placement[34,35]. Brimacombe reported functional failure in two patients each with an enlarged epiglottides[36]. Evans reported failed placement secondary to impaction with an asymptomatic anterior epiglottic cyst[37]. Aziz et al reported failure secondary to large cervical osteophytes which produced a posterior pharyngeal swelling (Forestier's disease)[38]. Where oropharyngeal pathology does not prevent successful placement or function the LMA may be a reasonable airway option, particularly when used awake or for airway rescue. It may be more appropriate to use alternative insertion techniques depending on the nature of the pathology, e.g. it has been suggested that use of a laryngoscope is suitable for patients with gross tonsillar hypertrophy[32]. The LMA has been successfully used for airway rescue in patients with quinsy[39], Ludwig's angina[40] and a thyroglossal tumor[41].

Laryngotracheal pathology

The LMA has been used both electively and for airway rescue in patients with laryngotracheal pathology. In this situation, placement is not generally impaired, but function may be impeded depending on the type/extent of the pathology and the degree of additional airway distortion produced by the inflated LMA cuff. Unlike the tracheal tube, the LMA cannot bypass laryngotracheal pathology, but it does allow the vocal cords and tracheobronchial tree to be observed fiberoptically whilst the patient is ventilated and with minimal interference in the pathological process. Thus the LMA has a role in both diagnosis and management. In this regard, it has been used in the assessment and management of stridor[42,43], in infants with airway problems in whom conventional laryngoscopy/bronchoscopy failed to provide an adequate diagnosis[44], and in children with laryngomalacia/tracheobronchomalacia[45,46]. In this latter situation, the LMA may not be the first choice for airway management since it cannot prevent collapse of the airways[47–49]. The LMA may be more useful for rigid infraglottic pathology and has been used for elective surgery in a child[27] and adult[28,50] with tracheal stenosis. In these cases minimal interference with airflow and lack of further tracheal damage is essential. However, Kokkinis and Papageorgiou reported failure of the LMA in two patients with tracheal stenosis following respiratory arrest where tracheal intubation had failed[51]. The

LMA has been used successfully following failed intubation in patients with laryngeal polyposis[40,52]. Samet et al have reported the successful passage of a rigid bronchoscope via the LMA to view the glottis and larynx of a neonate with stridor[53]. The LMA has been used to maintain the airway whilst a tracheal tumor was resected using a fiber-optic guided laser (D. Ferson, personal communication, 1996).

Non-fasted patients

The role of the LMA in non-fasted patients is primarily as a backup when other forms of airway management have failed and has been widely reported (see Chapter 14, *Unpredicted difficult airway*). Interestingly, there have been no documented cases of aspiration occurring in this situation. The extent to which the application of cricoid pressure has prevented this is unknown. The LMA has also been used electively in non-fasted patients. Asai has reported the use of the LMA as an aid to awake intubation and for rapid sequence induction in non-fasted patients[54]. Brimacombe and Berry have pointed out that insertion of the LMA in the awake patient with a full stomach could be a potent stimulus for vomiting, placing the topicalized patient at risk of aspiration. The risk/benefits of this technique mean that it should perhaps be confined to patients with anticipated intubation difficulty[55,56]. The planned use of the LMA for acute appendicitis has been reported[57,58], but is not recommended[59].

Burns patients

The LMA has been used for dressing changes in patients with facial burns or where contractures have led to difficulty in airway management[60–62]. Praskiko and Shrestha reported its use in 22 children undergoing reconstructive surgery, including two who were known impossible intubations[63]. The LMA is also more suitable than the tracheal tube for repeat anesthesia and avoidance of suxamethonium is a further advantage where burns are extensive since hyperkalemia is avoided.

References

1 Metabolic and nutritional disorders. In: Stoelting RK, Dierdorf SF, eds. *Anesthesia and co-existing disease*. New York: Churchill Livingstone, 1993;375–392.

2 Rocke DA, Murray WB, Rout CC, Gouws E. Relative risk analysis of factors associated with difficult intubation in obstetric anesthesia. *Anesthesiology* 1992;77:67–73.

3 Illing L, Duncan PG, Yip R. Gastro-oesophageal reflux during anaesthesia. *Can J Anaesth* 1992;**39**:466–470.

4 Hardy JF, Lepage Y, Bonneville Chouinard N. Occurrence of gastroesophageal reflux on induction of anaesthesia does not correlate with the volume of gastric contents. *Can J Anaesth* 1990;**37**:502–508.

★ 5 Godley M, Ramachandra AR. Use of LMA for awake intubation for Caesarean section. *Can J Anaesth* 1996;**43**:299–302.
Case report where LMA used as an airway intubator in an awake grossly obese obstetric patient.

6 Brain AIJ. *The Intavent laryngeal mask – instruction manual.* London: Intavent, 1991;1–58.

★ 7 Verghese C, Smith TGC, Young E. Prospective survey of the use of the laryngeal mask airway in 2359 patients. *Anaesthesia* 1993;**48**:58–60.
Large survey of LMA practice including its use in obese patients.

★ 8 Brimacombe J. Positive pressure ventilation with the size 5 LMA. *J Clin Anesth* (in press).
Prospective study of 179 patients managed with the size 5 LMA. Included 52 obese patients (body mass index 30–50) and the incidence of problems was similar to acceptable weight and overweight patients (body mass index 25–30).

9 Gunawardene RD. Laryngeal mask and patients with chronic respiratory disease. *Anaesthesia* 1989;**44**:531.

10 Brain AIJ. The laryngeal mask in patients with chronic respiratory disease. *Anaesthesia* 1989;**44**:790–791.

11 Stoelting RK, Dierdorf SF, McCammon RL. Obstructive airways disease. In: *Anesthesia and co-existing disease*. New York: Churchill Livingstone, 1988;195–226.

12 Brimacombe J, Sher M, Laing D, Berry A. The laryngeal mask airway: a new technique for fiberoptic guided vocal cord biopsy. *J Clin Anesth* 1996;**8**:273–275.

13 Divatia JV, Sareen R, Upadhye SM, Sharma KS, Shelgaonkar JR. Anaesthetic management of tracheal surgery using the laryngeal mask airway. *Anaesth Intens Care* 1994;**22**:69–73.

14 Slinger P, Robinson R, Shennib H, Benumof JL, Eisenkraft JB. Alternative technique for laser resection of a carinal obstruction. *J Cardiothoracic Anesth* 1992;**6**:749–755.

15 Brimacombe J, Newell S, Swainston R, Thompson J. A potential new technique for awake fibreoptic bronchoscopy – use of the laryngeal mask airway. *Med J Aust* 1992;**156**:876–877.

16 Du Plessis MC, Marshall Barr A, Verghese C, Lyall JRW. Fibreoptic bronchoscopy under general anaesthesia using the laryngeal mask airway. *Eur J Anaesthesiol* 1993;**10**:363–365.

17 Brimacombe J, Tucker P, Simons S. The laryngeal mask airway for awake diagnostic bronchoscopy – a study of 200 consecutive patients. *Eur J Anaesthesiol* 1995;**12**:357–361.

18 Polaner DM. The use of heliox and the laryngeal mask airway in a child with an anterior mediastinal mass. *Anesth Analg* 1996;**82**:208–210.

19 Buzzetti V, Cigada M, Solca M, Iapichino G. Use of the laryngeal mask airway during fibreoptic bronchoscopy. *Intens Care World* 1996;**13**:72–74.

20 Bautista Casasnovas A, Estevez Martinez E, Buznego Sanchez R, Rodriguez Perez E, Cabanas Gancedo R, Varela Cives R. [Pediatric fiber bronchoscopy. A propos 55 children examined]. *An Esp Pediatr* 1993;**39**:313–316.

21 Yamauchi M. Use of the LM in patients with pneumothorax. *J Clin Anesth (Rinsho-Masui)* 1993;**17**:239–240.

22 Arosio EM, Conci F. Use of the laryngeal mask airway for respiratory distress in the intensive care unit. *Anaesthesia* 1995;**50**:635–636.

23 Aoyagi M. Application of the laryngeal mask airway in ICU. *40th Meeting of the Japanese Society of Anesthesiology, Iwate Prefectual Hall, Japan, 22 April 1993,* pp.6–7 (Abstract).

24 Taylor JC, Bell GT. An asthmatic weaned from a ventilator using a laryngeal mask. *Anaesthesia* 1995;**50**:454–455.

25 Lonnqvist PA. Successful use of laryngeal mask airway in low-weight expremature infants with bronchopulmonary dysplasia undergoing crotherapy for retinopathy of the premature. *Anesthesiology* 1995;**83**:422–424.

★ 26 Ferrari LR, Goudsouzian NG. The use of the laryngeal mask airway in children with bronchopulmonary dysplasia. *Anesth Analg* 1995;**81**:310–313.
Study of 27 former premature infants with bronchopulmonary dysplasia undergoing general anesthesia for open eye vitrectomy with either the tracheal tube or LMA. The incidence of postoperative complications was lower in the LMA group and patients were discharged earlier. Shows the value of the LMA in patients with mild chronic respiratory disease.

27 Asai T, Fujise K, Uchida M. Use of the laryngeal mask in a child with tracheal stenosis. *Anesthesiology* 1991;**75**:903–904.

28 Asai T, Fujise K, Uchida M. Laryngeal mask and tracheal stenosis. *Anaesthesia* 1993;**48**:81.

29 Albertsen P, Eschen C, Verder H. Laryngeal mask used as a guideway for brief access to the intratracheal space in premature infants. *8th International Workshop on Surfactant Replacement, Oslo, 20–22 May 1993* (Abstract).

30 Langenstein H, Moller F, Krause R, Kluge R, Vogelsang H. Die Handhabung der Larynxmaske bei Augenoperationen. *Congress on Anaesthesia in Eye Surgery, Congress-Centrum Stadtpark, Hannover, 10–11 May 1996* (Abstract).

31 Maltby JR, Loken RG, Beriault MT, Archer DP. Laryngeal mask airway with mouth opening less than 20 mm. *Can J Anaesth* 1995;**42**:1140–1142.

32 van Heerden PV, Kirrage D. Large tonsils and the laryngeal mask airway. *Anaesthesia* 1989;**44**:703.

33 Collier C. A hazard with the laryngeal mask airway. *Anaesth Intens Care* 1991;**19**:301.

34 Kadota Y, Oda T, Yoshimura N. Application of a laryngeal mask to a fiberoptic bronchoscope-aided tracheal intubation. *J Clin Anesth* 1992;**4**:503–504.

35 Brimacombe J, Berry A. Mallampati grade and laryngeal mask placement. *Anesth Analg* 1996;**82**:1112–1113.

36 Brimacombe J. Analysis of 1500 laryngeal mask uses by one anaesthetist in adults undergoing routine anaesthesia. *Anaesthesia* 1996;**51**:76–80.

37 Evans A. Difficulty in inserting a laryngeal mask airway. *Anaesthesia* 1995;**50**:468–469.

38 Aziz ES, Thompson AR, Baer S. Difficult laryngeal mask insertion in a patient with Forestier's disease. *Anaesthesia* 1995;**50**:370.

39 Brimacombe J, Berry A, van Duren P. Use of a size 2 laryngeal mask airway to relieve life threatening hypoxia in an adult with quinsy. *Anaesth Intens Care* 1993;**21**:475–476.

40 King CJ, Davey AJ, Chandradeva K. Emergency use of the laryngeal mask airway in severe upper airway obstruction caused by supraglottic oedema. *Br J Anaesth* 1995;**75**:785–786.

41 Dalrymple G, Lloyd E. Laryngeal mask: a more secure airway than intubation? *Anaesthesia* 1992;**47**:712–713.

42 McNamee CJ, Meyns B, Pagliero KM. Flexible bronchoscopy via the laryngeal mask: a new technique. *Thorax* 1991;**46**:141–142.

43 Brimacombe J. The laryngeal mask airway – use in the management of stridor. *Anaesth Intens Care* 1992;**20**:117–118.

44 Maroof M, Khan RM, Cooper T, Siddique MS, Saqib N. Post thyroidectomy vocal cord examination using LMA aided fiberoscopy. *Anesthesiology* 1993;**79**:A1083 (Abstract).

45 Smith TGC, Whittet H, Heyworth T. Laryngomalacia – a specific indication for the laryngeal mask. *Anaesthesia* 1992;**47**:910.

46 Lawson R, Lloyd-Thomas AR. Three diagnostic conundrums solved using the laryngeal mask airway. *Anaesthesia* 1993;**48**:790–791.

47 Brimacombe J, Berry A, Wilson IG. Use of the laryngeal mask airway in children with laryngotracheal pathology. *Br J Anaesth* 1993;**71**:172–173.

48 Wilson IG. The laryngeal mask airway in paediatric practice. *Br J Anaesth* 1993;**70**:124–125.

49 Asai T, Morris S. The laryngeal mask and patients with 'collapsible' airways. *Anaesthesia* 1994;**49**:169–170.

50 Greatorex RA, Denny NM. Application of the laryngeal mask airway to thyroid surgery and the preservation of the recurrent laryngeal nerve. *Ann Roy Coll Surg Engl* 1991;**73**:352–354.

51 Kokkinis K, Papageorgiou E. Failure of the laryngeal mask airway (LMA) to ventilate patients with severe tracheal stenosis. *Resuscitation* 1995;**30**:21–22.

52 Pennant JH, Gajraj NM, Yamanouchi KJ. The laryngeal mask airway and laryngeal polyposis. *Anesthesiology* 1994;**78**:1206–1207.

53 Samet A, Talmon Y, Frankel R, Simon K. A new diagnostic approach to congenital stridor using a laryngeal mask airway and rigid endoscope. *J Laryngol Otol* 1994;**108**:1076–1077.

54 Asai T. Use of the laryngeal mask for tracheal intubation in patients at increased risk of aspiration of gastric contents. *Anesthesiology* 1992;**77**:1029–1030.

55 Benumof JL. Laryngeal mask airway – indications and contraindications. *Anesthesiology* 1992;**77**:843–846.

56 Brimacombe J, Berry A, Asai T. The use of the laryngeal mask airway as an aid to intubation in patients at risk of aspiration. *Anesthesiology* 1993;**78**:1197–1198.

57 Banos G, Cortes J, Vidal MI, Alvarez J. Experiencia de 100 pacientes anestesiados ventilados con mascarilla laringea. *Rev Esp Anestesiol Reanim* 1992;**39**:246–249.

58 Cristalli A, Rezzani S. La maschera laringea in chirurgia generale. *Minerva Anestesiol* 1995;**61**:23–27.

59 Brimacombe J, Berry A, Spong L. Esta indicada la mascarilla laringea en la cirugia abdominal baja? *Rev Esp Anestesiol Reanim* (in press).

60 Russell R, Judkins KC. The laryngeal mask airway and facial burns. *Anaesthesia* 1990;**45**:894.

61 Thomson KD, Ordman AJ, Parkhouse N, Morgan BD. Use of the Brain laryngeal mask airway in anticipation of difficult tracheal intubation. *Br J Plast Surg* 1989;**42**:478–480.

62 Shrestha BM, Basnyat NB. Experience with the laryngeal mask airway in Nepal. *Today's Anaesthetist* 1993;**8**:133–134.

63 Prasiko D, Shrestha BM. Laryngeal mask airway in pediatric burn contractures in Nepal. *11th World Congress of Anesthesiology, Sydney, 14–20 April 1996, Abstract Handbook* p.119 (Abstract).

12 Advanced uses: techniques

Endoscopy

The LMA lies at the crossroads of the gastrointestinal and respiratory tracts, facing into, but not penetrating, their respective sphincters. Both sphincters – the glottic and the upper esophageal – can be bypassed using the LMA as a guide.

Respiratory tract

Instruments passed through the tube of the LMA are guided towards the trachea and in this respect the LMA has been used for laryngobronchoscopy[1–3], respiratory tract surgery[4–6] and the management of the difficult airway[7]. Fiberoptic intubation is generally quicker and more effective with the LMA than with other airway intubators. Hagberg et al have shown that when compared with the Ovassapian airway[8], the LMA was a more successful aid to fiberoptic intubation in both awake and anesthetized patients[9]. Darling et al showed that the split LMA was superior to the Berman II airway intubator[10]. Murray and Renfrew have shown that pulmonary ventilation is more effective during fiberoptic intubation with the split LMA than with the Berman II airway[11]. Maroof showed that both experienced and inexperienced fiberoptic bronchoscopists could rapidly locate the laryngeal inlet using the split LMA[12]. The time taken to locate the laryngeal inlet using a fiberoptic scope passed through the LMA or William's airway intubator was similar[13]. The LMA can accommodate a larger fiberoptic scope (FOS) than the corresponding sizes of FLMA or tracheal tube. Brimacombe and Dunbar-Reid have shown that the mean flow resistance was 2.3 times higher with the FLMA compared with the LMA, 2.1 times higher with the tracheal tube compared with the LMA, and 1.2 times lower with the tracheal tube compared with the FLMA[14]. There are numerous advanced endoscopic techniques used to facilitate intubation via the LMA. These are discussed in Chapter 14.

Gastrointestinal tract

Instruments passed behind the LMA tend to pass posterior to the mask and into the upper gastrointestinal tract. The LMA synchronously shields the glottis from impaction with instruments passed behind the cuff. Most gastrointestinal endoscopic procedures are performed with sedation and topical spray, usually avoiding the need for airway support; in others there is an aspiration risk (for example endoscopy for hematemesis) and in such cases the LMA is contraindicated. In patients considered to be at low risk of aspiration the LMA could be utilized either as part of a sedation/ local anesthetic technique or under general anesthesia. Brimacombe has reported use of the LMA as a guide to the gastrointestinal tract in an awake and an anesthetized patient for placement of a gastroscope and nasogastric tube where conventional methods had failed[15]. Gajraj has reported its use in children undergoing esophagogastroduodenoscopy under general anesthesia[16]. Jeong et al reported a case of difficult passage of a nasogastric tube with the LMA in situ – the reasons for this difficulty were unclear[17].

Prolonged use

Prolonged anesthesia is commonly regarded as an indication for tracheal intubation and pulmonary ventilation[18,19], although this is theoretical. The reasons given are that intubation secures the airway and ventilation prevents respiratory fatigue and failure. Intubation and ventilation, however, carry with them a significant morbidity[20-22] and could perhaps be avoided in many circumstances. The feasibility of prolonged spontaneous ventilation anesthesia has increased recently as a result of improvements in clinical monitoring. Respiratory failure and fatigue can be detected and appropriate measures taken[23]. As a result of these advances, intubation may only be indicated to obtain a secure airway rather than to facilitate ventilation.

The LMA may further facilitate prolonged spontaneous ventilation anesthesia because it provides an effortless clear airway whilst avoiding the hazards of intubation and the use of muscle relaxants[24]. Also, when used as part of a balanced regional technique, the LMA will permit a lighter plane of general anesthesia than the tracheal tube, hence reducing exposure to the volatile agent[25]. In addition, it has been suggested that the LMA may be better than a tracheal tube regarding lung function since it allows more normal physiology to be maintained[24,26,27].

There are three issues to consider with respect to the use of the LMA during prolonged anesthesia with spontaneous ventilation: (1) is respiratory function impaired in the perioperative period? (2) does the LMA damage the pharynx when in situ for prolonged periods? and (3) do the risks of aspiration in ‘fasting’ patients increase during prolonged anesthesia with the LMA? Some limited data is available which addresses these questions.

1. Brimacombe and Shorney reported use of the LMA for 8 h in a young healthy patient using a spontaneous ventilation/epidural technique and found no demonstrable deterioration in respiratory function or evidence of respiratory fatigue either during or after the procedure[28] as measured by arterial blood gases, spirometry, and continuous respiratory pattern analysis using an extensometer or 'rubbery ruler'[29–31]. This work has been repeated in a further four patients with similar results[32].
2. Miura et al[33] and Brimacombe and Berry[34] reported that there was no increase in the incidence of sore throat following procedures lasting 1–2 h. Hamakawa, however, has suggested that there may be an increased incidence of sore throats for procedures over 3 h[35], but there is no evidence that the LMA damages the pharynx over periods of up to 24 h. Operations of more than 6 h duration have resulted in no adverse pharyngeal sequelae[28,32,36–39]. In addition, several authors have incidentally noted the use of the LMA for between 3 and 5 h and did not report any associated problems[27,40–45]. The LMA has been used in the ICU to provide respiratory support for 10–24 h with no apparent problems[46,47]. However, a small area of pharyngeal necrosis was noted when the semi-inflated LMA was left in situ for 8 days in the ICU (L Costa e Silva, personal communication, 1996).
3. Procedures lasting over 2 h are associated with a higher incidence of regurgitation than shorter procedures[48] in intubated ventilated patients, and gastric volume increases during surgery[49]. The risk of aspiration in prolonged peripheral or superficial surgery with either PPV or spontaneous ventilation (SV) has not been quantified. One patient aspirated 2 h into elective surgery with the LMA when anesthesia was too light[50]. A further patient who was not fasted aspirated after 1.5 h[51]. There have been no other reports linking regurgitation and aspiration with prolonged use.

Although there is little evidence that there is a significant problem with tracheal intubation for prolonged periods in healthy adult patients, the LMA may offer some modest advantages in terms of anesthetic depth and minor morbidity. These advantages must be weighed against any potential increased risk of aspiration associated with the LMA in 'fasting' patients. The maximum duration for which the LMA can be safely used is not yet known, but a limit of 2 h has been suggested based on the possible increased risk of aspiration and pharyngeal morbidity[52]. Asai considers it prudent not to use the LMA for prolonged procedures until controlled studies show that it is safe[52]. Brimacombe and co-workers suggest that this is a suitable technique in 'fasting' healthy patients undergoing surgery to the extremities[28,32]. Its use in older patients or those with moderate systemic or respiratory disease is unclear. Nishida reported airway obstruction and facial edema during a 4 h LMA anesthetic in a 3-year-old which rapidly resolved when the LMA was removed[53]. It was postulated that this was due to venous congestion. Further controlled comparative studies are required before any substantial conclusions can be drawn.

In summary, there is increasing evidence that the LMA may be safe for planned procedures in ASA 1–2 patients lasting 4–8 h in the hands of experienced LMA users[28,32,54–57] and possibly longer[46,47]. It would seem a particularly reasonable option when used as part of a balanced regional technique. The risk/benefit ratio of spontaneous versus controlled ventilation has not yet been determined. Use of the LMA for prolonged procedures should not be undertaken by inexperienced LMA users. If the LMA is used for prolonged periods, respiratory function must be closely monitored and any problems associated with its use should be reported. Cuff pressure control and monitoring, and frequent fiberoptic assessment of position should be performed. Anesthetic depth must be sufficient to prevent recurrent swallowing and regurgitation[36].

Non-supine position

Use of the LMA in the lithotomy, jack-knife, Trendelenburg and prone positions should be considered advanced techniques. The safety of the LMA in these positions has not been demonstrated in large controlled trials, although it can be inferred from several large studies[55,58–60]. The LMA would appear to be safe for use in the lateral position[61]. However, when moving patients from the supine to lateral position, adequate anesthetic depth must be maintained. Minor gynecological procedures such as D&C and cervical diathermy are routinely carried out with the face mask and the LMA would seem to be a reasonable alternative once some experience has been gained in the supine position.

In the lithotomy and Trendelenburg positions there is a theoretical increased risk of regurgitation, but this is unsubstantiated. El Mikatti et al studied 90 patients managed with the LMA and found that regurgitation of dye occurred in 1/30 patients in the Trendelenberg position and 1/30 in the lithotomy position compared with 0/30 in the supine position[62]. The safety of the LMA in the lithotomy position plus Trendelenburg tilt and intra-abdominal insufflation is less clear, but studies assessing its use for gynecological laparoscopy indicated that it may be safe if intra-abdominal pressures are kept below 25 cm H_2O and tilt <15 degrees[63,64] (see Chapter 13, *Gynecological laparoscopy*). Use of the LMA in the prone position is similarly controversial[65,66] but has been widely reported[58–60,67–73], including in spinal surgery[74]. The prone position may be associated with an increased risk of regurgitation, but not necessarily aspiration[48,75] since the regurgitated fluid will readily flow out of the LMA tube. Milligan has reported its safe use in 300 prone patients[60]. Herrick and Kennedy, however, reported a 3.5% (11/313) incidence of airway obstruction in children managed with the standard LMA in the prone position[58]. This was easily corrected and may have been related to kinking. One possible advantage of the LMA is that patients may position themselves in the prone position preinduction and the LMA inserted with the head to the side[73]. This may reduce the incidence of back problems during repositioning under anesthesia.

Awake insertion

Insertion of the LMA under topical anesthesia has been widely reported[1,3,39,40,76–86]. It has the advantage of there being ‘no bridges burnt’ when used in the anticipated difficult airway. Topicalization is required to obtund upper airway reflexes and sedation may be necessary in some patients. Topicalization may be achieved as for awake tracheal intubation[87], but preparation of the nose is not required. Superior laryngeal nerve block[88] and injection of local anesthesia via a cricothyroid puncture[1,3] may occasionally be useful adjuncts to awake insertion, but are rarely required. Even when topicalization is adequate, passage and inflation of the LMA into the hypopharynx may be uncomfortable, like swallowing an oversized food bolus, but once in position it is generally well tolerated[1,89]. It has been suggested that LMA insertion may be aided by active swallowing and by partial inflation of the cuff; the dynamics of insertion in the awake patient may differ from those under anesthesia. It is likely that lower cuff volumes will be required in awake patients due to the increased pharyngeal tone. In a prospective study of 50 patients undergoing awake diagnostic bronchoscopy, LMA insertion was achieved with topical anesthesia and sedation in all patients within three attempts (72% at first attempt)[1]. A direct view of the cords was achieved in 92% and all bronchoscopies were successfully performed. A larger follow-up study showed that the technique was successful in 199/200 patients. Reported complications included gagging (16%), coughing (10–12%), excessive salivation (6%) and recurrent swallowing (13–18%)[1,3,83]. These problems were surmounted with further topical anesthesia or sedation. Gagging and coughing may predispose to regurgitation, particularly in the sedated patient. This may not be a problem in the fasted patient, but may compromise the technique in the non-fasted patient[90]. Superior laryngeal nerve blocks have been used to aid insertion in awake and anesthetized patients[88]. There have been no comparative studies of the awake LMA technique with awake intubation or awake nasal fiberoptic diagnostic bronchoscopy. Further work is required to determine the best technique for LMA insertion in the awake patient.

The 'awake' technique has been used in infants with difficult airways[91-93], for neonatal resuscitation[94,95] and drug administration[96]. In neonatal resuscitation, reflexes are weak or absent before respiration is established, so in this situation LMA insertion is easily accomplished without topicalization. The success rate of placement and the incidence of complications in awake children are unknown. Awake insertion of the FLMA has been reported by Maltby et al in a patient with mouth opening of 18 mm[39].

Drug dispersal

The LMA has been used to administer nebulized salbutamol during anesthesia in a patient with acute bronchospasm[97]. Albertsen et al inserted the size 1 LMA in six premature babies with respiratory distress syndrome and passed a thin catheter via the LMA into the trachea[96]. After administration of surfactant, the catheter was withdrawn and the baby briefly ventilated through the LMA for improved drug dispersal. The advantage of the technique was that it allowed minimal handling of the babies while avoiding repeat tracheal intubation. Alexander and Smith investigated the possibility of blindly passing a preformed cannula into the trachea via the LMA for the purposes of drug administration during cardiopulmonary resuscitation (CPR) and found the success rate to be only 18% despite good positioning of the LMA[98].

Tracheal tube/LMA exchange

Coughing and gagging on the tracheal tube at the end of the anesthetic may result in acute hemodynamic changes, elevation of intracranial and intraocular pressure, and hypoxia. This may be particularly undesirable in patients with cardiorespiratory disease or in those undergoing intracranial, intraocular or major head and neck surgery. To date, the only approaches to the avoidance of such coughing are the use of opioids and tracheal extubation with the patient deeply anesthetized. There are problems with both and some authors consider that exchanging the tracheal tube for the LMA offers a possible solution[99]. The main benefit of such an exchange is that it facilitates a smooth emergence from anesthesia and allows the vocal cords to be observed. Airway exchange must take place while the patient is either anesthetized or paralyzed and is not recommended if the patient is at risk of aspiration. Should placement of the LMA fail the trachea may be re-intubated. Surgical procedures where a smooth emergence are important include: open eye surgery, head and neck surgery, neurosurgery, suspension laryngoscopy[100] and in patients with cardiorespiratory disease[100,101]. Observation of the vocal cords may be of assistance following thyroid surgery[102–105] or vocal cord biopsy[106]. Data from three small series suggests that the tracheal tube/LMA exchange may be suitable for selected otoneurosurgical[101], neurosurgical[99] and carotid endarterectomy[107] patients.

Elective exchange of an adequately functioning LMA for a tracheal tube may be required intraoperatively if contraindications for LMA usage develop such as a change in aspiration risk, e.g. conversion from diagnostic laparoscopy to laparotomy, or increased ventilatory requirements. Intubation may be conducted via the LMA or following removal. Unplanned anesthesia lasting more than 2 h is probably not an indication for LMA/tracheal tube exchange[32]. Indeed, the process of exchanging airway devices may itself increase the risk of regurgitation.

References

1 Brimacombe J, Newell S, Swainston R, Thompson J. A potential new technique for awake fibreoptic bronchoscopy – use of the laryngeal mask airway. *Med J Aust* 1992;**156**:876–877.

★ 2 Du Plessis MC, Marshall Barr A, Verghese C, Lyall JRW. Fibreoptic bronchoscopy under general anaesthesia using the laryngeal mask airway. *Eur J Anaesthesiol* 1993;**10**:363–365.
Prospective study of 140 patients undergoing diagnostic bronchoscopy via the LMA under general anesthesia. The technique was successful in 139 and there were no major complications.

★ 3 Brimacombe J, Tucker P, Simons S. The laryngeal mask airway for awake diagnostic bronchoscopy – a study of 200 consecutive patients. *Eur J Anaesthesiol* 1995;**12**:357–361.
Retrospective study of 200 patients undergoing diagnostic bronchoscopy via the LMA under topical anesthesia and sedation. The technique was successful in 199 patients and complication rates were similar to those reported for transnasal awake bronchoscopy with no fatalities directly attributable to the LMA technique and a 3% incidence of major perioperative complications.

4 Slinger P, Robinson R, Shennib H, Benumof JL, Eisenkraft JB. Alternative technique for laser resection of a carinal obstruction. *J Cardiothoracic Anesth* 1992;**6**:749–755.

5 Divatia JV, Sareen R, Upadhye SM, Sharma KS, Shelgaonkar JR. Anaesthetic management of tracheal surgery using the laryngeal mask airway. *Anaesth Intens Care* 1994;**22**:69–73.

6 Sher M, Brimacombe J, Laing D. Anaesthesia for laser pharyngoplasty – a comparison of the tracheal tube versus reinforced laryngeal mask airway. *Anaesth Intens Care* 1995;**23**:149–154.

7 Brimacombe J, Berry A, Brain A. The laryngeal mask airway. In: Sandler AN, Doyle DJ, eds. *The difficult airway I.* Philadelphia: WB Saunders, 1995;411–437.

8 Ovassapian A, Mesnick PS. The art of fiberoptic intubation. In: Sandler AN, Doyle DJ, eds. *The difficult airway I.* Philadelphia: WB Saunders, 1995;391–409.

9 Hagberg C, Abramson D, Chelly J. A comparison of fiberoptic orotracheal intubation using two different intubating conduits. *Anesthesiology* 1995;**83**:A1220 (Abstract).

10 Darling JR, Keohane M, Murray JM. A split laryngeal mask as an aid to training in fibreoptic tracheal intubation. A comparison with the Berman II intubating airway. *Anaesthesia* 1993;**48**:1079–1082.

11 Murray JM, Renfrew CW. Arterial carbon dioxide tensions during fiberoptic tracheal intubation: a comparison of the split laryngeal mask with the Berman II airway. *Anesth Analg* 1995;**81**:1311–1312.

12 Maroof M, Khan RM, Khan H, Stewart J, Mroze C. Evaluation of a modified laryngeal mask airway as an aid to fibre optic intubation (FOI). *Anesthesiology* 1992;77:A1062 (Abstract).

13 Crichlow A, Locken R, Todesco J. The laryngeal mask airway and fibreoptic laryngoscopy. *Can J Anaesth* 1992;**39**:742–743.

★ **14** Brimacombe J, Dunbar-Reid K. The effect of introducing fibreoptic bronchoscopes on gas flow in laryngeal masks and tracheal tubes. *Anaesthesia* 1996;**51**:923–928.
Laboratory study assessing the effect of different size of fiberoptic scopes of gas flow. This study shows that flow is better with the LMA than with either the tracheal tube or flexible LMA.

★ **15** Brimacombe J. The laryngeal mask airway for access to the upper gastrointestinal tract. *Anesthesiology* 1996;**84**:1009–1010.
Two case reports of LMA usage for access to the upper gastrointestinal tract, firstly as an aid to awake gastroscopy and secondly to facilitate placement of a nasogastric tube during anesthesia.

16 Gajraj NM. Use of the laryngeal mask airway during oesophago-gastro-duodenoscopy. *Anaesthesia* 1996;**51**:991.

17 Jeong J, Yang H, Cho H. Clinical investigation of laryngeal mask airway. *J Kor Soc Anesthesiol* 1993;**25**:708–718.

18 Fell D. The practical conduct of anaesthesia. In: Aitkinhead AR, Smith G, eds. *Textbook of anaesthesia*. Edinburgh: Churchill Livingstone, 1990;349–362.

19 Nagi H, Brimacombe J. LMA and swallowing. *Anaesth Intens Care* 1992;**20**:116–117.

20 Harmer M. Complications of tracheal intubation. In: Latto IP, Rosen M, eds. *Difficulties in tracheal intubation.* London: Baillière Tindall, 1987;36–48.

21 Mushin WW, Rendell-Baker L, Thompson PW, Mapleson WW (eds) Physiological aspects. In *Automatic ventilation of the lungs*. Oxford: Blackwell Scientific, 1980;1–32.

22 Ng WS. Pathophysiological effects of tracheal intubation. In: Latto IP, Rosen M, eds. *Difficulties in tracheal intubation.* London: Baillière Tindall, 1984;12–35.

23 Sackner M, Krieger B. Non-invasive respiratory monitoring. In: Scharf SM, Cassidy S, eds. *Heart and lung interactions in health and disease.* New York: Marcel Dekker, 1989;663–805.

24 White DC. The laryngeal mask – a non-invasive airway. *Eur J Anaesthesiol* 1991;**4**:1–4.

25 Wilkins CJ, Cramp PG, Staples J, Stevens WC. Comparison of the anesthetic requirement for tolerance of laryngeal mask airway and endotracheal tube. *Anesth Analg* 1992;**75**:794–797.

26 Leach AB, Alexander CA. The laryngeal mask – an overview. *Eur J Anaesthesiol* 1991;**4**:19–31.

27 Brain AIJ. The development of the laryngeal mask – a brief history of the invention, early clinical studies and experimental work from which the laryngeal mask evolved. *Eur J Anaesthesiol* 1991;**4**:5–17.

★ **28** Brimacombe J, Shorney N. The laryngeal mask airway and prolonged balanced anaesthesia. *Can J Anaesth* 1993;**40**:360–364.
Case report of an 8 h procedure in a young healthy patient using a spontaneous ventilation/epidural technique. There was no demonstrable deterioration in respiratory function or evidence of respiratory fatigue either during or after the procedure, and no sore throat.

29 Brimacombe J. Noninvasive monitoring of tidal volume with an extensometer: laboratory and clinical studies. *Anaesth Intens Care* 1993;**21**:62–66.

30 Brimacombe J, Macfie A, Masters A. The extensometer – use in spontaneously ventilating awake volunteers. *Anaesthesia* 1993;**47**:871–877.

31 Brimacombe J, Macfie A, McCrirrick A. The extensometer – potential application in anaesthesia and intensive care. *Anaesthesia* 1991;**46**:756–761.

32 Brimacombe J, Archdeacon J. The laryngeal mask airway for unplanned prolonged procedures. *Can J Anaesth* 1995;**42**:1176.

33 Miura M. Problems during insertion of the laryngeal mask airway and postoperative pharyngalgia. *40th Meeting of the Japanese Society of Anesthesiology, Iwate Prefectual Hall, Japan, 22 April 1993*, pp.2–3 (Abstract).

34 Brimacombe J, Berry A. Laryngeal mask airway cuff pressure and position during anaesthesia lasting 1–2 hours. *Can J Anaesth* 1994;**41**:589–593.

35 Hamakawa T. Sore throat after the use of the LM. *J Clin Anesth (Rinsho-Masui)* 1993;**17**:245–246.

36 Brimacombe J. Laryngeal mask anaesthesia and recurrent swallowing. *Anaesth Intens Care* 1991;**19**:275–276.

37 Brain AIJ. *The laryngeal mask – instruction manual.* London: Intavent, 1990;1–38.

38 Yamauchi M. Use of the LM in patients with pneumothorax. *J Clin Anesth (Rinsho-Masui)* 1993;**17**:239–240.

38 Maltby JR, Loken RG, Beriault MT, Archer DP. Laryngeal mask airway with mouth opening less than 20 mm. *Can J Anaesth* 1995;**42**:1140–1142.

40 Maltby JR, Loken RG, Watson NC. The laryngeal mask airway: clinical appraisal in 250 patients. *Can J Anaesth* 1990;**37**:509–513.

41 Brain AI, McGhee TD, McAteer EJ, Thomas A, Abu Saad MA, Bushman JA. The laryngeal mask airway. Development and preliminary trials of a new type of airway. *Anaesthesia* 1985;**40**:356–361.

42 Miranda AF, Reddy SVG. Controlled ventilation with Brain laryngeal mask. *Med J Malaysia* 1991;**45**:65–69.
43 Collier C. A hazard with the laryngeal mask airway. *Anaesth Inten Care* 1991;**19**:301.
44 Janssens M, Marechal J. The laryngeal mask – Liege experience. *Acta Anaesthesiol Belg* 1991;**42**:199–206.
45 Costa e Silva L, Brimacombe J. The laryngeal mask airway for stereotactic implantation of fetal hypophysis. *Anesth Analg* 1996;**82**:430–431.
46 Aoyagi M. Application of the laryngeal mask airway in ICU. *40th Meeting of the Japanese Society of Anesthesiology, Iwate Prefectual Hall, Japan, 22 April 1993,* pp.6–7 (Abstract).
47 Arosio EM, Conci F. Use of the laryngeal mask airway for respiratory distress in the intensive care unit. *Anaesthesia* 1995;**50**:635–636.
48 Blitt CD, Gutman HL, Cohen DD, Weisman H, Dillon JB. 'Silent' regurgitation and aspiration during general anaesthesia. *Anesth Analg* 1970;**49**:707–713.
49 Hester AW, Heath ML. Pulmonary acid aspiration syndrome: should prophylaxis be routine? *Br J Anaesth* 1977;**49**:595–599.
50 Maroof M, Khan RM, Siddique MS. Intraoperative aspiration pneumonitis and the laryngeal mask airway. *Anesth Analg* 1993;**77**:409–410.
51 Wilkinson PA, Cyna AM, MacLeod DM, Campbell JR, Criswell J, John R. The laryngeal mask: cautionary tales. *Anaesthesia* 1990;**45**:167–168.
52 Asai T, Morris S. The laryngeal mask airway: its features, effects and role. *Can J Anaesth* 1994;**41**:930–960.
53 Nishida Y. A complication associated with the use of the LM. *J Clin Anesth (Rinsho-Masui)* 1991;**15**:802.
54 Brimacombe J. Analysis of 1500 laryngeal mask uses by one anaesthetist in adults undergoing routine anaesthesia. *Anaesthesia* 1996;**51**:76–80.
55 Verghese C, Brimacombe J. Survey of laryngeal mask usage in 11 910 patients – safety and efficacy for conventional and nonconventional usage. *Anesth Analg* 1996;**82**:129–133.
56 Fujii T, Watanabe S, Taguchi N, Takeshima R. Airway protection by the laryngeal mask during various neck positions and during protracted surgeries: sealing to dye placed in the pharynx. *Anesth Analg* 1996;**82**:S118 (Abstract).
57 Langenstein H, Moller F, Krause R, Kluge R, Vogelsang H. Die Handhabung der Larynxmaske bei Augenoperationen. *Congress on Anaesthesia in Eye Surgery, Congress-Centrum Stadtpark, Hannover, 10–11 May 1996* (Abstract).
58 Herrick MJ, Kennedy DJ. Airway obstruction and the laryngeal mask airway in paediatric radiotherapy. *Anaesthesia* 1992;**47**:910.
59 Verghese C, Smith TGC, Young E. Prospective survey of the use of the laryngeal mask airway in 2359 patients. *Anaesthesia* 1993;**48**:58–60.
60 Milligan KA. Laryngeal mask in the prone position. *Anaesthesia* 1994;**49**:449.
61 Chen CH, Lin CC, Tan PP. [Clinical experience of laryngeal mask airway in lateral position during anesthesia]. *Acta Anaesthesiol Sin* 1995;**33**:31–34.
62 El Mikatti N, Luthra AD, Healy TEJ, Mortimer AJ. Gastric regurgitation during general anaesthesia in different positions with the laryngeal mask airway. *Anaesthesia* 1995;**50**:1053–1055.
63 Goodwin APL, Rowe WL, Ogg TW. Day case laparoscopy – a comparison of two anaesthetic techniques using the laryngeal mask during spontaneous breathing. *Anaesthesia* 1992;**47**:892–895.
64 Swann DG, Spens H, Edwards SA, Chestnut RJ. Anaesthesia for gynaecological laparoscopy – a comparison between the laryngeal mask airway and tracheal intubation. *Anaesthesia* 1993;**48**:431–434.
65 Lim W, Cone AM. Laryngeal mask and the prone position. *Anaesthesia* 1994;**49**:542.
66 Fisher JA, Ananthanarayan C, Edelist G. Role of the laryngeal mask in airway management. *Can J Anaesth* 1992;**39**:1–3.
67 Ngan Kee WD. Laryngeal mask airway for radiotherapy in the prone position. *Anaesthesia* 1992;**47**:446–447.
68 Sidhu VS. The laryngeal mask airway for anaesthesia in the prone position. *Anaesth Intens Care* 1992;**20**:119.
69 Elias M. Laryngeal mask airway and radiotherapy in the prone position. *Anaesthesia* 1992;**47**:1005.
70 Coyne BJ. The use of the laryngeal mask airway in day case and short stay surgery. *Ir J Med Sci* 1990;**159**:185–186.
71 Poltronieri J. [The laryngeal mask]. *Ann Fr Anesth Reanim* 1990;**9**:362–366.
72 Doyle DJ. Clinical applications of the laryngeal mask airway. *Contemporary Anaesth* 1993;**4**:8–15.
73 McCaughey W, Bhanumurthy S. Laryngeal mask placement in the prone position. *Anaesthesia* 1993;**48**:1104–1105.
74 Zanetti G. La maschera laringea in ortopedia. *Minerva Anestesiol* 1995;**61**:57–58.
75 Turndorf H, Rodis ID, Clark TS. 'Silent' regurgitation during anaesthesia. *Anesth Analg* 1974;**53**:700–703.
76 Brimacombe JR. LMA in awake fibreoptic bronchoscopy. *Anaesth Intens Care* 1991;**19**:472.
77 Brimacombe J. The laryngeal mask airway – use in the management of stridor. *Anaesth Intens Care* 1992;**20**:117–118.
78 Asai T. Use of the laryngeal mask for tracheal intubation in patients at increased risk of aspiration of gastric contents. *Anesthesiology* 1992;**77**:1029–1030.
79 Ferguson C, Herdman M, Evans K, Hayes M, Cole PV. Flow resistance of the laryngeal mask in awake subjects. *Br J Anaesth* 1991;**66**:400P (Abstract).

80 McCrirrick A, Pracilio JA. Awake intubation: a new technique. *Anaesthesia* 1991;**46**:661–663.

81 Carey MF, Smith J, Cooney CM. Laryngeal mask to aid tracheal intubation. *Anaesthesia* 1991;**46**:1083.

82 Asai T. Fiberoptic tracheal intubation through the laryngeal mask airway in an awake patient with cervical spine instability. *Anesth Analg* 1993;**77**:404.

83 Alberge MC, Rabarijoana A, Macchi P, Pulcini A, Aime-Raucoules M, Grimaud D. Use of the laryngeal mask airway for bronchoscopy in awake patients with respiratory insufficiency. *Anesthesiology* 1994;**81**:A1462 (Abstract).

84 Theroux MC, Kettrick RG, Khine HH. Laryngeal mask airway and fiberoptic endoscopy in an infant with Schwartz–Jampel syndrome. *Anesthesiology* 1995;**82**:605.

85 King CJ, Davey AJ, Chandradeva K. Emergency use of the laryngeal mask airway in severe upper airway obstruction caused by supraglottic oedema. *Br J Anaesth* 1995;**75**:785–786.

86 Godley M, Ramachandra AR. Use of LMA for awake intubation for Caesarean section. *Can J Anaesth* 1996;**43**:299–302.

87 Benumof JL. Management of the difficult adult airway – with special emphasis on awake tracheal intubation. *Anesthesiology* 1991;**75**:1087–1110.

88 Dasey N, Mansour N. Coughing and laryngospasm with the laryngeal mask. *Anaesthesia* 1989;**44**:865.

89 Brimacombe J, Berry A. Active swallowing to aid LMA insertion in awake patients. *Anesth Analg* 1994;**78**:1029.

90 Brimacombe J, Berry A. The role of the laryngeal mask airway for failed tracheal intubation in the patient with a 'Full Stomach'. *Anesth Analg* 1994;**78**:818–819.

91 Denny NM, Desilva KD, Webber PA. Laryngeal mask airway for emergency tracheostomy in a neonate. *Anaesthesia* 1990;**45**:895.

92 Markakis DA, Sayson SC, Schreiner MS. Insertion of the laryngeal mask airway in awake infants with the Robin sequence. *Anesth Analg* 1992;**75**:822–824.

93 Johnson CM, Sims C. Awake fibreoptic intubation via a laryngeal mask in an infant with Goldenhar's syndrome. *Anaesth Intens Care* 1994;**22**:194–197.

94 Paterson SJ, Byrne PJ, Molesky MG, Seal RF, Finucane BT. Neonatal resuscitation using the laryngeal mask airway. *Anesthesiology* 1994;**80**:1248–1253.

95 Brimacombe J, Gandini D. Resuscitation of neonates with the laryngeal mask – a caution. *Pediatrics* 1995;**95**:453–454.

96 Albertsen P, Eschen C, Verder H. Laryngeal mask used as a guideway for brief access to the intratracheal space in premature infants. *8th International Workshop on Surfactant Replacement, Oslo, 20–22 May 1993* (Abstract).

97 Spain BT, Riley RH. Salbutamol via the laryngeal mask airway for relief of bronchospasm. *Anaesthesia* 1992;**47**:1107.

98 Alexander R, Smith G. Laryngeal mask airway (LMA) and tracheal route for drug administration in resuscitation. *Third Congress of the European Resuscitation Council, Seville, Spain, 6–8 June 1996,* p.56 (Abstract).

★ **99** Costa e Silva L, Brimacombe J. Tracheal tube/laryngeal mask exchange for emergence. *Anesthesiology* 1996;**85**:218. *Pilot study of 10 patients undergoing major neurosurgery in whom the tracheal tube was exchanged for the LMA at the end of the procedure to facilitate smooth emergence.*

100 Briggs RJS, Bailey P, Howard DJ. The laryngeal mask: a new type of airway in anesthesia for direct laryngoscopy. *Otolaryngol Head Neck Surg* 1992;**107**:603–605.

101 Nair I, Bailey PM. Use of the laryngeal mask for airway maintenance following tracheal extubation. *Anaesthesia* 1995;**50**:174–175.

102 Maroof M, Siddique M, Khan RM. Post-thyroidectomy vocal cord examination by fibreoscopy aided by the laryngeal mask airway. *Anaesthesia* 1992;**47**:445.

103 Rowbottom SJ, Morton CPJ. Diagnostic fibreoptic bronchoscopy using the laryngeal mask. *Anaesthesia* 1991;**46**:161.

104 Maroof M, Khan RM, Cooper T, Siddique MS, Saqib N. Post thyroidectomy vocal cord examination using LMA aided fiberoscopy. *Anesthesiology* 1993;**79**:A1083 (Abstract).

105 Stott S, Riley R. Visualising the airway after thyroidectomy. *Anaesth Intens Care* 1994;**22**:121.

106 Brimacombe J, Sher M, Laing D, Berry A. The laryngeal mask airway: a new technique for fiberoptic guided vocal cord biopsy. *J Clin Anesth* 1996;**8**:273–275.

107 Costa e Silva L, Brimacombe J. The laryngeal mask for carotid endarterectomy. *J Cardiothoracic and Vascular Anesthesia* 1996;**10**:972–973.

13 Advanced uses: surgery

Educational issues

Many advanced uses of the LMA require cooperation between anesthesiologist and surgeon to optimize benefit and minimize risk. It is recommended that surgeons and their assistants working in close proximity with the device become familiar with its merits and demerits[1]. A surgical learning curve is likely and simpler advanced uses such as ear and nose surgery should be introduced before proceeding to more complex advanced procedures such as adenotonsillectomy, laser pharyngoplasty and vocal cord biopsy. The use of the LMA for ear, nose and throat (ENT), head, neck and dental surgery has been the subject of four reviews[1-4].

Shared access

LMA versus FLMA

The decision to use the LMA or FLMA will primarily depend on the requirements for surgical access and the experience of the anesthesiologist. If there are no special requirements, the standard LMA will be the most appropriate choice since work of breathing is lower[5] and it may be marginally easier to insert. For surgical procedures to the mouth, pharynx, lower face, neck, upper thorax, and whenever drapes threaten the stability of the standard LMA or a tonsillar gag is required, the FLMA is better suited. The design differences between the two devices have already been discussed (see Chapter 4, *The standard laryngeal mask airway* and *The flexible laryngeal mask airway*). Important practical differences are that rotation of the LMA mask in the hypopharynx is easily detected by observation of the black line, but with the FLMA this only serves to indicate rotation of the tube. The stability of the LMA is influenced by the method of fixation and head/neck position. FLMA stability is independent of these factors[6], but displacement may be more difficult to recognize. Christie has suggested using a foam 'V-pack' (Dentmed, Bristol, UK) to stabilize the FLMA internally during dental procedures and facilitate the recovery of teeth fragments[7]. The device is inserted on the palatal aspect of the FLMA taking care not to displace the mask caudally.

Presurgical assessment

Once insertion is complete, the anesthesiologist should verify that the LMA is functioning adequately and ensure that the oropharyngeal leak pressure is at least

10 cm H_2O (see Chapter 6, *Cuff inflation*). It is not necessary to provoke leaks deliberately by excessive bag inflation, provided the lungs can be normally inflated without leaks occurring. Provided the seal is not compromised, soiling should not occur in head and neck surgery even if the mouth were to become completely filled with fluid. If there is any doubt about its position or functional integrity, the LMA should be repositioned or an alternative airway management technique utilized. Both surgeon and anesthesiologist should inspect the oral cavity to note the position of the LMA in the mouth. It is useful to mark the tube at the level of the teeth so that displacement might be more easily detected. The LMA/FLMA tubing can be loosely fixed with a cotton tie, but the silicone tube may be damaged if this is too tight. If continuous suction is applied, a traditional gauze throat pack is not routinely required. Provided the seal is not compromised, soiling should not occur. Traditional gauze throat packs are usually unnecessary except perhaps in dental surgery where there is a possible risk of dental fragments becoming wedged behind the cuff. Care is needed with instruments such as gags and suckers to maintain cuff integrity. Ravalia and Steele have suggested using a suction catheter positioned in the groove between the stem and mask as an alternative to a throat pack[8]. The catheter is placed in the midline prior to cuff inflation and placed on continuous low grade suction during the procedure.

Bite blocks and tonsillar gags

Excessive mouth opening and/or placement of a large bite block may cause the LMA/FLMA tube to obstruct. Particular vigilance is required during extraction when the surgeon applies downward pressure to the mandible[9]. This may produce partial airway obstruction in up to 10% of patients[9]. Several maneuvers have been described to relieve obstruction including forward displacement of the mandible, head extension and repositioning of the LMA[10]. If kinking of the FLMA tube occurs, this is likely to be related to previous damage and the device should be replaced. Heath and Sinnathamby report a 20% initial obstruction rate during use of the tonsillar gag in a series of 112 patients[11]. Only three patients, however, required subsequent intubation. Other authors have reported a mechanical obstruction rate of 2–18% which was readily corrected[12,13]. Care must be taken to prevent the blades of the gag compromising the LMA cuff (too large a blade) or kinking the dorsal aspect of the tube (too small a blade). Education of surgical staff is critical to successful use of the FLMA with a tonsillar gag. It is possible that a tonsillar gag specific to the FLMA could be designed.

Emergence

The LMA should be left in situ during recovery from oral surgery where it will continue to provide a clear airway and protect the respiratory tract. It is mandatory to insert the recommended bite guard before the patient wakes. Patients should ideally be recovered in the lateral position to allow the continual drainage of blood and secretions and complications will be minimized if patients are not disturbed during this period. However, care should be taken to position the patient while he or she is still under an adequate depth of anesthesia.

Ear and nose surgery

Several trials and anecdotal reports suggest that the LMA may be safely used for ear and nose surgery including tympanoplasty, rhinoplasty, septoplasty, submucosal resection, antral washouts, reduction of nasal fractures and nasal polypectomy[14-19]. Compared with the face mask, the LMA provides better perioperative oxygen saturation and improved surgical conditions for pediatric myringoplasty[20,21]. In a comparative trail of 41 adult patients undergoing rhinoplasty, the LMA was shown to be superior to the tracheal tube with less blood in the trachea and fewer emergence problems[18]. Care must be taken when placing the LMA or FLMA to prevent malposition and rotation and to test the effectiveness of the seal[22,23]. In one instance, aspiration of pus occurred secondary to malposition of the LMA in a patient with chronic sinusitis[24]. Where the LMA tube may interfere with the surgical field an FLMA should be used. Williams et al compared the FLMA and tracheal intubation in 66 patients for nasal surgery and found that airway maintenance and airway protection was equally effective in both groups[17]. The LMA provided superior conditions for emergence compared with the Guedel airway and face mask.

Dental surgery

Nasal mask anesthesia has traditionally been used for short dental procedures, but is associated with a high incidence of hypoxic events[25-27]. Tracheal intubation carries a significant morbidity related to airway trauma and the use of muscle relaxants[28,29]. A number of studies have looked at the use of the LMA for oral surgery including simple extraction[30,31] and removal of impacted wisdom teeth[9,10,28]. Young reported a series of 421 dental anesthetics using the standard LMA[10]. An unobstructed airway was achieved in 81% of patients, in 17% temporary obstruction occurred which was relieved by a variety of maneuvers and in 2% obstruction was persistent, but judged acceptable for the short duration of these operations. Bailie et al compared the use of the LMA with the nasal mask in 50 children presenting for dental outpatient single tooth extraction[31]. There was no difference between the two groups as regards surgical access, difficulty of extraction or bleeding. George and Sanders compared the FLMA, LMA and nasal mask for single tooth extraction in 78 ASA 1–2 children and found a significantly higher incidence of arrhythmias, airway obstruction and desaturation with the nasal mask[27]. Overall anesthesia time was similar. The FLMA is better suited for dental surgery and Goodwin et al compared uncuffed nasal tracheal intubation using suxamethonium with the FLMA in 60 patients undergoing extraction of impacted third molars[28]. There was a higher incidence of technical anesthetic difficulty, postoperative muscle pains and readmission for excessive bleeding in the tracheal tube group. Noble and Wooler recommend the use of the LMA in dental chair anesthesia[30]. Quinn et al compared nasotracheal intubation with the FLMA for dentoalveolar surgery in 100 patients and found that the FLMA provided satisfactory conditions for both anesthesia and surgery, but vigilance with the airway was required, especially at the time of extraction[9]. Partial airway obstruction occurred in 10% of patients with the FLMA during extraction. Thirty-eight per cent of patients undergoing nasal intubation had epistaxis and in 6% blood was identified in the trachea. No patient in the FLMA group aspirated blood. There were no differences in the incidence of perioperative oxygen saturation or postoperative complications. The high incidence of sore throat with the FLMA (60%) may have been related to the use of a throat pack or inexperience with the device.

Other oral surgery

The LMA has been used for several other forms of oral surgery. This includes removal of a cyst at the base of the tongue[32], suture of a torn uvula[32], repair of cleft palate[33–35], fixation of mandibular fractures (followed failed intubation)[36], revision of a cheek flap (following failed face mask ventilation)[37], Burkitt's lymphoma[38], excision of a tongue tumor[39], glossopexy (following failed gaseous induction)[40], quinsy[41] and laser pharyngoplasty[42].

Adenotonsillectomy

The tonsils are easily accessible when the LMA/FLMA is correctly positioned and there is increasing evidence supporting the use of the FLMA for adenotonsillectomy where it offers potential advantages over the tracheal tube (especially the uncuffed tracheal tube) in terms of tracheal soiling and recovery characteristics[12,13,43–46]. In some centers the FLMA has become the preferred technique. For example, at the Royal National Throat, Nose and Ear Hospital, UK, the FLMA is utilized by 60% of anesthesiologists for adenotonsillectomy[45].

It is possible to use the standard LMA for adenotonsillectomy[47–49], but the lumen of the tube is frequently occluded by the tonsillar gag. Dubreuil et al compared the LMA, face mask and tracheal tube in a random prospective trail of 89 children undergoing adenoidectomy and found that oxygen saturation was better with the LMA[43]. Versichelen et al studied 60 children undergoing adenoidectomy and myringoplasty with the LMA and found insertion easy and a low incidence of complications, but felt that the FLMA would be more suitable[47].

Insertion of the LMA is sometimes difficult in patients with large tonsils[33,50]. However, insertion of the FLMA is usually easy since it can be moved between the tonsils[12,13,49]. It has been suggested that a laryngoscope may be useful when placing the LMA in patients with tonsillar hypertrophy[33,50]. Webster et al compared the tracheal tube and FLMA in 109 children and demonstrated that the FLMA is a safe alternative to tracheal intubation for adenotonsillectomy[13]. In the early part of the study, when experience was being gained, the FLMA was abandoned in five patients in favor of tracheal intubation before the start of surgery due to difficulty in placement. The incidence of stridor and laryngeal spasm was lower with the FLMA than with the tracheal tube following surgery. Similarly Williams and Bailey compared the FLMA and tracheal tube in 104 patients for adenotonsillectomy[12]. They found that the FLMA did not interfere with surgical access, resisted compression and protected the lower airway from contamination and blood. Recovery was less eventful in the FLMA group with less obstruction and better airway acceptance. In a follow-up survey Williams and Bailey report no major complications in over 650 uses for adenotonsillectomy[45]. Fiani et al demonstrated fewer episodes of bronchospasm, laryngeal spasm, nasal bleeding and desaturation in a randomized trial comparing the FLMA with the tracheal tube[44]. The FLMA was successfully placed in 13/14 patients. Studies by Hackmann[51] and Webster et al[52] have shown that there is no direct evidence that the LMA is superior to the tracheal tube for adenotonsillectomy in terms of outcome.

One of the authors (JB) has noted that some surgeons are using hand held CO_2 lasers to obtain hemostasis of the tonsillar bed in children. Care must be taken to ensure that laser safety requirements are met. The LMA has been used to secure the airway of a patient with a massive postoperative bleed from the tonsillar bed following a uvulo-palato-pharyngoplasty[53].

Laser surgery

The LMA has been successfully used during tunable dye laser surgery to the face[54,55], Nd–YAG laser surgery to the trachea[56] and carina[57], and CO_2 laser surgery to the soft palate[58] and tonsillar bed.

Safety

The energy density for port wine facial surgery is insufficient to damage the LMA[54,55,59]. Laser respiratory tract surgery is conducted via an incision in the neck[56] or through a flexible fiberoptic bronchoscope, minimizing the risk of a direct hit[57]. Accidental impact, however, is more likely during laser surgery to the oropharynx[58]. Safety may be increased by wrapping the tube in protective foil[60] or by using a laser-resistant sheath[61]. The weakest point of the LMA/FLMA is the cuff[62]. Filling the cuff with air will reduce the chance of ignition, but nitrous oxide readily diffuses into the cuff during nitrous oxide/oxygen anesthesia[63]. It would be possible to fill the cuff with saline or a methylene blue solution to facilitate early detection of perforation and to prevent flaming, but any residual fluid remaining in the cuff may result in cuff rupture during autoclaving[64] and may be uneconomical. The use of wet gauze swabs over the cuff have already been reported during laser pharyngoplasty[58]. The inspired oxygen concentration should be reduced to maintain SaO_2 >95% and nitrous oxide should be avoided where possible. During laser surgery to the oropharynx, gas leaks should be prevented by using spontaneous ventilation or maintaining airway pressure below leak pressures during positive pressure ventilation (PPV)[55]. Use of the CO_2 laser at power densities below 2.25×10^3 W cm^{-2} appears to be safe with the LMA and FLMA[62,65,66], but further studies are required to confirm this (see Chapter 4, *Laser*).

Laser pharyngoplasty

Laser pharyngoplasty is a relatively new technique used in the treatment of palatal flutter and involves controlled laser burns to the nasal and oral surfaces of the soft palate, a process which takes about 10–30 min and can be conducted on a day case basis[67]. Patients undergoing laser pharyngoplasty tend to have difficult airways due to their underlying airway problem[68,69] and the associated risk factors of being overweight, middle-aged males[70]. Sher et al compared the FLMA with the tracheal tube for laser pharyngoplasty in 165 patients using a PPV technique and showed significantly more airway problems with the tracheal tube at induction and during recovery[42]. Recommendations for use of the FLMA for laser pharyngoplasty are given in Table 13.1.

Table 13.1 Recommended anesthetic management for laser pharyngoplasty

1. Atropine with the premed
2. Preoxygenation
3. Propofol 2.5 mg kg^{-1}
4. FLMA insertion
5. Functional assessment – reposition if leak
6. Nondepolarizing muscle relaxant
7. O_2/air/isoflurane to keep Sao_2 >95%
8. Keep airway pressures <20 cm H_2O
9. Insertion of mouth gag
10. Repeat functional assessment
11. Place moist gauze over LMA cuff
12. Proceed with surgery
13. Transfer patient to the trolley and place in left lateral position
14. Reverse neuromuscular blockade
15. Insert bite guard
16. Discontinue anesthetic
17. Remove FLMA when opening mouth to command

Reproduced from reference 42 with permission from the Australian Society of Anesthesiologists: *Anesthesia and Intensive Care.*

Major head and neck surgery

The LMA may be useful for some forms of major surgery to the head and neck, but the requirements for a totally secure airway tend to support the continued use of tracheal intubation either via the nasal or oral route. The LMA cannot be used for major pharyngeal surgery or where surgery might cause displacement of the bowl from the hypopharynx. Laryngeal spasm can occur with the LMA in situ[71] and may occur during neck dissection if the patient is not paralyzed[72].

If used for major head and neck surgery, surgeons must be warned that neck anatomy may be slightly altered and that excessive neck pressure might displace the cuff. There have been two occasions on which the LMA cuff was damaged during neck surgery. Hardingham reported that following successful excision of a branchial cyst, the surgeon found a deeper, nonpulsatile cyst under considerable tension, with fine blood vessels and nerves traversing its wall. Fine needle aspiration revealed that the 'pharyngocele' was, in fact, the cuff of the LMA![73] Similarly Kalapac et al reported biopsy of a 'hard, rubbery mass' in the left neck close to the deep cervical lymph nodes[74]. On both occasions there was partial loss of airway control. These incidents confirm the need for ongoing communication between anesthesiologist and surgeon and of the potential dangers of using the LMA during neck dissection. The authors strongly recommend that surgeons working in close proximity with the device become familiar with its merits and demerits. Anesthesiologists in their turn must inform surgeons when the LMA has implications for the surgical procedure. In most instances of major head and neck surgery the requirements for a totally secure airway tend to support the continued use of tracheal intubation either via the nasal or oral route. The FLMA has been used for major head and neck surgery lasting 9 h in a patient with a known difficult airway[75].

Carotid endarterectomy

Sustained increases in blood pressure above normal levels are undesirable in patients undergoing carotid endarterectomy since hypertension may contribute to cerebral edema, particularly in diseased areas of the brain with altered ability to autoregulate cerebral blood flow[76]. Chronic hypertension is present in 60–80% of these patients and many experience exaggerated intraoperative fluctuations in arterial blood pressure which may also contribute to myocardial ischemia in patients with coronary artery disease[77,78]. Maintaining hemodynamic stability is an important goal of anesthesia management. In this regard tracheal intubation is not ideal since it is associated with a 25–50% increase in pulse rate and blood pressure[79]. Furthermore, patients frequently cough during emergence, precipitating acute changes in arterial and venous blood pressures and threatening the surgical site. Strategies aimed at solving this problem include use of lidocaine spray, intravenous antihypertensives, or deep extubation followed by face mask ventilation.

Costa e Silva and Brimacombe have reported use of the LMA for carotid endarterectomy[80]. In three patients it was exchanged for the tracheal tube to facilitate smooth emergence and in the fourth it was used for the entire procedure following failed intubation. No patient coughed or gagged during emergence and blood pressure/pulse rate remained within ±15% of baseline values during placement and emergence. Antihypertensives were not required during these phases. The LMA utilized for the procedure was not displaced by the surgeon and did not interfere with the surgical field. There were no perioperative cardiovascular or cerebrovascular complications.

Tracheostomy

The LMA does not preclude access to the anterior neck and tracheostomy can be readily performed with the LMA in situ. The most common circumstance precipitating this is following successful placement of the LMA in the 'cannot intubate, cannot ventilate' situation where prolonged airway security is required[81-91]. Its use in this situation is appropriate since it might be the only means of providing oxygen whilst the procedure is performed. The LMA may also be used for elective tracheostomy provided there are no contraindications to its use such as high inflation pressures, airway pathology or existence of an aspiration risk. The LMA has also been used for fiberoptic guided percutaneous tracheostomy in the intensive care unit where it allows PPV and synchronous views of the trachea without interfering with the surgical field[53,92]. The technique is limited to fasted patients with normal lung compliance and minimal glottic edema[53,92–94]. There are no trials comparing the LMA with other techniques for percutaneous tracheostomy, such as use of a rigid bronchoscope[95].

Microlaryngeal surgery

The position of the LMA normally precludes its use for procedures distal to the tonsils, but fiberoptic guided microlaryngeal surgery may be performed through the LMA[96] including injection of polytetrafluoroethylene (Teflon) into the vocal cords. A further possible use is as an alternative to suspension laryngoscopy for fiberoptic vocal cord biopsy in patients with minor laryngeal pathology and with no evidence of infraglottic airway obstruction[97]. By avoiding tracheal intubation and the suspension laryngoscope, trauma to soft tissues may be reduced[98] and the hypertensive response attenuated[99]. The LMA also facilitates a smooth emergence from anesthesia compared with the tracheal tube and allows the operator to continually observe the vocal cords throughout emergence. Other potential benefits are reliable airway control, an improved view of the vocal cords, ease of progression to bronchoscopy and reduced surgical time. It would seem a particularly useful technique in patients where the avoidance of the pressor response is a concern or in whom an adequate view cannot be obtained with a suspension microlaryngoscope. A technique of using the LMA for microlaryngeal surgery has been described by Briggs et al in which conventional suspension microlaryngoscopy was performed using a Venturi jet and the LMA was utilized to facilitate smooth induction and recovery, but removed for the procedure[100].

Tracheal/carinal surgery

Slinger et al reported the use of the LMA for laser resection of a carinal obstruction[57]. It was felt that the LMA allowed an optimal compromise between laser fire safety and maintenance of oxygenation/ventilation, particularly important in patients with severely compromised airways. In some of these patients formal ventilation may be difficult or undesirable, or they may be unable to tolerate the increased work of respiration during fiberoptic bronchoscopy via a tracheal tube. Similar advantages were also noted by Divatia et al when using the LMA for resection of a tracheal tumor[56]. Ferson has reported the use of the LMA for laser surgery to a variety of respiratory tract tumors (D Ferson, personal communication, 1996). The value of these applications, however, is unclear since compared with the rigid bronchoscope, the view through the fiberscope is less satisfactory and bleeding or airway collapse will be difficult to treat[101]. The LMA has been used for the placement of an expandable metallic tracheal stent[102], as a blocker during tracheoplasty[103] and for insertion of a Montgomery T-tube[104].

Thyroid/parathyroid/thymic surgery

A UK survey reported that up to 8% of anesthesiologists were using the LMA for thyroid/parathyroid surgery[105]. One notable advantage is that the dynamic view of the larynx afforded by the LMA and the avoidance of muscle relaxants may help prevent recurrent laryngeal nerve injury[72,106–108]; this concept has been supported in two recent studies[109,110]. Goldik et al[109] studied 50 patients and Hobbiger et al 97 patients[110] and both groups found a zero incidence of recurrent laryngeal nerve dysfunction. This compares with the usual injury rate of approximately 4%[111,112]. The technique involves continual fiberoptic observation of the vocal cords and use of a nerve stimulator to locate the recurrent laryngeal nerve where it is not readily identified by dissection. Care must be taken to keep the LMA tube away from the surgical site. Not all authors support the use of the LMA for thyroid surgery. Charters et al have urged caution when the LMA is used in this area since sudden loss of the airway secondary to laryngeal spasm or displacement can occur and rapid correction of problems may be difficult[113,114]. Some of these problems may be overcome by paralyzing the patient, but viewing the vocal cords will be less useful. At the Royal Berkshire Hospital, UK, the most common technique used over a 3-year period is to paralyze and ventilate patients with the LMA and view the cords through it following reversal at the end of the procedure. It has been suggested that the LMA may be the airway of choice for thyroid surgery where the trachea is grossly deviated or narrowed since it may prevent further tracheal damage[106]. Alternatively, the LMA may not be suitable for patients with weakened tracheal rings since it cannot prevent collapse of the airway[115] and its use should perhaps be limited to patients with small tumors[116]. Several authors have suggested that the LMA could replace the tracheal tube at the conclusion of surgery to enable observation of the vocal cords fiberoptically during the recovery period[117-120] (see Chapter 12, *Tracheal tube/LMA exchange*). Palomba et al have reported the successful use of the LMA in 22 patients with myasthenia gravis undergoing thymectomy[121].

Ophthalmic surgery

The LMA has been used in both elective[105,122-140] and emergency eye surgery[105,141-143]. Balog et al reported the use of the LMA in 139 children undergoing day case extraocular surgery including strabismus repair, examination under anesthesia, gonioscopy and nasolacrimal duct probing, eyelid repair, scleral/conjunctival procedures, electroretinography, foreign body removal and enucleation[135]. In one patient the LMA could not be placed and in two further patients was replaced with a tracheal tube. There were no other complications associated with its use and no child required hospital admission. More controversial is the use of the LMA for intraocular surgery[144]. The potential advantages of the LMA for intraocular surgery are that it offers better control over intraocular pressure at insertion and provides a smooth, cough-free recovery[122,123,130,134], theoretically minimizing the risk of suture displacement. It may also shorten overall operating room time and make patients more comfortable post-operatively. This is achieved at the expense of a possible increased risk of displacement, the fact that a full valsalva can occur since the cords are not penetrated, and the LMA is less suitable for PPV. Although displacement of the LMA can occur[133,144], it is rare and preventable if guidelines for use are followed[145] (Table 13.2).

The safety and efficacy of the LMA for ophthalmic surgery has been suggested by two large audit surveys[137,138]. Wainwright reported a series of 1877 patients undergoing anesthesia for a wide range of ophthalmic surgery with the LMA, including 1498 intraocular procedures (cataract, trabeculectomy, vitreoretinal surgery)[137]. Of these 1424 were ventilated and 455 patients breathed spontaneously. No patient had any clinical signs of aspiration. The author considered the LMA not only to be safe, but a great improvement for patients undergoing general anesthesia for ophthalmic surgery. Langenstein et al used the LMA in 792 patients undergoing eye surgery and found the device safe and effective in 98%[138]. In 14 patients the device was not considered effective due to excessive leak or high end-tidal CO_2 and there were three complications: two patients developed gastric insufflation and one had excessive bronchial secretions. The authors also showed that the device was safe for procedures lasting up to 4 h and was beneficial to patients with cardiorespiratory disease. The LMA/PPV technique has been successfully used in over 1000 patients undergoing intraocular surgery from other series[128,144,146] and comparative studies with the tracheal tube draw favorable general conclusions[122–125,132,134]. Myint et al consider that spontaneous ventilation with a laryngeal mask is an acceptable alternative to controlled ventilation with tracheal intubation for elective intraocular surgery, but consider controlled ventilation/muscle relaxation via the LMA to be the optimal technique[136].

The LMA has been used in the management of ophthalmic splash injuries[147]. The proximal end of the LMA tube is placed under or connected to a tap and the flow adjusted. The inflated cuff is then placed around the eye socket with the tip pressed into the bridge of the nose, thus allowing the eye to be continually irrigated. Care must be taken to ensure that the LMA utilized for this purpose has been autoclaved and is not a source of further contamination or injury.

Table 13.2 Recommendations for use of the LMA during open eye surgery

1. All patients should be paralyzed and ventilated and the level of neuromuscular blockade carefully monitored. Spontaneous ventilation anesthesia via the LMA in the patient with an open eye is not recommended for routine use.
2. The ease with which the patient can be ventilated should be carefully assessed prior to surgery, including capnometry and tidal volume monitoring, and the pressure at which the cuff leaks should be determined. The position of the LMA can also be verified using a fiberoptic scope. Where faultless ventilation is not achieved, the LMA should be substituted with a tracheal tube. Peak airway pressures should be maintained below 20 cm H_2O to minimize the risk of gastric dilatation and operating room pollution.
3. Good communication with the ophthalmic surgeon is essential to minimize the risk of LMA displacement. The LMA should be fixed firmly with the tube bent caudally over the chin to avoid impingement on the surgical field or the FLMA used.
4. The LMA should preferably be left in situ until the patient is fully awake.
5. There is no place for the LMA in the nonfasted patient with a penetrating eye injury other than for airway rescue.

Remote and repeat anesthesia

The LMA would appear to have a particular role in remote anesthesia for repeat radiotherapy[148–152], radiological imaging[153–158] and burns dressings[159]. Herrick and Kennedy used the LMA in 313 patients and found that 3.5% of children developed airway obstruction in the prone position prior to commencement of treatment; this obstruction was easily corrected[148]. By comparison the authors experienced airway obstruction on 2.1% (11/525) using a Guedel-type airway adapted for insufflation, but on two occasions this occurred during treatment necessitating interruption of irradiation. Moylan and Luce reported the successful use of the FLMA in 145 children who underwent 2500 radiotherapy procedures with no major complication[160]. Patients undergoing daily radiotherapy will benefit from avoidance of the morbidity associated with repeated tracheal intubation which can produce subglottic mucosal damage[161].

Gynecological laparoscopy

Prior to the availability of the LMA, opinion was polarized as to the most suitable anesthetic technique for gynecological laparoscopy. Many authors considered that tracheal intubation and ventilation were mandatory to reduce the risk of aspiration and hypoventilation. Others argued that spontaneous ventilation with a face mask was a safe technique in experienced hands and with a skilled surgeon. Advocates of the face mask also point out that minor morbidity is reduced with the face mask and that the risk of awareness is minimized if muscle relaxation is avoided. The LMA has added a further dimension to the debate and this subject has been reviewed by Brimacombe and Berry[162].

Pre-LMA studies

The changes in hemodynamic and respiratory function associated with intraperitoneal CO_2 insufflation and Trendelenburg tilt have been investigated extensively and found to be relatively insignificant[163]. However, there is a paucity of data regarding the incidence of regurgitation during laparoscopy and how it is influenced by tilt, pressure, mode of ventilation and airway type. Duffy measured pharyngeal pH and reported a 2.2% (2/93) incidence of regurgitation in intubated ventilated patients, but patients were given atropine[164] and placed in steep Trendelenburg tilt[165]. Carlsson and Islander using a similar technique showed that regurgitation occurred in 20% of emergency laparoscopies[166]. Kurer and Welch reported no episodes of regurgitation in 120 patients, 50% of whom were managed with the face mask and spontaneous ventilation[167]. Epidemiological evidence from large series shows a very low incidence of aspiration. The Royal College of Obstetricians and Gynaecologists, UK, reported no aspiration events and one episode of regurgitation from 50 048 patients of whom an estimated 10% were managed with a face mask[168,169]. Wong and Nkana reported 15 000 face mask anesthetics[170] and Scott 2000[171] with no aspiration events. It seems that the lower esophageal sphincter is capable of rapid adaptive responses to changes in intragastric pressure during laparoscopy with maximum intraperitoneal pressures of

30 cm H_2O and 10–15 degree head down tilt, and that barrier pressure is increased or maintained[172]. Roberts and Goodman reported no episodes of reflux, as determined by an esophageal pH probe, in 63 women undergoing gynecological laparoscopy[173]. Raised intra-abdominal pressure and Trendelenburg tilt do not therefore necessarily increase the risk of regurgitation[172].

LMA studies

A postal survey of consultants employed by the South East Thames Regional Health Authority, UK, revealed that approximately 40% used the LMA for gynecological laparoscopy[105]. A similar survey of current practice in Wales showed that 23% of consultants and 34% of nonconsultants were prepared to use the LMA during anesthesia for laparoscopic clip sterilization[174]. Others report even higher usage rates[175]. Considering the large numbers of patients and the fact that recommendations already exist to intubate and ventilate[168], there is a remarkable lack of data demonstrating its efficacy and safety. Regurgitation of dye has been reported in 1/16 patients undergoing laparoscopy[176]. There has been one report of pulmonary aspiration in a patient who underwent elective laparoscopic sterilization with a PPV technique[177]. Published trials are limited in terms of patient numbers and method of assessment of regurgitation, but they suggest that the LMA is a safe technique[178,179]. The results of large-scale epidemiological studies have recently become available and support the finding of controlled trials. Brimacombe[180] and Malins and Cooper[181] used the LMA in 3000 laparoscopy patients without producing major complications. Verghese and Brimacombe reported its use in 1469 laparoscopy patients and no aspiration or regurgitation events occurred[175]. Complication rates were comparable to more conventional LMA usage.

The safety of anesthesia for gynecological laparoscopy probably depends largely on short operative time, close intraoperative monitoring and the experience of both anesthesiologist and surgeon[167]. Regardless of the concerns of sore throat and incomplete reversal of muscle relaxant, the aim of anesthesia for laparoscopy must be to minimize risk of aspiration and life threatening dysrhythmias. Proving that a technique meets these criteria is logistically difficult; further larger studies comparing the LMA with the tracheal tube and face mask are required to better indicate the degree of tilt, the duration of procedure and patient type for which the technique may be regarded as reasonably 'safe'. The physiological and clinical data available to determine the suitability of the LMA are inadequate, but it would seem that there are reasonable grounds for experienced clinicians to use the LMA provided certain guidelines are considered. Further proof is required before widespread adoption of these techniques can be recommended. Suggested guidelines for use of the LMA during laparoscopy are given in Table 13.3.

Lower abdominal surgery

Some forms of elective lower abdominal surgery, such as hysterectomy, suprapubic prostatectomy and elective appendectomy, may be of sufficient low risk to warrant use of the LMA, although this remains unproven[183]. Traction on the upper abdominal

Table 13.3 Suggested guidelines for use of the LMA during laparoscopy

1. Experienced LMA user
2. Meticulous selection of patients – fasted, no history of esophageal reflux; normal lung compliance
3. Surgeon aware that the LMA is being used?
4. Select correct size of LMA: size 4 >50 kg
5. Insert the LMA when anesthetic depth is adequate ± muscle relaxation (mivacurium, rorcuronium suitable)
6. Use standard insertion technique to achieve optimal placement of the LMA
7. Either SV or PPV – use tidal volume 8–10 ml kg^{-1}
8. Either total intravenous anesthesia or volatile agent (avoid halothane)
9. Adhere to '15' rule: <15 degrees tilt; <15 cm H_2O IAP; <15 min duration
10. Avoid inadequate anesthesia or muscle relaxation during surgery
11. Reverse muscle relaxant prior to termination of general anesthesia
12. Avoid disturbance of the patient during emergence

Key: IAP=intra-abdominal pressure; SV = spontaneous ventilation.

Reproduced with permission from reference 182, *Ambulatory Surgery*.

organs may reduce compliance and increase intragastric pressure. Stimulation of the peritoneum may increase the incidence of coughing, which is frequently associated with regurgitation[184,185]. There is no evidence to suggest that use of the LMA for lower abdominal elective surgery is unsafe. Indeed, Verghese and Brimacombe reported the use of the LMA for gynecological laparotomy in 644 patients with a similar complication rate to more conventional usage[175]. The authors considered that controlled trials of the LMA versus the tracheal tube were warranted. Kumagai et al reported the successful use of the LMA versus the tracheal tube for major gynecological surgery in 80 patients undergoing balanced regional anesthesia in which the incidence of postoperative nausea and vomiting was similar[186]. Palomba et al reported the successful use of the LMA in 19 patients for total abdominal hysterectomy[121]. Harada and Namiki reported the successful use of the LMA plus an epidural in 95 patients undergoing elective lower abdominal surgery[187]. Whenever lower abdominal surgery is being performed it is important to ensure adequate anesthetic depth to prevent coughing during peritoneal stimulation and to protect the airway by tracheal intubation if upper abdominal organs are to be manipulated[188].

Upper abdominal surgery

It was reported that approximately 5% of anesthesiologists in the South East Thames Region, UK, considered the LMA suitable for laparoscopic cholecystectomy and laparotomy[150]. Sofair[189] has used the LMA for laparoscopic cholecystectomy in a professional singer with a potentially difficult airway, but this decision has been critisised by Brimacombe and Berry[190]. Verghese and Brimacombe have reported the uneventful use of the LMA for laparoscopic cholecystectomy, open cholecystectomy, colectomy, anterior resection and elective aortic aneurysm repair[175]. Similarly Okazaki reported no episodes of aspiration in 120 elderly patients undergoing cholecystecomy or transverse resection of the colon using balanced regional anesthesia[191]. Palomba et al have reported using the LMA in 135 patients for major abdominal or vascular surgery in combination with spinal or epidural anesthesia[121]. Lauretti et al used the LMA for seven patients undergoing renal transplantation in combination with a thoracic epidural[192]. The manufacturer and the majority of authors, including the inventor, do not consider the LMA appropriate for upper abdominal surgery, even in skilled hands, despite possible benefits in terms of postoperative respiratory function[175,183,190]. It has been shown that 60% of patients undergoing upper abdominal surgery have stomach contents that put them at risk of aspiration[193]. One large study (before the LMA was available) has demonstrated an increased likelihood of aspiration in patients undergoing upper abdominal surgery[194] and aspiration is known to be more likely in the elderly[184]. Using the LMA, severe aspiration has occurred following elective open cholecystectomy[195,196]. Both aspiration and ventilatory difficulties may occur during laparoscopic cholecystectomy, making the LMA even less suitable for this procedure[197]. The risk of regurgitation during upper abdominal surgery was recently highlighted by Brimacombe[188]. A 54-year-old patient regurgitated during a total abdominal hysterectomy when she was subjected to a sudden examination of her upper abdominal organs. Aspiration did not occur because a new LMA prototype designed to divert regurgitated fluids from the airway was being used for airway management[198].

Cardiothoracic surgery

The LMA in its present form is unsuitable for cardiothoracic surgery because of the requirements for high airway pressures. Llagunes et al have suggested using the LMA in cardiac surgery as an alternative to the face mask following induction of anesthesia and prior to tracheal intubation to minimize the risk of gastric distension with the face mask[199]. Seung and Kim used the LMA as an alternative to tracheal intubation in a patient with sick sinus syndrome undergoing thyroidectomy[200]. Peck et al have used the LMA for pediatric patients undergoing cardiac catheterization studies[201]. It has also been used for cardiac surgery where tracheal intubation failed[82,202,203] and following failed placement of a double lumen tracheal tube during thoracotomy[204]. The LMA has also been used for mediastinoscopy[205], but Asai and Morris have warned that the LMA cannot provide adequate airway control if the trachea is compressed and is therefore unsuitable for this procedure[206]. It has been used to provide pressure support ventilation in the post anesthesia care unit following a upper lobectomy in a man with severe reactive airway disease[207] and in four patients during one lung anesthesia following thoracotomy[208].

Polaner has reported use of the LMA for administration of anesthesia in an asthmatic child with an anterior mediastinal mass using 20% oxygen in helium (Heliox) to improve air flow[209]. The LMA was chosen because a conventional mask would have been awkward to use so close to the surgical field. It also allowed the maintenance of a relatively secure airway with spontaneous ventilation and minimized lower airway irritation that could have been precipitated by a tracheal tube, thus decreasing the risk of bronchospasm in a susceptible patient. Hattamer and Dodds reported a similar case[210]. One lung ventilation could theoretically be achieved via the LMA using a fiberoptically placed bronchial blocker.

Minimally invasive neurosurgery

Minimally invasive neurosurgery is a relatively new field with few trials assessing the suitability of various anesthetic techniques[211]. The LMA may be useful since it provides a secure airway in a potentially difficult situation, without the need for more complex methods, and allows anesthesia to be lightened for neurological testing. The LMA also avoids the need for head extension and airway instrumentation and allows controlled ventilation. Induction of anesthesia with the stereotactic frame in situ is potentially hazardous since both face mask ventilation and tracheal intubation may be difficult, but the LMA has been successfully placed following application of the stereotactic frame and induction of anesthesia[212,213]. It is important that the facility exists for rapid removal of the stereotactic frame and that patients are preoxygenated and not paralyzed prior to placement. Placement of the LMA is possible from the front where access from above is limited by the frame. The technique is simple, but should be practiced on normal patients first. The anesthesiologist stands below and to the side of the patient's head[213] (see Chapter 19, *Thumb insertion technique*). The tongue is pulled below the lower lip by an assistant and the tip of the fully deflated mask is pressed into the hard palate using the thumb (thus the thumb from below substitutes the index finger from above used in the standard recommended technique). The mask is then pressed against the curve of the hard palate and posterior oropharynx until the LMA passes down into the hypopharynx. The LMA has been used for stereotactic implantation of fetal substantia nigra into parkinsonian patients, a procedure which may take 3–4 h[213], for stereotactic brain biopsy[212] and for stereotactic neurosurgery in children[214]. The role of the LMA for minimally invasive and major neurosurgery has been discussed in a review of airway management for neuroanesthesia by Spiekermann et al[215].

Major neurosurgery

Coughing and gagging on the tracheal tube may result in acute hemodynamic changes and elevation of intracranial pressure[216]. These are particularly undesirable in patients undergoing intracranial surgery who need to be woken mid-procedure for assessment or during routine emergence from anesthesia. Hagberg et al have reported use of the LMA in four pediatric patients for awake craniotomy for excision of epileptic foci[217]. Anesthesia is discontinued mid-surgery and the LMA removed for cortical mapping of language assessment. Anesthesia is then recommenced and the LMA re-inserted. Costa e Silva and Brimacombe have exchanged the tracheal tube for the LMA at the end of 10 major neurosurgical procedures (intracranial aneurysm repair and tumor removal) in adults to facilitate a smooth emergence[218]. No patient coughed during emergence or removal and there were no adverse events. The rate pressure product varied by less than 15% of pre-exchange baseline values in all patients during the exchange, subsequent emergence and LMA removal. Conci et al reported the successful use of the LMA in 54 ASA 1–4 patients undergoing a wide range of elective and emergency neurosurgical procedures[158]. Ferson et al have reported the elective use of the LMA as an airway intubator in a patient with a posterior cerebellar tumor. They suggest that an additional indication for use of the LMA may be for the prevention of increased intracranial pressure during general anesthesia by avoiding laryngoscopy (D Ferson, personal communication, 1996). A similar case has been reported by Costa e Silva and Brimacombe (L Costa e Silva, personal communication, 1996).

Electroencephalographic mapping procedures

Ammar and Towley have suggested using the LMA for electroencephalographic mapping procedures in which electrodes are passed through the foramen ovale in the preoperative assessment of patients suffering from temporal lobe epilepsy[219]. The procedure is impossible with a face mask and tracheal intubation is not required for such a short procedure.

Bronchoscopy

Fiberoptic bronchoscopy is usually performed transnasally under local anesthesia and sedation, or occasionally under general anesthesia via a tracheal tube[220]. Advantages of the awake transnasal route include the ability to dynamically assess the upper airway combined with the avoidance of general anesthesia. Arterial desaturation and hemorrhage from the nose are the main drawbacks. Several modifications of the face mask have been developed which may improve oxygenation and provide guidance for the fiberoptic scope for adults[221–223] and children[224]. These modified face masks are well tolerated by patients, but probably provide a less effective airway than the LMA. General anesthesia via a tracheal tube provides good operating conditions and maintenance of oxygenation and is commonly used in high risk cases[225], but has all the attendant disadvantages of general anesthesia in a patient with poor lung function and associated cardiovascular disease. These disadvantages may be less with the general anesthesia/ LMA technique, although this is unproven.

The LMA allows easy location of the glottis whilst maintaining ventilation and oxygenation[226–228]. Diagnostic bronchoscopy has been performed down the LMA in both awake[229–231] and anesthetized patients[118,232–241], and in children[232,235,237,239,240,242,243], including transbronchial biopsy[229,233,238,239]. Du Plessis et al reported the successful use of the LMA in 139/140 patients for diagnostic bronchoscopy under general anesthesia[238]. Brimacombe et al have studied the use of the LMA for awake diagnostic bronchoscopy in 50 patients[229]. This study has been extended to 200 patients in which the technique was successful in 99.5% of patients[230]. Complication rates were similar to those reported for transnasal awake bronchoscopy with no fatalities directly attributable to the LMA technique and a 3% incidence of major perioperative complications. Mortality rates vary from 0.01 to 0.5% and major complications from 0.08 to 5%[220,244–248]. Recent guidelines published by the British Thoracic Society for care during bronchoscopy state that arterial oxygen saturation should be maintained at 90% or greater[249]. It is interesting to note that only three patients desaturated below 90% in this series. It was suggested that the technique may have a role where respiratory function is critically impaired. Buzzetti et al successfully used the LMA for fiberoptic bronchoscopy in three immunocompromised patients (orthoptic liver transplant and

Hodgkin's lymphoma) with respiratory failure and five single lung transplant patients during their long-term follow-up after surgery (a total of 25 bronchoscopies)[241].

The LMA has also been used to extract a bronchial foreign body in a child[242] and to perform bronchial lavage in a 3.3 kg infant following failed rigid bronchoscopy[243]. Interestingly, in the latter case the tracheal tube would have been too small to allow the passage of a fiberoptic scope, although a 2.2 mm fiberoptic scope has recently become available[250]. Samet et al have successfully passed a rigid bronchoscope via the LMA to facilitate diagnosis of congenital stridor[251].

References

1 Brimacombe J, Berry A. The laryngeal mask airway for dental surgery – a review. *Aust Dent J* 1995;**40**:10–14.

2 Brimacombe J, Berry A. Use of the laryngeal mask airway in otolaryngology. *J Otolaryngol* 1995;**24**:125–133.

3 Nair I, Bailey PM. Review of uses of the laryngeal mask in ENT anaesthesia. *Anaesthesia* 1995;**50**:898–900.

4 Ruby RRF, Webster AC, Morley-Forster PK, Dain S. Laryngeal mask airway in paediatric otolaryngologic surgery. *J Otolaryngol* 1996;**24**:288–291.

5 Al-Hasani A. Resistance to constant air flow imposed by the standard laryngeal mask, the reinforced laryngeal mask airway and RAE tubes. *Br J Anaesth* 1993;**71**:594–596.

6 Brain AIJ. *The Intavent laryngeal mask – instruction manual.* London: Intavent, 1991;1–58.

7 Christie IW. A means of stabilising laryngeal mask airways during dental procedures. *Anaesthesia* 1996;**51**:604.

8 Ravalia A, Steele A. Reinforced laryngeal mask airway and nasal surgery. *Anaesthesia* 1996;**51**:286.

★ 9 Quinn AC, Samaan A, McAteer EM, Moss E, Vucevic M. The reinforced laryngeal mask airway for dento-alveolar surgery. *Br J Anaesth* 1996;**77**:185–188.
Randomized prospective study of 100 patients comparing the flexible LMA with the RAE tube for dentoalveolar surgery. Showed that the devices performed the same, but epistaxis and aspiration of blood more common with the RAE tube and transient airway obsruction more common with the flexible LMA.

★ 10 Young TM. The laryngeal mask in dental anaesthesia. *Eur J Anaesthesiol* 1991;**4**:53–59.
Early report of LMA usage for dental surgery in 421 patients. Showed that 2% had persistent partial airway obstruction. Was published before the availability of the flexible LMA.

11 Heath ML, Sinnathamby SW. The reinforced laryngeal mask airway for adenotonsillectomy. *Br J Anaesth* 1994;**72**:728–729.

★ 12 Williams PJ, Bailey PM. Comparison of the reinforced laryngeal mask airway and tracheal intubation for adenotonsillectomy. *Br J Anaesth* 1993;**70**:30–33.
Randomized prospective study of 104 patients undergoing adenotonsillectomy with the flexible LMA or tracheal tube. Showed that emergence was smoother and there was less aspiration of blood with the flexible LMA.

★ 13 Webster AC, Morley-Forster PK, Dain S, et al. Anaesthesia for adenotonsillectomy: a comparison between tracheal intubation and the armoured laryngeal mask airway. *Can J Anaesth* 1993;**40**:1171–1177.
Randomized prospective study of 110 patients undergoing adenotonsillectomy with the flexible LMA or tracheal tube. Showed the LMA to be superior and found there was a learning curve with the technique.

14 Ebata T, Nishiki S, Masuda A, Amaha K. Anaesthesia for Treacher Collins syndrome using a laryngeal mask airway. *Can J Anaesth* 1991;**38**:1043–1045.

15 Daum RE, O'Reilly BJ. The laryngeal mask airway in ENT surgery. *J Laryngol Otol* 1992;**106**:28–30.

16 Bing J. Masque larynge pour reduction de fracture du nez. *Ann Fr Anesth Reanim* 1991;**10**:494.

★ 17 Williams PJ, Thompsett C, Bailey PM. Comparison of the reinforced laryngeal mask airway and tracheal intubation for nasal surgery. *Anaesthesia* 1995;**50**:987–989.
Prospective study of 65 patients undergoing nasal surgery with the tracheal tube (removed deep) versus FLMA (removed awake). Showed that the FLMA had better emergence characteristics. Recommend leaving FLMA in situ.

18 Rheineck Leyssius AT, Vos RJ, Blommesteijn R, Kalkman CJ. Use of the laryngeal mask airway versus orotracheal intubation to secure a patient airway in rhinoplastic surgery. *Anesthesiology* 1994;**81**:A1293 (Abstract).

19 Dain SL, Webster AC, Morley-Forster P, Ruby R, Weberpals J, Cook MJ. Propofol for insertion of the laryngeal mask airway for short ENT procedures in children. *Anesth Analg* 1996;**82**:S83 (Abstract).

20 Johnston DF, Wrigley SR, Robb PJ, Jones HE. The laryngeal mask airway in paediatric anaesthesia. *Anaesthesia* 1990;**45**:924–927.

21 Watcha MF, Garner FT, White PF, Lusk R. Laryngeal mask airway vs face mask and Guedel airway during pediatric myringotomy. *Arch Otolaryngol Head Neck Surg* 1994;**120**:877–880.

22 Ravalia D, Kumar N. Rotation of reinforced laryngeal mask airway. *Anaesthesia* 1994;**49**:541–542.

23 Brain AIJ. Rotation of reinforced laryngeal mask airway. *Anaesthesia* 1994;**49**:542.

24 Terada H, Ootaka H, Ohta S, Suzuki MI. Airway obstruction due to pus from sinusitis during the use of the LM. *J Clin Anesth (Rinsho-Masui)* 1993;**17**:673–674.

25 Bone ME, Galler D, Flynn PJ. Arterial oxygen saturation during general anaesthesia for paediatric dental extractions. *Anaesthesia* 1987;**42**:879–882.

26 Allen NA, Rowbotham DJ, Nimmo WS. Hypoxaemia during outpatient dental anaesthesia. *Anaesthesia* 1989;**44**:509–511.

27 George JM, Sanders GM. The reinforced laryngeal mask in paediatric outpatient dental surgery. *11th World Congress of Anesthesiology, Sydney, 14–20 April 1996, Abstract Handbook*, p.477 (Abstract).

28 Goodwin A, Ogg TW, Lamb W, Adlam D. The reinforced laryngeal mask airway in dental day surgery. *Ambulatory Surg* 1993;**1**:31–35.

29 Latto IP. Management of difficult intubation. In: Latto IP, Rosen M, eds. *Difficulties in tracheal intubation*. London: Baillière Tindall, 1987;99–141.

30 Noble H, Wooller DJ. Laryngeal masks and chair dental anaesthesia. *Anaesthesia* 1991;**46**:591.

31 Bailie R, Barnett MB, Fraser JF. The Brain laryngeal mask – a comparative study with the nasal mask in paediatric dental outpatients. *Anaesthesia* 1991;**46**:358–360.

32 Brain AI, McGhee TD, McAteer EJ, Thomas A, Abu Saad MA, Bushman JA. The laryngeal mask airway. Development and preliminary trials of a new type of airway. *Anaesthesia* 1985;**40**:356–361.

33 Mason DG, Bingham RM. The laryngeal mask airway in children. *Anaesthesia* 1990;**45**:760–763.

34 Beveridge ME. Laryngeal mask anaesthesia for repair of cleft palate. *Anaesthesia* 1989;**44**:656–657.

35 Zagnoev M, McCloskey J, Martin T. Fiberoptic intubation via the laryngeal mask airway. *Anesth Analg* 1994;**78**:813–814.

36 Allen JG, Flower EA. The Brain laryngeal mask. An alternative to difficult intubation. *Br Dent J* 1990;**168**:202–204.

37 Judkins KC. When the chips are down – the laryngeal mask in anger. *Anaesthesia* 1993;**48**:353.

38 Stott SA. Use of the laryngeal mask airway in the developing world. *Anaesthesia* 1993;**48**:450.

39 Kadota Y, Oda T, Yoshimura N. Application of a laryngeal mask to a fiberoptic bronchoscope-aided tracheal intubation. *J Clin Anesth* 1992;**4**:503–504.

40 Mecklem D, Brimacombe J, Yarker J. Glossopexy in Pierre Robin sequence using the laryngeal mask airway. *J Clin Anesth* 1995;**7**:267–269.

41 Brimacombe J, Berry A, van Duren P. Use of a size 2 laryngeal mask airway to relieve life threatening hypoxia in an adult with quinsy. *Anaesth Intens Care* 1993;**21**:475–476.

★ **42** Sher M, Brimacombe J, Laing D. Anaesthesia for laser pharyngoplasty – a comparison of the tracheal tube versus reinforced laryngeal mask airway. *Anaesth Intens Care* 1995;**23**:149–154.
Unblinded comparative study of the flexible LMA and tracheal tube for laser pharyngoplasty. Demonstrates fewer airway problems with the FLMA.

43 Dubreuil M, Cros AM, Boudey C, Esteben D, Milacic M. Is adenoidectomy in children safer with laryngeal mask than with facial mask or with endotracheal intubation. *Abstract of presentation at Bordeaux International Congress, 2–3 July 1992* (Abstract).

44 Fiani N, Scandella C, Giolitto N, Prudhomme G, Leon A. Comparison of reinforced laryngeal mask vs endotracheal tube in tonsillectomy. *Anesthesiology* 1994;**81**:A491 (Abstract).

45 Williams PJ, Bailey PM. The reinforced laryngeal mask airway for adenotonsillectomy. *Br J Anaesth* 1994;**72**:729.

46 Puig C, Parizot P, Hayem C, et al. Masque larynge pour adenoidectomie chez l'enfant. *SPAR conference September* 1992;R161 (Abstract).

47 Versichelen L, Van Der Schueren G, Mergaert C, Rolly G. The use of the laryngeal mask airway during short lasting ENT surgery in children. *Abstract of presentation at Bordeaux International Congress, 2–3 July 1992* (Abstract).

48 Tachoires D, Andres J. Laryngeal mask and tonsilectomies. *Abstract of presentation at Bordeaux International Congress, 2–3 July 1992* (Abstract).

49 Alexander CA. A modified Intavent laryngeal mask for ENT and dental anaesthesia. *Anaesthesia* 1990;**45**:892–893.

50 van Heerden PV, Kirrage D. Large tonsils and the laryngeal mask airway. *Anaesthesia* 1989;**44**:703.

51 Hackmann T. Anaesthesia for adenotonsillectomy. *Can J Anaesth* 1994;**41**:757–758.

52 Webster AC, Morley PK, Dain S, Ganapathy S. Anaesthesia for adenotonsillectomy. *Can J Anaesth* 1994;**41**:758.

53 Brimacombe J, Clarke G, Simons S. The laryngeal mask airway for endoscopic guided percutaneous tracheostomy. *Anaesthesia* 1994;**49**:358–359.

54 Garbin GS, Bogetz MS, Grekin RC, Frieden IJ. The laryngeal mask as an airway during laser treatment of port wine stains. *Anesthesiology* 1992;**75**:A953 (Abstract).

55 Epstein RH, Halmi W. Oxygen leakage around the laryngeal mask airway during laser treatment of port wine stains in children. *Anesthesiology* 1993;**79**:A1154 (Abstract).

56 Divatia JV, Sareen R, Upadhye SM, Sharma KS, Shelgaonkar JR. Anaesthetic management of tracheal surgery using the laryngeal mask airway. *Anaesth Intens Care* 1994;**22**:69–73.

57 Slinger P, Robinson R, Shennib H, Benumof JL, Eisenkraft JB. Alternative technique for laser resection of a carinal obstruction. *J Cardiothoracic Anesth* 1992;**6**:749–755.

58 Brimacombe J, Sher M, Berry A. The reinforced laryngeal mask airway for laser pharyngoplasty. *Anaesthesia* 1993;**48**:1105.

59 McCulloch T, Jones MR, O'Neill A. Safety of the laryngeal mask with the flash-pumped dye laser. *11th World Congress of Anesthesiology, Sydney, 14–20 April 1996, Abstract Handbook*, p.615 (Abstract).

60 Sosis MB. Evaluation of five metallic tapes for protection of endotracheal tubes during CO_2 laser surgery. *Anesth Analg* 1989;**68**:392–393.

61 Sosis MB, Dillon F. Prevention of CO_2 laser-induced endotracheal tube fires with the Laser-Guard protective coating. *J Clin Anesth* 1992;**4**:25–27.

62 Brimacombe J. The incendiary characteristics of the laryngeal and reinforced laryngeal mask airway to CO_2 laser strike – a comparison with two polyvinyl chloride tracheal tubes. *Anaesth Intens Care* 1994;**22**:694–697.

63 Lumb AB, Wrigley MW. The effect of nitrous oxide on laryngeal mask cuff pressure. In vitro and in vivo studies. *Anaesthesia* 1992;**47**:320–323.

64 Biro P. Damage to laryngeal masks during sterilisation. *Anesth Analg* 1993;**77**:1079.

65 Pennant JH, Gajraj NM. Lasers and the laryngeal mask airway. *Anaesthesia* 1994;**49**:448–449.

66 Brimacombe J, Sher M. The laryngeal mask airway for laser surgery to the pharynx. *Anaesthesia* 1994;**49**:1009.

67 Tully A, Brantiscano T, Loring SH, Engel LA. Influence of posterior cricoarytenoid muscle activity on pressure-flow relationship of the larynx. *J Appl Physiol* 1991;**70**:2252–2258.

68 Andoh K, Shima T, Tajima T, Hoshi K, Hashimoto Y. [Perioperative management of uvulopalatopharyngoplasty for the obstructive sleep apnea patient]. *Masui* 1992;**41**:140–144.

69 Dodds C, Ryall DM. Tonsils, obesity and obstructive apnoea. *Br J Hosp Med* 1992;**47**:62–66.

70 Rose DK, Cohen MM. The airway: problems and predictions in 18 500 patients. *Can J Anaesth* 1994;**41**:372–383.

71 McCrirrick A, Ramage DT, Pracilio JA, Hickman JA. Experience with the laryngeal mask airway in two hundred patients. *Anaesth Intens Care* 1991;**19**:256–260.

72 Tanigawa K, Inoue Y, Iwata S. Protection of recurrent laryngeal nerve during neck surgery: a new combination of neurotracer, laryngeal mask airway, and fiberoptic bronchoscope. *Anesthesiology* 1991;**74**:966–967.

73 Hardingham M, Hills MM. Laryngeal mask. *Br Med J* 1993;**306**:580–581.

74 Kalapac S, Donald S, Brimacombe J. Laryngeal mask biopsy! *Anaesth Intens Care* 1996;**24**:283.

75 Maltby JR, Loken RG, Beriault MT, Archer DP. Laryngeal mask airway with mouth opening less than 20 mm. *Can J Anaesth* 1995;**42**:1140–1142.

76 Stoelting RK, Miller RD. Central nervous system disease. In: *Basics of anesthesia*. New York: Churchill Livingstone, 1994;331–341.

77 Smith JS, Roizen MF, Cahalan MK. Does anesthetic technique make a difference? Augmentation of systolic blood pressure during carotid end-arterectomy: effects of phenylephrine versus light anesthesia and of isoflurane versus halothane on the incidence of myocardial ischemia. *Anesthesiology* 1988;**69**:846.

78 Asiddao CB, Donegan JH, Whitesell RC, Kalbfeisch JH. Factors associated with perioperative complications during carotid endarterectomy. *Anesth Analg* 1982;**61**:631.

79 Ng WS. Pathophysiological effects of tracheal intubation. In: Latto IP, Rosen M, eds. *Difficulties in tracheal intubation*. London: Baillière Tindall, 1984;12–35.

★ **80** Costa e Silva L, Brimacombe J. The laryngeal mask for carotid endarterectomy. *J Cardiothoracic and Vascular Anesth* 1996;**10**:972–973.
Report of LMA usage for carotid endarterectomy in four patients.

81 Thomson KD. Laryngeal mask airway for elective tracheostomy. *Anaesthesia* 1992;**47**:76.

82 Foster SJ, Clowes NW. Laryngeal mask airway for coronary artery bypass grafting. *Anaesthesia* 1991;**46**:701.

83 Denny NM, Desilva KD, Webber PA. Laryngeal mask airway for emergency tracheostomy in a neonate. *Anaesthesia* 1990;**45**:895.

84 Calder I, Ordman AJ, Jackowski A, Crockard HA. The Brain laryngeal mask airway. An alternative to emergency tracheal intubation. *Anaesthesia* 1990;**45**:137–139.

85 Dalrymple G, Lloyd E. Laryngeal mask: a more secure airway than intubation? *Anaesthesia* 1992;**47**:712–713.

86 Lee JJ, Yau K, Barcroft J. LMA and respiratory arrest after anterior cervical fusion. *Can J Anaesth* 1993;**40**:395–396.

87 Pennant JH, Gajraj NM, Yamanouchi KJ. The laryngeal mask airway and laryngeal polyposis. *Anesthesiology* 1994;**78**:1206–1207.

88 Wheatley RS, Stainthorp SF. Intubation of a one-day-old baby with the Pierre–Robin syndrome via a laryngeal mask. *Anaesthesia* 1994;**49**:733.

89 Pennant JH, Gajraj NM, Griffith K. Puncture of the laryngeal mask airway cuff. *Anaesthesia* 1994;**49**:448.

90 Weinberger J, Tanna N. Use of Intavent Laryngeal Mask Airway. *J Otolaryngol* 1994;**23**:73.

91 Dalmeida RE, Mayhew J, Gallagher T, Herring LE. The laryngeal mask airway: a must in the obstetric suite. *J Clin Anesth* (in press).

92 Dexter TJ. The laryngeal mask airway: a method to improve visualisation of the trachea and larynx during fibreoptic assisted percutaneous tracheostomy. *Anaesth Intens Care* 1994;**22**:35–39.

93 Dexter TJ. Laryngeal oedema, a marker of an 'at risk' airway. *Anaesthesia* 1994;**49**:826.

94 Ip-Yam C, Shaw S. The laryngeal mask airway and endoscopic guided percutaneous tracheostomy. *Anaesthesia* 1994;**49**:733–734.

95 Brimacombe J, Clarke G. Rigid bronchoscope: a possible new option for percutaneous dilatational tracheostomy. *Aesthesiology* 1995;**83**:647–648.

96 Brain AIJ. The development of the laryngeal mask – a brief history of the invention, early clinical studies and experimental work from which the laryngeal mask evolved. *Eur J Anaesthesiol* 1991;**4**:5–17.

★ 97 Brimacombe J, Sher M, Laing D, Berry A. The laryngeal mask airway: a new technique for fiberoptic guided vocal cord biopsy. *J Clin Anesth* 1996;**8**:273–275.
Pilot study of 10 patients undergoing vocal cord biopsy via the LMA. Showed minimal hemodynamic responses during the procedure. Adequate samples obtained in all patients.

98 Lee SK, Hong KH, Choe H, Song HS. Comparison of the effects of the laryngeal mask airway and endotracheal intubation on vocal function. *Br J Anaesth* 1993;**71**:648–650.

99 Wilson IG, Fell D, Robinson SL, Smith G. Cardiovascular responses to insertion of the laryngeal mask. *Anaesthesia* 1992;**47**:300–302.

100 Briggs RJS, Bailey P, Howard DJ. The laryngeal mask: a new type of airway in anesthesia for direct laryngoscopy. *Otolaryngol Head Neck Surg* 1992;**107**:603–605.

101 Benumof JL. The rigid bronchoscope: gold standard technique for laser resection of a carinal tumour. *J Cardiothoracic Anesth* 1992;**6**:753.

102 Catala JC, Garcia-Pedrajas F, Carrera J, Monedero P. Placement of an endotracheal device via the laryngeal mask airway in a patient with tracheal stenosis. *Anesthesiology* 1996;**84**:239–240.

103 Eckhardt III WF, Forman S, Denman W, Grillo HC, Muehrcke D. Another use for the laryngeal mask airway – as a blocker during tracheoplasty. *Anesth Analg* 1995;**80**:622–624.

104 Uchiyama M, Yoshino A. Insertion of the Montgomery T-tube. *Anaesthesia* 1995;**50**:476–477.

105 Akhtar TM, Shankar RK, Street MK. Is Guedel's airway and facemask dead? *Today's Anaesthetist* 1994;**9**:56–58.

106 Greatorex RA, Denny NM. Application of the laryngeal mask airway to thyroid surgery and the preservation of the recurrent laryngeal nerve. *Ann Roy Coll Surg Engl* 1991;**73**:352–354.

107 Akhtar TM. Laryngeal mask airway and visualisation of vocal cords during thyroid surgery. *Can J Anaesth* 1991;**38**:140.

108 Premachandra DJ. Application of the laryngeal mask airway to thyroid surgery and the preservation of the recurrent laryngeal nerve. *Ann Roy Coll Surg Engl* 1992;**74**:226.

109 Goldik Z, Lazarovici H, Baron E, Heifetz M, Krausz M, Cohen O. Continuous fibreoptic video laryngoscopy through the laryngeal mask during thyroidectomy. *Br J Anaesth* 1995;**74**:13 (Abstract).

110 Hobbiger HE, Allen JG, Greatorex RG, Denny NM. The laryngeal mask airway for thyroid and parathyroid surgery. *Anaesthesia* 1996;**51**:972–974.

111 Ready AR, Barnes J. Complications of thyroidectomy. *Br J Anaesth* 1994;**81**:1555–1556.

112 Marthensson H, Terins J. Recurrent laryngeal nerve palsy in thyroid gland surgery related to operations and nerves at risk. *Arch Surg* 1985;**120**:475–477.

113 Charters P, Cave-Bigley D. Application of the laryngeal mask airway to thyroid surgery and the preservation of the recurrent laryngeal nerve. *Ann Roy Coll Surg Engl* 1992;**74**:225–226.

114 Charters P, Cave-Bigley D, Roysam CS, Tanigawa K, Inoue Y, Iwata S. Should a laryngeal mask be routinely used in patients undergoing thyroid surgery? *Anesthesiology* 1991;**75**:918–919.

115 Wade JSH. Respiratory obstruction in thyroid surgery. *Ann Roy Coll Surg Engl* 1980;**62**:15–24.

116 Asai T, Morris S. The laryngeal mask airway: its features, effects and role. *Can J Anaesth* 1994;**41**:930–960.

117 Maroof M, Siddique M, Khan RM. Post-thyroidectomy vocal cord examination by fibreoscopy aided by the laryngeal mask airway. *Anaesthesia* 1992;**47**:445.

118 Rowbottom SJ, Morton CPJ. Diagnostic fibreoptic bronchoscopy using the laryngeal mask. *Anaesthesia* 1991;**46**:161.

119 Maroof M, Khan RM, Cooper T, Siddique MS, Saqib N. Post thyroidectomy vocal cord examination using LMA aided fiberoscopy. *Anesthesiology* 1993;**79**:A1083 (Abstract).

120 Stott S, Riley R. Visualising the airway after thyroidectomy. *Anaesth Intens Care* 1994;**22**:121.

121 Palomba R, Scibelli G, De Robertis E, Bardari G. Laryngeal mask airway use in clinical anaesthesia: our trends. *10th Postgraduate Course in Critical Care Medicine, Trieste, Italy, 13–19 November 1995* (Abstract).

122 Denny NM, Gadelrab R. Complications following general anaesthesia for cataract surgery: a comparison of the laryngeal mask airway with tracheal intubation. *J Roy Soc Med* 1993;**86**:521–522.

123 Holden R, Morsman CD, Butler J, Clark GS, Hughes DS, Bacon PJ. Intra-ocular pressure changes using the laryngeal mask airway and tracheal tube. *Anaesthesia* 1991;**46**:922–924.

124 Akhtar TM, McMurray P, Kerr WJ, Kenny GNC. A comparison of laryngeal mask airway with tracheal tube for intra-ocular ophthalmic surgery. *Anaesthesia* 1992;**47**:668–671.

125 Watcha MF, White PF, Tychsen L, Steven JL. Comparative effects of laryngeal mask airway and endotracheal tube insertion on intraocular pressure in children. *Anesth Analg* 1992;**75**:355–360.

126 Verghese C, Smith TGC, Young E. Prospective survey of the use of the laryngeal mask airway in 2359 patients. *Anaesthesia* 1993;**48**:58–60.

127 Watcha MF, White PF, Tyschen L, Stevens JL. Comparison of intraocular pressure changes with laryngeal mask or tracheal tube insertion. *Anesthesiology* 1992;**77**:A1175 (Abstract).

128 Daum REO, Downes RN, Vardy S. Day-stay cataract surgery under general anaesthesia. *Today's Anaesthetist* 1992;7:24–28.

129 Nathanson MH, Ferguson C, Nancekievill DG. Airway maintenance for short ophthalmological procedures in children. *Anaesthesia* 1992;**47**:542.

130 Thomson KD. The effect of the laryngeal mask airway on coughing after eye surgery under general anaesthetic. *Ophthalmic Surg* 1992;**23**:630–631.

131 Thomson JPS. Eye movement during cataract surgery. *Anaesth Intens Care* 1993;**21**:376.

132 Lamb K, James MFM, Janicki PK. The laryngeal mask airway for intraocular surgery: effects on intraocular pressure and stress responses. *Br J Anaesth* 1992;**69**:143–147.

133 Ripart J, Cohendy R, Eledjam JJ. The laryngeal mask airway and intraocular surgery. *Br J Anaesth* 1993;**70**:704.

134 Barclay K, Wall T, Wareham K, Asai T. Intra-ocular pressure changes in patients with glaucoma – comparison between the laryngeal mask airway and tracheal tube. *Anaesthesia* 1994;**49**:159–162.

135 Balog CC, Bogetz MS, Good WH, Way WL, Hoyt CS. The laryngeal mask is an ideal airway for many outpatient pediatric ophthalmologic procedures. *Anesth Analg* 1994;**78**:S17 (Abstract).

★ 136 Myint Y, Singh AK, Peacock JE, Padfield A. Changes in intra-ocular pressure during general anaesthesia. A comparison of spontaneous breathing through a laryngeal mask with positive pressure ventilation through a tracheal tube. *Anaesthesia* 1995;**50**:126–129.

Prospective study of 40 patients suggesting that spontaneous ventilation via the FLMA is suitable for intraocular surgery provided anesthetic depth is adequate.

137 Wainwright AC. Positive pressure ventilation and the laryngeal mask airway in ophthalmic anaesthesia. *Br J Anaesth* 1995;**75**:249–250.

138 Langenstein H, Moller F, Krause R, Kluge R, Vogelsang H. Die Handhabung der Larynxmaske bei Augenoperationen. *Congress on Anaesthesia in Eye Surgery, Congress-Centrum Stadtpark, Hannover, 10–11 May 1996* (Abstract).

139 Barontini G, Scarani F, Negri M. Uso della maschera laringea in chirurgia oculistica. *Minerva Anestesiol* 1995;**61**:3–6.

140 Janke EL, Fletcher JE, Lewis IH. Anaesthetic management of the Kenny–Caffey syndrome using the laryngeal mask. *Paediatr Anaesth* 1996;**6**:235–238.

141 Fuchs K, Kukule I, Knoch M, Wiegand W. Larynxmaske versus Intubation bei erschwerten Intubationsbedingungen beim Franceschetti–Zwahlen–Klein-Syndrom (Treacher–Collins-Syndrom). *Anaesthesiol Intensivmed Notfalmed Schmerzther* 1993;**28**:190–192.

142 Alexander R. The laryngeal mask airway and ocular surgery. *Can J Anaesth* 1993;**40**:901–902.

143 Milligan KA. Laryngeal mask in the prone position. *Anaesthesia* 1994;**49**:449.

144 McCartney CA, Wilkinson DJ, Rabey PG, et al. The laryngeal mask airway and intra-ocular surgery. *Anaesthesia* 1992;**47**:445–446.

145 Brimacombe J, Berry A. The laryngeal mask airway for intra-ocular surgery. *Anaesthesia* 1993;**48**:827.

146 Haden RM, Pinnock CA, Campbell RL. The laryngeal mask for intraocular surgery. *Br J Anaesth* 1993;**71**:772.

147 Brimacombe J, Aebersold R, Smith J. The laryngeal mask for ophthalmic splash injuries. *Today's Anaesthetist* 1996;**11**:52.

148 Herrick MJ, Kennedy DJ. Airway obstruction and the laryngeal mask airway in paediatric radiotherapy. *Anaesthesia* 1992;**47**:910.

149 Marjot R. Trauma to the posterior pharyngeal wall caused by a laryngeal mask airway. *Anaesthesia* 1991;**46**:589–590.

150 Waite K, Filshie J. The use of a laryngeal mask airway for CT radiotherapy planning and daily radiotherapy. *Anaesthesia* 1990;**45**:894.

151 Taylor DH, Child CSB. The laryngeal mask for radiotherapy in children. *Anaesthesia* 1990;**45**:690.

152 Leach AB, Alexander CA. The laryngeal mask – an overview. *Eur J Anaesthesiol* 1991;**4**:19–31.

153 Langton JA, Wilson I, Fell D. Use of the laryngeal mask airway during magnetic resonance imaging. *Anaesthesia* 1992;**47**:532.

154 Rafferty C, Burke AM, Cossar DF, Farling PA. Laryngeal mask and magnetic resonance imaging. *Anaesthesia* 1990;**45**:591–592.

155 Van Obbergh LJ, Muller G, Zeippen B, Dooms G. Propofol (P) infusion (I) and laryngeal mask (LMA) for magnetic resonance imaging (MRI) in children. *Anesthesiology* 1992;**77**:A1177 (Abstract).

156 Puig C, Parizot P. [Laryngeal mask in anesthesia for magnetic resonance imaging in children (letter)]. *Ann Fr Anesth Reanim* 1992;**11**:608.

157 Stevens JE, Burden G. Reinforced laryngeal mask airway and magnetic resonance imaging. *Anaesthesia* 1994;**49**:79–80.

158 Conci F, Arosio M, Gramegna M, Rota E, Boselli L. La maschera laringea in neurochirurgia, neuroradiologia e neurorianimazione. *Minerva Anestesiol* 1995;**61**:17–21.

159 Russell R, Judkins KC. The laryngeal mask airway and facial burns. *Anaesthesia* 1990;**45**:894.

160 Moylan SL, Luce MA. The reinforced laryngeal mask airway in paediatric radiotherapy. *Br J Anaesth* 1993;**71**:172.

161 Harmer M. Complications of tracheal intubation. In: Latto IP, Rosen M, eds. *Difficulties in tracheal intubation.* London: Baillière Tindall, 1987;36–48.

162 Brimacombe J, Berry A. Airway management during gynaecological laparoscopy – is it safe to use the laryngeal mask airway? *Ambulatory Surg* 1995;**3**:65–70.

163 Tang CS, Tsai LK, Lee TH, et al. [The hemodynamic and ventilatory effects between Trendelenburg and reverse Trendelenburg position during laparoscopy with CO_2-insufflation]. *Ma Tsui Hsueh Tsa Chi* 1993;**31**:217–224.

164 Cotton BR, Smith G. Single and combined effects of atropine and metoclopramide on the lower oesophageal sphincter pressure. *Br J Anaesth* 1981;**53**:869–874.

165 Duffy BL. Regurgitation during pelvic laparoscopy. *Br J Anaesth* 1979;**51**:1089–1090.

166 Carlsson C, Islander G. Silent gastropharyngeal regurgitation during anesthesia. *Anesth Analg* 1981;**60**:655–657.

167 Kurer FL, Welch DB. Gynaecological laparoscopy: clinical experiences of two anaesthetic techniques. *Br J Anaesth* 1984;**56**:1207–1211.

168 *Gynaecological laparoscopy: The report of the working party of the confidential enquiry into gynaecological laparoscopy.* London: The Royal College of Obstetricians and Gynaecologists, 1978.

169 Scott DB. Regurgitation during laparoscopy. *Br J Anaesth* 1980;**52**:559.

170 Wong HC, Nkana CA. In the real world. In: Wetchler BV, ed. *Anesthesia for ambulatory surgery.* Philadelphia: Lippincott, 1985;357–395.

171 Scott DB. Some effects of peritoneal insufflation of carbon dioxide at laparoscopy. *Anaesthesia* 1970;**25**:590.

172 Jones MJ, Mitchell RW, Hindocha N. Effect of increased intra-abdominal pressure during laparoscopy on the lower esophageal sphincter. *Anesth Analg* 1989;**68**:63–65.

173 Roberts CJ, Goodman NW. Gastro-oesophageal reflux during elective laparoscopy. *Anaesthesia* 1990;**45**:1009–1011.

174 Dingley J, Asai T. Insertion methods of the laryngeal mask airway. A survey of current practice in Wales. *Anaesthesia* 1996;**51**:596–599.

★ **175** Verghese C, Brimacombe J. Survey of laryngeal mask usage in 11 910 patients – safety and efficacy for conventional and nonconventional usage. *Anesth Analg* 1996;**82**:129–133.
Prospective survey of 11 910 LMA anesthetics which includes over 2000 patients undergoing either lower abdominal surgery or gynecological laparoscopy. There was no difference in complication rates compared with more conventional usage.

176 Akhtar TM, Street MK. Risk of aspiration with the laryngeal mask. *Br J Anaesth* 1994;**72**:447–450.

177 Wilkinson PA, Cyna AM, MacLeod DM, Campbell JR, Criswell J, John R. The laryngeal mask: cautionary tales. *Anaesthesia* 1990;**45**:167–168.

178 Goodwin APL, Rowe WL, Ogg TW. Day case laparoscopy – a comparison of two anaesthetic techniques using the laryngeal mask during spontaneous breathing. *Anaesthesia* 1992;**47**:892–895.

179 Swann DG, Spens H, Edwards SA, Chestnut RJ. Anaesthesia for gynaecological laparoscopy – a comparison between the laryngeal mask airway and tracheal intubation. *Anaesthesia* 1993;**48**:431–434.

180 Brimacombe J. Laparoscopy and the laryngeal mask airway. *Br J Anaesth* 1994;**73**:121.

181 Malins AF, Cooper GM. Laparoscopy and the laryngeal mask airway. *Br J Anaesth* 1994;**73**:121.

182 Brimacombe J, Berry A. The role of the laryngeal mask airway for failed tracheal intubation in the patient with a 'Full Stomach'. *Anesth Analg* 1994;**78**:818–819.

183 Brimacombe J. The laryngeal mask airway for abdominal surgery. *J Clin Exp Med* 1994;**171**:949–951.

184 Warner MA, Warner WE, Webber JG. Clinical significance of pulmonary aspiration during the perioperative period. *Anesthesiology* 1993;**78**:56–62.

185 Vanner RG. Gastro-oesophageal reflux and regurgitation during general anaesthesia for termination of pregnancy. *Int J Obstet Anesth* 1992;**1**:123–128.

186 Kumagai A, Iwasaki H, Kawana S, Namiki A. Laryngeal mask airway does not reduce the incidence of post-operative nausea and vomiting after gynaecological surgery. *Anesth Analg* 1996;**81**:S255 (Abstract).

187 Harada Y, Namiki A. Incidence of sore throat after endotracheal intubation is not different from that after use of the laryngeal mask airway. *11th World Congress of Anesthesiology, Sydney, 14–20 April 1996, Abstract Handbook*, p.511 (Abstract).

188 Brimacombe J. Airway protection with the new laryngeal mask prototype. *Anaesthesia* 1996;**51**:602–603.

189 Sofair E. Preanesthetic assessment – the professional singer with a difficult airway. *Anesthesiol News* 1993;**June**:4–10.

190 Brimacombe J, Berry A. Lennon, laparoscopic cholecystectomy and the laryngeal mask airway. *Anesthesiol News* 1995;4–5.

191 Okazaki H. Use of the laryngeal mask for adult patients. *J Clin Exp Med* 1992;**12**:869–868.

192 Lauretti GR, Garcia LV, De Mattos AL, Slullitel A. Anestesia epidural continua e mascare laringea para transplant renal. *Rev Brasil Anestesiol* 1995;**44**:CBA 203.

193 Hester AW, Heath ML. Pulmonary acid aspiration syndrome: should prophylaxis be routine? *Br J Anaesth* 1977;**49**:595–599.

194 Olsson GL, Hallen B, Hambraeus Jonzon K. Aspiration during anaesthesia: a computer-aided study of 185 358 anaesthetics. *Acta Anaesthesiol Scand* 1986;**30**:84–92.

195 Griffin RM, Hatcher IS. Aspiration pneumonia and the laryngeal mask airway. *Anaesthesia* 1990;**45**:1039–1040.

196 Riddell PL, Philpott B, Brain AIJ, Krapez JR, Griffin RM, Hatcher IS. Aspiration pneumonia and the laryngeal mask airway. *Anaesthesia* 1991;**46**:418–419.

197 Marco AP, Yeo CJ, Rock P. Anesthesia for a patient undergoing laparoscopic cholecystectomy. *Anesthesiology* 1990;**73**:1268–1270.

198 Brain AIJ, Verghese C, Strube P, Brimacombe J. A new laryngeal mask prototype – preliminary evaluation of seal pressures and glottic isolation. *Anaesthesia* 1995;**50**:42–48.

199 Llagunes J, Rodriguez-Hesles C, Aguar F. Laryngeal mask airway in cardiac surgery. *Can J Anaesth* 1994;**41**:1016.

200 Seung IS, Kim DW. Laryngeal mask airway – general anaesthesia with laryngeal mask airway for operation of a patient with sick-sinus syndrome. *J Kor Soc Anesthesiol* 1993;**26**:820–822.

201 Peck D, Holland R, Merry A. Paediatric cardiac catheterisation and the laryngeal mask airway. *Anaesth Intens Care* 1995;**23**:643–644 (Abstract).

202 White A, Sinclair M, Pillai R. Laryngeal mask airway for coronary artery bypass grafting. *Anaesthesia* 1991;**46**:1083.

203 White A, Sinclair M, Pillai R. Laryngeal mask airway for coronary artery bypass grafting. *Anaesthesia* 1991;**46**:234.

204 Riley RH, Swan HD. Value of the laryngeal mask airway during thoracotomy. *Anesthesiology* 1992;**77**:1051.

205 West KJ, Ahmed MI. The laryngeal mask airway in mediastinoscopy. *Anaesthesia* 1993;**48**:826–827.

206 Asai T, Morris S. The laryngeal mask and patients with 'collapsible' airways. *Anaesthesia* 1994;**49**:169–170.

207 Groudine SB, Lumb PD, Sandison MR. Pressure support ventilation with the laryngeal mask airway: a method to manage severe reactive airway disease postoperatively. *Can J Anaesth* 1995;**42**:341–343.

208 Groudine SB, Lumb PD. Noninvasive ventilatory support with the laryngeal mask airway. *Am J Anesthesiol* 1996;124–128.

209 Polaner DM. The use of heliox and the laryngeal mask airway in a child with an anterior mediastinal mass. *Anesth Analg* 1996;**82**:208–210.

210 Hattamer SJ, Dodds TM. Use of the laryngeal mask airway to manage a patient with anterior mediastinal mass. *Anesth Analg* 1995;**80**:SCA139 (Abstract).

211 Steen SN, Zelman V, Arven P, Baijat P, Apuzzo MLJ. Techniques and refinements of anaesthesia for stereotaxy. In: Apuzzo MLJ, ed. *Brain surgery: complication avoidance and management*. Los Angeles: Churchill Livingstone, 1993.

212 Graham D. Another use for the laryngeal mask airway. *Anaesthesia* 1995;**50**:368–369.

213 Costa e Silva L, Brimacombe J. The laryngeal mask airway for stereotactic implantation of fetal hypophysis. *Anesth Analg* 1996;**82**:430–431.

214 Boisson C, Camboulives J, Som SP, Regis J, Peragut JC. Propofol et masque larynge pour neuroradiochirurgie stereotaxique en pediatrie (Gamma Unit). *SFAR 36e Congres National, Paris, 30 September–2 October 1994* (Abstract).

215 Spiekermann BF, Stone DJ, Bogdonoff DL, Yemen TA. Airway management in neuroanaesthesia. *Can J Anaesth* 1996;**43**:820–834.

216 Shapiro HM, Drummond JC. Neurosurgical anesthesia. In: Miller RD, ed. *Anesthesia*. Melbourne: Churchill Livingstone, 1995;1897–1946.

217 Hagberg C, Berry J, Haque S. The laryngeal mask for awake craniotomy in pediatric patients. *Anesthesiology* 1995;**83**:A184 (Abstract).

218 Costa e Silva L, Brimacombe J. Tracheal tube/laryngeal mask exchange for emergence. *Anesthesiology* 1996;**85**:218.

219 Ammar T, Towley RM. The laryngeal mask airway. *Anaesthesia* 1990;**45**:75.

220 Simpson FG, Arnold AG, Purvis A, Belfield PW, Muers MF, Cooke NJ. Postal survey of bronchoscopic practice by physicians in the United Kingdom. *Thorax* 1986;**41**:311–317.

221 Rogers SN, Benumof JL. New and easy techniques for fiberoptic endoscopy-aided tracheal intubation. *Anesthesiology* 1983;**59**:569–572.

222 Patil V, Stehling LC, Zauder HL, Koch JP. Mechanical aids for fiberoptic endoscopy. *Anesthesiology* 1982;**57**:69–70.

223 Higgins MS, Marco AP. An aid to oral fiberoptic intubation. *Anesthesiology* 1996;77:1236–1237.

224 Frei FJ, Wengen DF, Rutishauser M, Ummenhofer W. The airway endoscopy mask: useful device for fibreoptic evaluation and intubation of the paediatric airway. *Paediatr Anaesth* 1995;5:319–324.

225 Matsushima Y, Jones RL, King EG, Moysa G, Alton JDM. Alterations in pulmonary mechanics and gas exchange during routine fiberoptic bronchoscopy. *Chest* 1984;**86**:184–188.

226 Crichlow A, Locken R, Todesco J. The laryngeal mask airway and fibreoptic laryngoscopy. *Can J Anaesth* 1992;**39**:742–743.

227 Darling JR, Keohane M, Murray JM. A split laryngeal mask as an aid to training in fibreoptic tracheal intubation. A comparison with the Berman II intubating airway. *Anaesthesia* 1993;**48**:1079–1082.

228 Maroof M, Khan RM, Khan H, Stewart J, Mroze C. Evaluation of a modified laryngeal mask airway as an aid to fibre optic intubation (FOI). *Anesthesiology* 1992;**77**:A1062 (Abstract).

229 Brimacombe J, Newell S, Swainston R, Thompson J. A potential new technique for awake fibreoptic bronchoscopy – use of the laryngeal mask airway. *Med J Aust* 1992;**156**:876–877.

230 Brimacombe J, Tucker P, Simons S. The laryngeal mask airway for awake diagnostic bronchoscopy – a study of 200 consecutive patients. *Eur J Anaesthesiol* 1995;**12**:357–361.

231 Alberge MC, Rabarijoana A, Macchi P, Pulcini A, Aime-Raucoules M, Grimaud D. Use of the laryngeal mask airway for bronchoscopy in awake patients with respiratory insufficiency. *Anesthesiology* 1994;**81**:A1462 (Abstract).

232 Walker RW, Murrell D. Yet another use for the laryngeal mask airway. *Anaesthesia* 1991;**46**:591.

233 McNamee CJ, Meyns B, Pagliero KM. Flexible bronchoscopy via the laryngeal mask: a new technique. *Thorax* 1991;**46**:141–142.

234 Maroof M, Siddique M, Khan RM. Difficult diagnostic laryngoscopy and bronchoscopy aided by the laryngeal mask airway. *J Laryngol Otol* 1992;**106**:722.

235 Smith TGC, Whittet H, Heyworth T. Laryngomalacia – a specific indication for the laryngeal mask. *Anaesthesia* 1992;**47**:910.

236 Dich-Neilsen JO, Nagel P. Flexible fibreoptic bronchoscopy via the laryngeal mask. *Acta Anaesthesiol Scand* 1993;**37**:17–19.

237 Cortes J, Franco A, Cid M, Vidal MI, Rabanal S. Uso de la mascarilla laringea para bronchoscopia fibroptica en un neonato con malformaciones faciales. *Revista Espanola* 1992;**39**:324–325.

238 Du Plessis MC, Marshall Barr A, Verghese C, Lyall JRW. Fibreoptic bronchoscopy under general anaesthesia using the laryngeal mask airway. *Eur J Anaesthesiol* 1993;**10**:363–365.

239 Lawson R, Lloyd-Thomas AR. Three diagnostic conundrums solved using the laryngeal mask airway. *Anaesthesia* 1993;**48**:790–791.

240 Bautista Casasnovas A, Estevez Martinez E, Buznego Sanchez R, Rodriguez Perez E, Cabanas Gancedo R, Varela Cives R. [Pediatric fiber bronchoscopy. A propos 55 children examined]. *An Esp Pediatr* 1993;**39**:313–316.

241 Buzzetti V, Cigada M, Solca M, Iapichino G. Use of the laryngeal mask airway during fibreoptic bronchoscopy. *Intens Care World* 1996;**13**:72–74.

242 Tatsumi K, Furuya H, Nagahata T, et al. [Removal of a bronchial foreign body in a child using the laryngeal mask]. *Masui* 1993;**42**:441–444.

243 Yahagi N, Kumon K, Tanigami H. Bronchial lavage with a fibreoptic bronchoscope via a laryngeal mask airway in an infant. *Anaesthesia* 1994;**49**:450.

244 Credle WFJ, Smiddy JF, Elliot RC. Complications of fiberoptic bronchoscopy. *Am Rev Resp Dis* 1974;**109**:67–72.

245 Suratt PM, Smiddy JF, Gruber B. Deaths and complications associated with fiberoptic bronchoscopy. *Chest* 1976;**69**:747–751.

246 Pereira W, Kovnat DM, Snider GL. A prospective comparative study of complications following fiberoptic bronchoscopy. *Chest* 1978;**73**:813–816.

247 Dresin RB, Albert RK, Talley PA, Kryger MH, Scoggin CH, Zwillich CW. Flexible fibreoptic bronchoscopy in the teaching hospital. *Chest* 1978;**74**:144–149.

248 Lukowsky GI, Ovchinnikov AA, Bilal A. Complications of rigid bronchoscopy under general anaesthesia and flexible fibreoptic bronchoscopy under topical anaesthesia. *Chest* 1981;**79**:316–321.

249 Harrison BDW. Guidelines for care during bronchoscopy. *Thorax* 1993;**48**:584.

250 Wrigley SR, Black AE, Sidhu VS. A fibreoptic laryngoscope for paediatric anaesthesia. A study to evaluate the use of the 2.2 mm Olympus (LF-P) intubating fibrescope. *Anaesthesia* 1995;**50**:709–712.

251 Samet A, Talmon Y, Frankel R, Simon K. A new diagnostic approach to congenital stridor using a laryngeal mask airway and rigid endoscope. *J Laryngol Otol* 1994;**108**:1076–1077.

14 Difficult airway

Overview

Difficult intubation

'There is one skill above all else that an anesthesiologist is expected to exhibit and that is to maintain the airway impeccably'[1]. Yet it is not always possible to succeed in every attempt at tracheal intubation or to prevent every accident. The incidence of airway problems during conventional intubation depends on the definition used[2]. Difficulty in tracheal intubation occurs in 1–3% of patients, depending on anesthetic experience[3], and intubation fails in 0.05–0.2%, being highest in the obstetric population[4,5]. Rose and Cohen, in a prospective survey of 18 500 patients, showed that tracheal intubation is not always easy, even in skilled hands, requiring three or more attempts in 2% of patients in urban teaching hospitals and with a failure rate of 0.3% using the laryngoscope[6]. The immediately life threatening 'cannot intubate, cannot ventilate' situation is rarer still, occurring in 0.01% of all anesthetics[7]. It is possible to predict a proportion of difficult airways using a variety of bedside tests, but even in optimum circumstances there is only a 22–80% chance of predicting difficult intubation[8–11] and there is large interobserver variability on the same patients[12].

The LMA does not reliably protect against aspiration and in this respect it is interesting to note that inability to successfully manage difficult airways is responsible for 30% of deaths totally attributable to anesthesia[13], whereas aspiration pneumonitis per se is an infrequent cause of anesthesia-related mortality. Eighty five per cent of all respiratory-related closed malpractice claims in the USA involve a brain-damaged or dead patient. Inadequate ventilation (33%), esophageal intubation (18%) and difficult tracheal intubation (17%) account for 68% of these claims[13]. Aspiration represents only 5% of respiratory claims against the anesthesiologist and is an uncommon adverse outcome of failed or difficult intubation[13].

Role of the LMA

The LMA has a role in the management of the difficult airway both as a substitute airway and as an aid to intubation and has been widely used in the management of the adult[14–64] (Table 14.1) and pediatric[25,65–83] difficult airway (see Chapter 16, *Pediatric difficult airway* and Table 16.1). The role of the LMA in difficult airway management has been the subject of several reviews[84–87]. The LMA is useful because it can generally

Table 14.1 Adult airway problems managed with the laryngeal mask airway

Acromegaly[*25*]	Motor vehicle accident[98]
Acute airway obstruction with HALO traction[55]	Nasopharyngeal hemorrhage[96]
Ankylosing spondylitis[40,*41*]	Neck contracture[44,95]
Ankylosis of temperomandibular joints[*61*]	Nonspecific congenital anomaly[25]
Calcinosos universalis[*25*]	Nonspecific difficult intubation[22,28,*29*,*30*,*31*,*32*,33,*34*,35–38,*39*]
Cervical spondylitis[*25*]	Oral tumor[23,*42*]
Cheek flap breakdown[90]	Ossification of the posterior longitudinal ligament[*23*]
Facial burns[43,91]	Percutaneous tracheostomy[57,58]
Failed obstetric intubation[14,15,*16*,17–21,92,93]	Post-op pharyngeal bleed[48,49]
Failed rigid bronchoscopy[51]	Quinsy[59]
Fractured jaw[54]	Rheumatoid arthritis[22,23,*24*,25,*26*,27,62]
Klippel–Feil syndrome[94]	Stridor[60]
Laryngeal edema[93]	Spinal tumor[*25*]
Limited mouth opening[95]	Tracheostomy[48,49,55,56,92]
Micrognathia[96]	Treacher Collins[53]
Micrognathia[47] (aid to blind nasal intubation)	Unstable neck[45,*46*]
Misplaced double lumen tube[52]	
Morbid obesity[*97*]	

Reference numbers in italic indicate that the LMA was also used as an airway intubator.

be inserted rapidly and accurately with a single attempt, is associated with a low incidence of tissue trauma, and is acceptable to patients requiring an awake intubation. It has also been shown that the LMA can accommodate a larger FOS than either the FLMA or tracheal tube at clinically useful ventilatory settings[88] (Figure 14.1). The difficulty in viewing the larynx which often underlies difficulty in intubation is irrelevant to LMA placement. It is therefore associated with a low risk/benefit ratio in a situation where there is a significant incidence of morbidity and mortality[13]. It is one of the three nonsurgical techniques currently recommended for use when an anesthetized patient can be neither intubated nor mask ventilated[86,89]. It is the only one of these three that is used in routine anesthesia. As such it can be practiced daily and the equipment is immediately available for use.

Placement in the abnormal airway

The success rate of LMA placement in the abnormal airway is unknown, but there are over 60 case reports (Tables 14.1 and 16.1) and four uncontrolled studies[23,25,64,99] to support the claim that LMA insertion is readily achieved in these patients. Kadota et al[23] and Silk et al[25] reported successful placement in 5/5 and 47/48 patients with predicted/known difficult airways respectively. Langenstein compared 30 patients with known abnormal airways with 50 normal patients and found LMA insertion successful in all but one patient who had limited mouth opening (10 mm)[64]. Ventilation was excellent and leak pressures were significantly higher in patients with neck radiotherapy compared with normal patients. Fiberoptic intubation was successful in all patients. Sher et al in an unblinded study of 165 patients compared insertion of the FLMA with the tracheal tube in patients undergoing laser surgery for severe snoring and found significantly fewer problems with FLMA insertion than with tracheal intubation (1.8 versus 11.6%)[99]. Although not directly assessed, the study population could be considered at high risk of having difficult airways.

Placement is probably independent of factors used to predict[100,101] or score[102] difficult intubation. McCrory and Moriarty studied 100 patients and found that LMA positioning was related to Mallampati grading[103]. The validity of this study has been questioned[104,105]. Asai found that 3/12 patients in whom LMA placement failed unexpectedly were subsequently difficult to intubate[106]. In a retrospective study of 272 patients Brimacombe and Berry found no correlation between Mallampati grade, ease of insertion or final fiberoptic position of the LMA[100]. This series included 29 grade III and three grade IV[5] patients. In a further study of 1500 adult patients undergoing LMA anesthesia in which Mallampati grades and fiberoptic scores were similarly obtained[101] there were 102 grade III and 13 grade IV. All failed placements occurred in Mallampati grades I or II. There was no correlation between fiberoptic scoring and Mallampati grade. Voyagis et al randomly allocated 435 patients to receive either a tracheal tube or LMA and found that LMA insertion was not more difficult in cases of suspected difficult intubation[107]. In a study of the size 5 LMA for positive pressure ventilation (PPV), Brimacombe showed that there was no correlation between fiberoptic score or Mallampati score and the pressure at which gastric insufflation or oropharyngeal leak occurred[108]. In all patients who were Mallampati

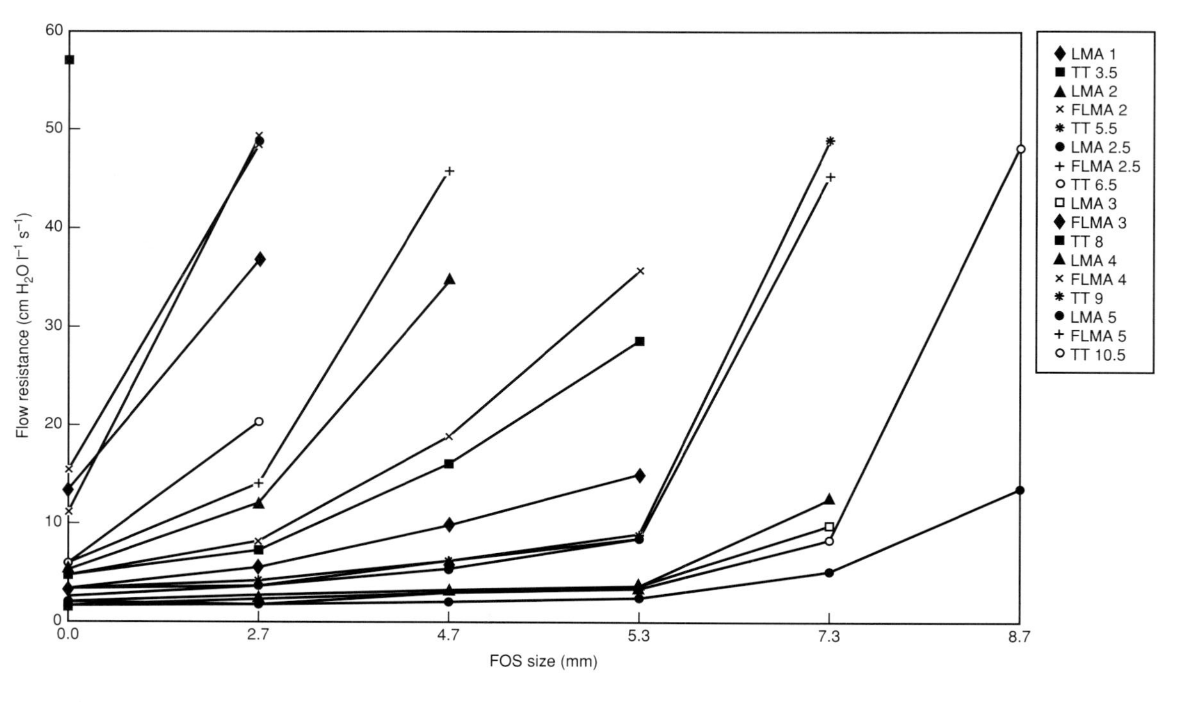

Figure 14.1 Flow resistance (cm H_2O l^{-1} s^{-1}) for the various sizes of laryngeal mask (LMA), the flexible laryngeal mask (FLMA) and tracheal tube (TT) with different sizes of fiberoptic scope (FOS) at peak flow rate of 0.5 l s^{-1}. Peak airway pressure = flow resistance × 0.5[88]. Reproduced with permission, *Anaesthesia*[88].

III LMA insertion was accomplished at the first attempt with fiberoptic scores of 3 and 4.

It has been argued that if it is difficult to see the uvula, palate and faucial pillars then blindly passing the LMA around the base of the tongue will also be difficult[103]. However, the correct path followed by the LMA during insertion is entirely posterior and parallels the process of deglutition with the index finger substituting the action of the tongue[109]. It relies on sliding the fully deflated cuff along the posterior palato-pharyngeal curve and avoiding anterior pharyngeal structures. A high Mallampati grade primarily implies that the base of the tongue is disproportionately large and this is probably irrelevant for most aspects of LMA placement[110]. It has also been suggested that the presence of an anterior larynx may make LMA insertion easier. Data from the prospective study of Mahiou et al looking at 362 patients showed that ease of insertion of the LMA did not correlate with Mallampati grade or Cormack and Lehane scoring[102]. The latter finding suggests that the position of the larynx has little bearing on LMA insertion.

Failed placement in the abnormal airway

There are several reports where LMA placement has failed in patients with difficult airways[19,25,93,94,99,111–114]. A number of patient factors may suggest difficult placement. Hyperextension of the neck may make placement more difficult by reducing the oropharyngeal angle to less than 90 degrees[114]. Laboratory work by Ishimura et al has very effectively illustrated this point[114] . Limited mouth opening, oropharyngeal pathology and cricoid pressure will impede placement by varying degrees depending on severity/force. The average distance between the upper and lower incisor teeth in patients with normal temporomandibular joint function is 47 mm with a range of 31–55 mm[115]. Maltby et al have reported successful insertion in patients with mouth opening of 12–18 mm[95]. Langenstein reported failed insertion in a patient with mouth opening of 10 mm[64]. Placement may be successful, but function inadequate, if there is glottic or subglottic pathology. Monso et al suggested that pre-induction fiberoptic nasendoscopy could be used to predict ease of insertion[116]. The authors examined 24 fit patients and found that there was an association between a posteriorly lying epiglottis at nasendoscopy and airway obstruction following LMA insertion. There was no association with large aryepiglottic folds or a large anteriorly placed epiglottis. The practical problems of this technique as a predictor of LMA insertion have been highlighted[117].

History

The potential of the new device for resuscitation and difficult airway management were appreciated shortly after its invention[118]. In February 1983, an early prototype was successfully used in a 114 kg male undergoing laparotomy who could not be intubated[42]. In 1984, writing in the *Archives of Emergency Medicine*, Brain offered the LMA as a possible new solution to airway problems in the emergency situation[119]. The following year, writing in *Anaesthesia*, Brain described its use in three cases of difficult intubation[28]. By 1985 it had been used in five patients with anticipated intubation difficulty. Fiberoptic investigation suggested the possibility of using the LMA as an airway intubator and in May/June of 1983 a prototype LMA with a 14 mm internal diameter (ID) was used to blindly intubate three patients with a size 9 mm tracheal tube (Figure 14.2)[118]. By April 1987 the LMA had been used in 21 patients in whom conventional intubation was difficult and in October 1987 it was successfully used for the first time in pediatric failed intubation[118]. In 1988, Smith reported the successful use of the LMA in 15 patients with juvenile rheumatoid arthritis[27]. In 1989, Chadd et al passed a gum elastic bougie down the LMA of two anesthetized patients and railroaded a tracheal tube after removal of the LMA[40]. The following year Allison and McCrory refined this technique by directing the bougie into the trachea under fiberoptic guidance[120]. Awake intubation via the LMA was first reported by McCrirrick and Pracilio in 1991[30]. In the same year a modification of the LMA, the split LMA, was described by Brimacombe and Johns; this overcame the problem of tracheal tube size limitation when the standard LMA was used as an airway intubator[121]. In 1993, the LMA was included in the American Society of Anesthesiologist's difficult airway algorithm. The role of the LMA in the ASA algorithm was extended in 1996[86].

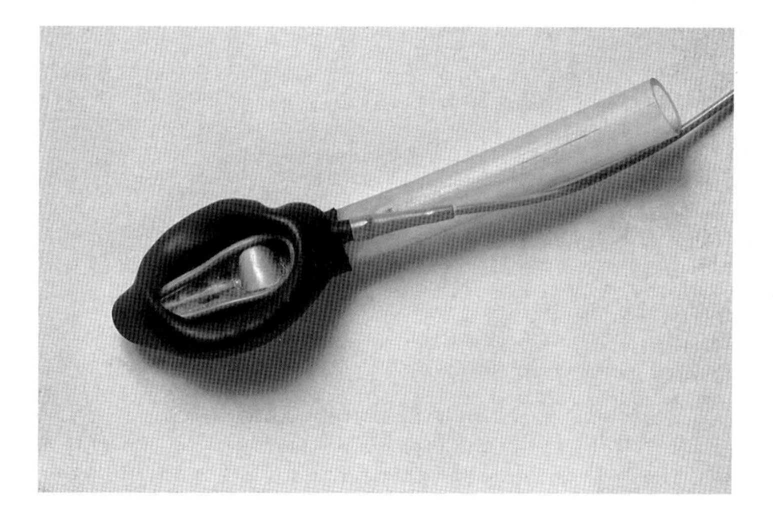

Figure 14.2 Early prototype intubating laryngeal mask (1983).

The LMA and the ASA difficult airway algorithm

The ASA algorithm was introduced in 1991 and has become the gold standard for the management of the difficult airway. At the time the algorithm was being researched (meta-analytical techniques) little was known about the LMA and, although recognized as a major advance in airway management, it was only included in the emergency airway management limb[89] (Figure 14.3). Five years later, however, the literature on and experience with the LMA had substantially increased to the extent that Benumof (who has been closely associated with development of the ASA

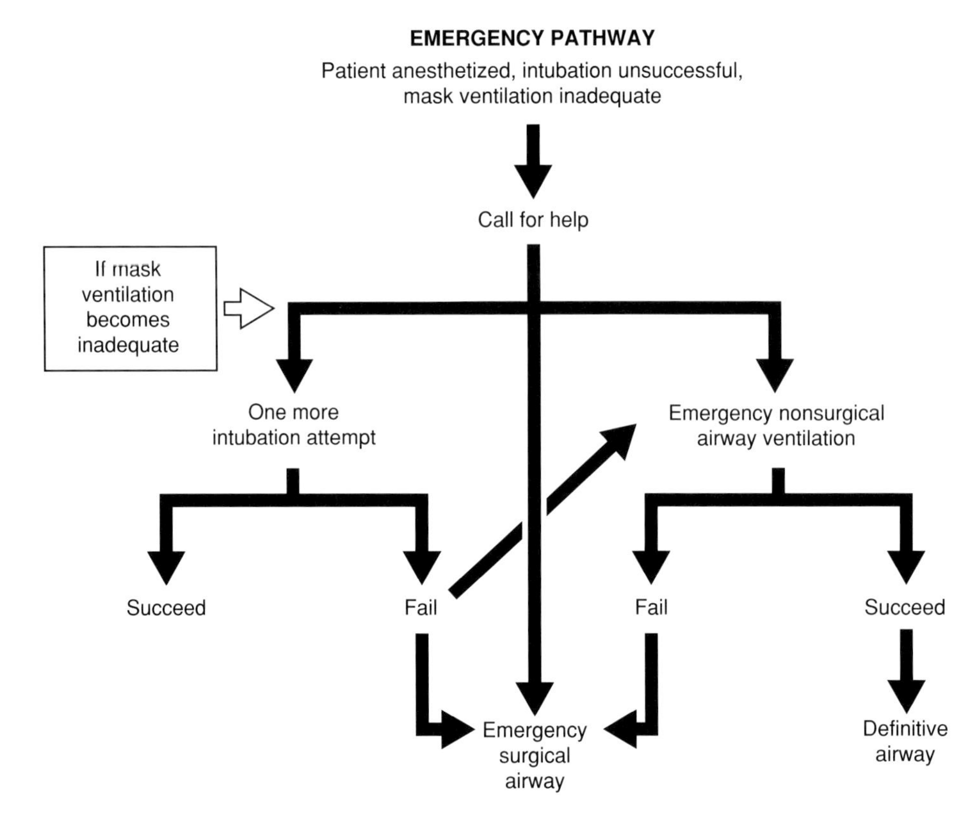

Figure 14.3 The place of the LMA in the original ASA algorithm.

algorithm) was able to review its multiple uses within the ASA difficult airway algorithm[86].

Benumof considers that by facilitating controlled ventilation and tracheal intubation the LMA can be placed in the airway algorithm in five places: (1) on the awake intubation limb of the algorithm as aid to tracheal intubation; (2) on the nonemergency pathway of the anesthetized limb as a definitive airway or (3) as an aid to tracheal intubation; (4) on the emergency anesthetized pathway as a life saving ventilatory device or (5) as an aid to tracheal intubation (Figure 14.4). He concluded:

> With multiple uses and multiple places of use, the LMA is an important option within the ASA difficult airway algorithm. More importantly, the clinical record of LMA use in 'cannot ventilate, cannot intubate' situations has been excellent, and in patients whose lungs cannot be ventilated because of supraglottic obstruction and whose trachea cannot be intubated due to unfavorable anatomy (but not periglottic pathology), the LMA should be immediately available and considered as the first treatment of choice.[86]

The LMA as a definitive airway

The LMA has been used as the definitive airway (i.e. the patient was not intubated after LMA insertion where circumstances have dictated) for the predicted[22,41–46,53,91,122] and the

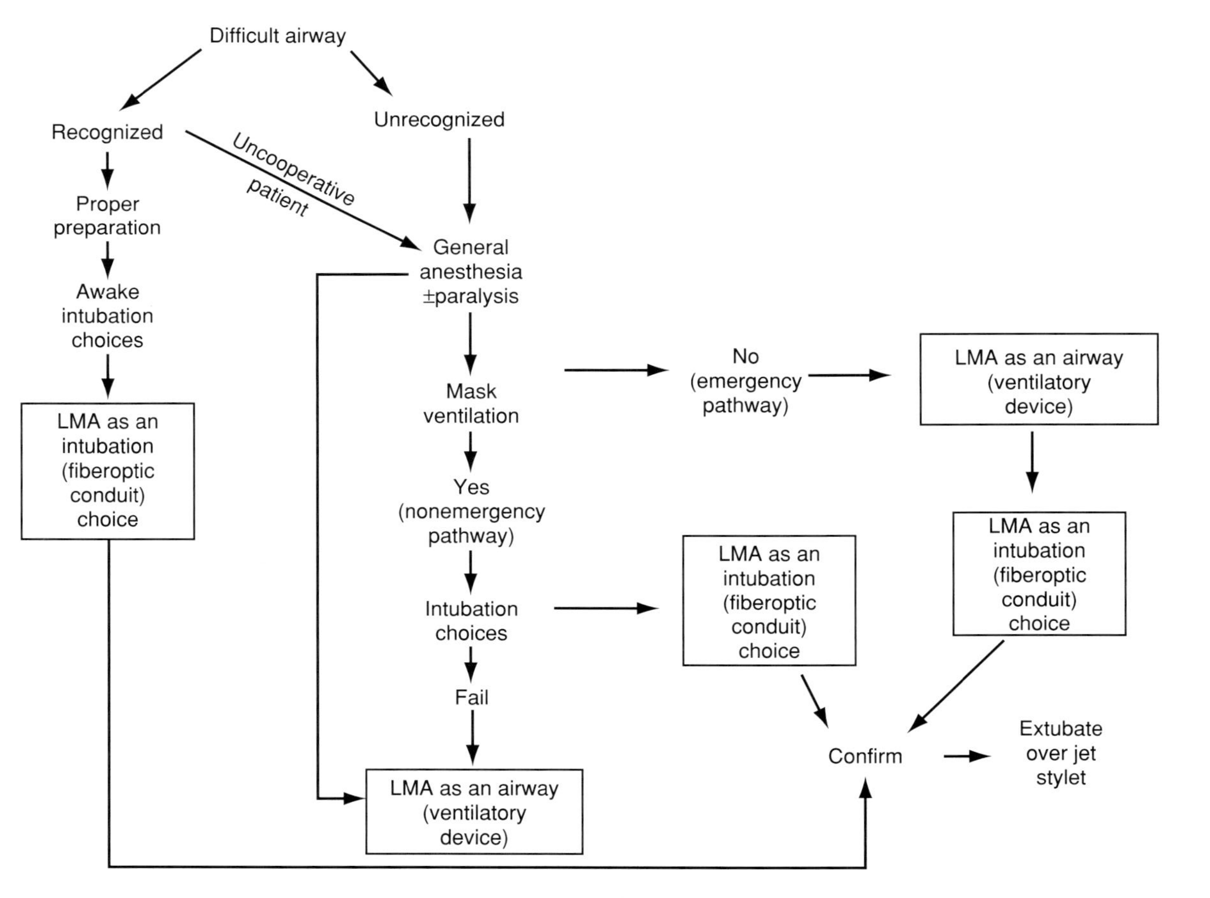

Figure 14.4 The place of the LMA in the new ASA algorithm[86]. Reproduced with permission, *Anesthesiology*.

unpredicted difficult airway[28,35–37,39,52,123], in both fasted[22,28,35–37,39,41–46,52,53,122] and non-fasted patients[14,16–21,26,28,55,98,123], and in children and neonates[65,67,69,70,72,74–79,82,124–131]. The LMA has been successfully used during failed intubation even when the cuff was punctured by sharp teeth during insertion[132]. It has also been used following accidental extubation in the left lumbar position[133].

The LMA as an aid to intubation (airway intubator)

The ease of access to the vocal cords and trachea and the ability to monitor adequacy of respiration and perform patient ventilation while intubating make the LMA useful as an aid to intubation. The curved LMA tube is shaped to direct the passage of a tracheal tube into the trachea and the 30 degree angle at which the tube enters the bowl was specifically designed for this purpose[118]. In up to 96% of cases the vocal cords will be visible directly below the aperture bars of the LMA when the standard technique is used[101,134] (Figure 14.5). In some patients, the vocal cord view may be obscured by a downfolded epiglottis, but this may be circumnavigated by manipulation of the fiberoptic scope. The authors have noted that it is occasionally possible to 'unfurl' the epiglottis by withdrawing and then re-inserting the inflated device by about 6 cm. Adejumo and Davies suggested that epiglottic obstruction may be relieved by digital elevation of anterior pharyngeal tissues followed by rotation of the LMA tube though 360 degrees[94]. Charters has warned that a 360 degree rotation with the LMA tip in the hypopharynx runs the risk of arytenoid dislocation[135]. For successful intubation, the pharyngolaryngeal reflexes must be sufficiently obtunded to allow passage of a tracheal tube. It is possible to use topical anesthesia for both LMA insertion and intubation via the LMA[136], or to insert the LMA under local anesthesia and use it to aid intubation following induction of general anesthesia[25]. Asai and others suggest that awake techniques are safer in the predicted difficult airway[137] (Figure 14.6).

Technical considerations

There are several device features to consider when using the LMA as an aid to intubation. Firstly, the internal diameter of the LMA tube will only accommodate a relatively small cuffed tracheal tube, but this is sufficient to ventilate most patients. If a larger bore tracheal tube is needed, several strategies have been suggested: the problem can be resolved by swapping for a larger tube by use of a tube changer[23,31,63,138–144] or bougie[30,40,120] following removal of the LMA; the LMA can be modified by splitting it ventrally[121]; a large internal diameter LMA may be utilized – the size 5 LMA will accept a 7.0 mm ID tracheal tube[145] and the size 3, 4 and 5 prototype intubating LMA will accommodate a size 8.0 mm ID tracheal tube[146] (Figure 14.7). Secondly, in patients with long necks the cuff of the tracheal tube may not be long enough to pass down the length of the LMA and then through the vocal cords[147]. The mean distance from the mask aperture bars (MAB) to the vocal cords is 3.6 cm in adults and when

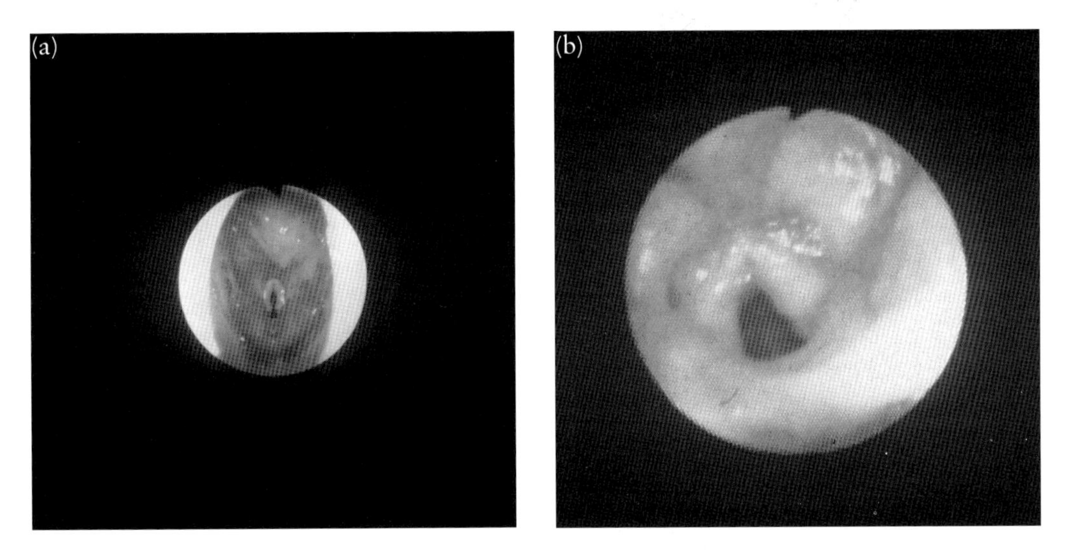

Figure 14.5 View of the vocal cords via the LMA from (a) above the mask aperture bars and (b) below the mask aperture bars.

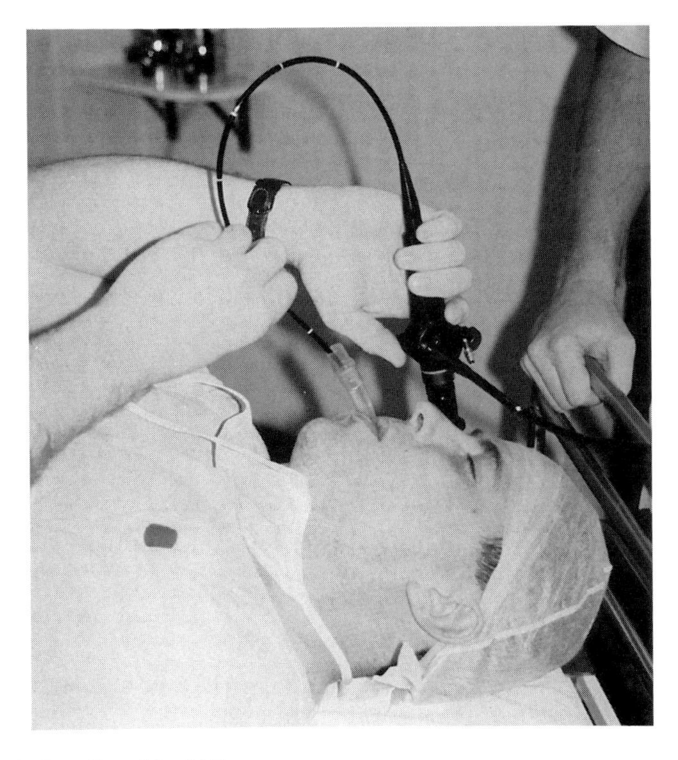

Figure 14.6 Awake insertion of the LMA.

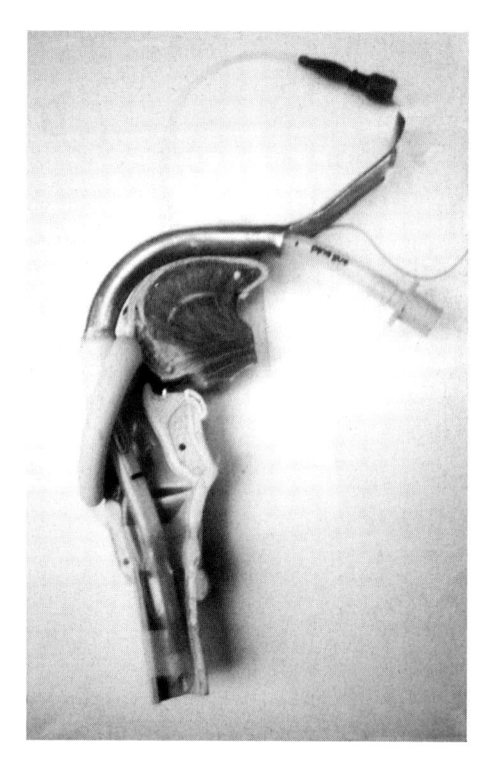

Figure 14.7 Recent prototype intubating LMA (1994).

the tracheal tube is inserted to its full length through the LMA the distance at the teeth will generally be about 21 cm. It has been suggested that the tracheal tube must protrude 9.5 cm beyond the MAB to ensure complete passage into the trachea[147]. It is useful to keep readily available the longer size 5–6 mm microlaryngeal tube (Mallindkrodt Medical, Athlone, Ireland) if more tracheal tube length is required[148]. Asai has suggested than a 6 mm reinforced tracheal tube might be more useful because of its flexibility and increased length (33 cm)[149]. Thirdly, removal of the LMA over the tracheal tube may be difficult following successful intubation. Removal of the LMA is probably unnecessary in most situations[150], but Breen considers it an important maneuver to facilitate a safe smooth awake extubation in the patient with the difficult airway[151]. If LMA removal is desired, it can be accomplished using a second tracheal tube as an extender[68,151–153], either Magill's[72] or Bulldog[151] forceps to hold the tracheal tube in place, or the LMA can be shortened[33,72,131,154], though the manufacturer does not recommend cutting the tube. An LMA with a tube shortened by 2 cm was commercially available in the UK, but production has been discontinued[155]. The prototype intubating LMA[146] and the preproduction device also have a shortened tube (see Chapter 17, *Intubating LMA*). Finally, some authors have suggested that the MAB may interfere with passage of instrumentation[33]. The simpler solution is to prime the LMA with the airway device by passing the tip just beyond the MAB prior to insertion. Removal of the MAB has been suggested, but the MAB prevent the epiglottis folding back into the tube and are sufficiently elastic to allow the passage of a well-lubricated tracheal tube[156]. Catala et al removed the MAB to facilitate passage of a tracheal stent[157]. Removal of the MAB, splitting or shortening of the standard device invalidate the device warranty (UK).

Blind techniques

The advantage of blind intubation is that it does not require availability of or familiarity with the fiberoptic scope or other intubating aid. The disadvantages are those of any blind technique in that it may be time consuming, misplacement may result in trauma, and there is a risk of esophageal intubation. Reported success rates for blind passage of a tracheal tube via the LMA vary between 30 and 93%[158–160] depending on technique, experience, the number of attempts taken, the equipment chosen and the application of cricoid pressure. The type of tracheal tube, the orientation of the tracheal tube bevel and manipulation of the patient's head and neck may affect success rates[160]. Heath found that blind passage of a size 6 cuffed tube was successful in 90% of anesthetized paralyzed patients. Cricoid pressure reduced the success rate to 56%[159]. Lim et al investigated the influence of the type of tracheal tube and positioning of the head on success rates for LMA assisted blind orotracheal intubation using a lubricated size 6 mm cuffed tracheal tube[160]. After a maximum of three attempts, success rates were 30% (Argyle), 93.3% (Portex) and 76.7% (Kendall Curity). The first attempt was performed in the 'sniffing the morning air' position and this was successful in 52% of successful intubations; the second attempt using extension at the atlanto-occipital joint was successful in a further 35% of successful intubations; the third attempt used varying degrees of neck flexion and extension at the atlanto-occipital joint. The LMA inventor recommends a two stage maneuver for blind intubation through the LMA: firstly, head extension to maximize the chance of the tube tip entering the laryngeal vestibule; secondly, when resistance is felt as the tube tip contacts the anterior wall of the larynx (approximately 3 cm) head and neck flexion to align the axes of the tracheal tube and the trachea. The object of this sequence is to enable one to negotiate the S-shaped route from the pharynx with minimal risk of trauma. Good lubrication, gentleness and use of a tube with a rounded bevel should further reduce this risk. Blind intubation via a prototype intubating LMA was found to be successful at the first or second attempt in 92% of patients[146]. The first attempt was made in the neutral position, the second with extension and the third with flexion of the guiding handle. Most of the failed placements occurred in the early part of the study, suggesting an early learning curve. Causes for failure included malalignment of the mask and glottic apertures leading to impaction or esophageal intubation (see Chapter 17, *Intubating LMA*). Langenstein[64] compared blind intubation via the LMA (mainly using an uncuffed tracheal tube) in patients with abnormal airways with that in patients with normal airways and showed that the success rates were similarly low in both (22 versus 19%).

Blind passage of a stylet or a bougie into the trachea is possible, followed by removal of the LMA and railroading of an appropriate size tracheal tube over the intratracheal device. Successful blind passage of a gum elastic bougie (GEB) has been reported in both awake[30] and anesthetized patients[40] and in both adults (84%)[120] and children (88%)[161]. Failures have also been reported[32,36,73,96,162,163]. Success may be increased by pointing the GEB tip anteriorly and then rotating it by 180 degrees when it enters the trachea[120]. Dean et al suggested that advancing the tip of the GEB through the midline shaft prior to LMA placement increases the success rate[164]. Although successful use has been reported for tube changers in awake[138] and anesthetized patients[142], two small trials have demonstrated success rates of 0[139] and 30%[140], the latter with prior good fiberoptic view of the cords through the LMA. Some tube changers are thicker and stiffer than the normal bougie, making them more likely to follow a posterior path and enter the esophagus[140]. Wafai et al have shown that success rates increase from 0 to 85% within three attempts if the tube changer tip is curved anteriorly[165].

Fiberoptic techniques

Fiberoptic guided techniques[166] have predictably higher success rates of over 90–100% at a single attempt, and intubation is usually rapidly achieved with minimal risk of trauma and esophageal intubation[23,25]. Optimal LMA placement will increase the chances of success by providing a better view of the vocal cords and improving the alignment of the tracheal tube with the tracheal lumen. Problems may arise when railroading the tracheal tube secondary to impaction with the MABs, the glottic inlet or anterior tracheal wall. A further cause of failure is the development of an S-bend in the fiberoptic scope. This may be corrected by withdrawal of the fiberoptic scope.

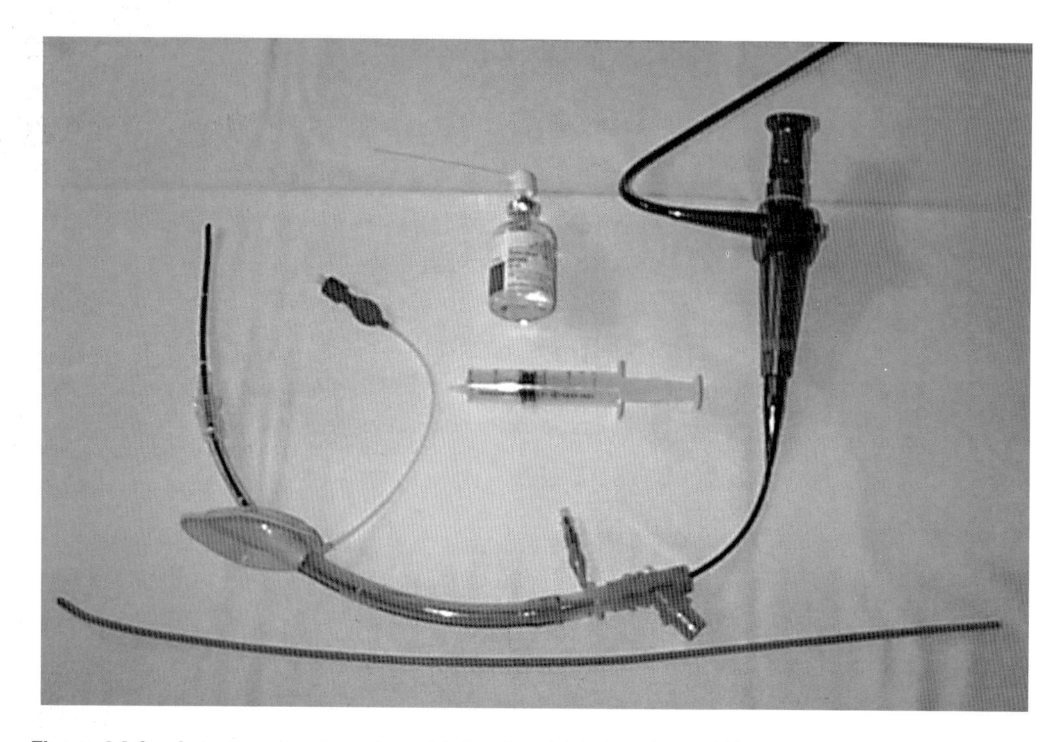

Figure 14.8 Selection of equipment used to facilitate intubation via the LMA.

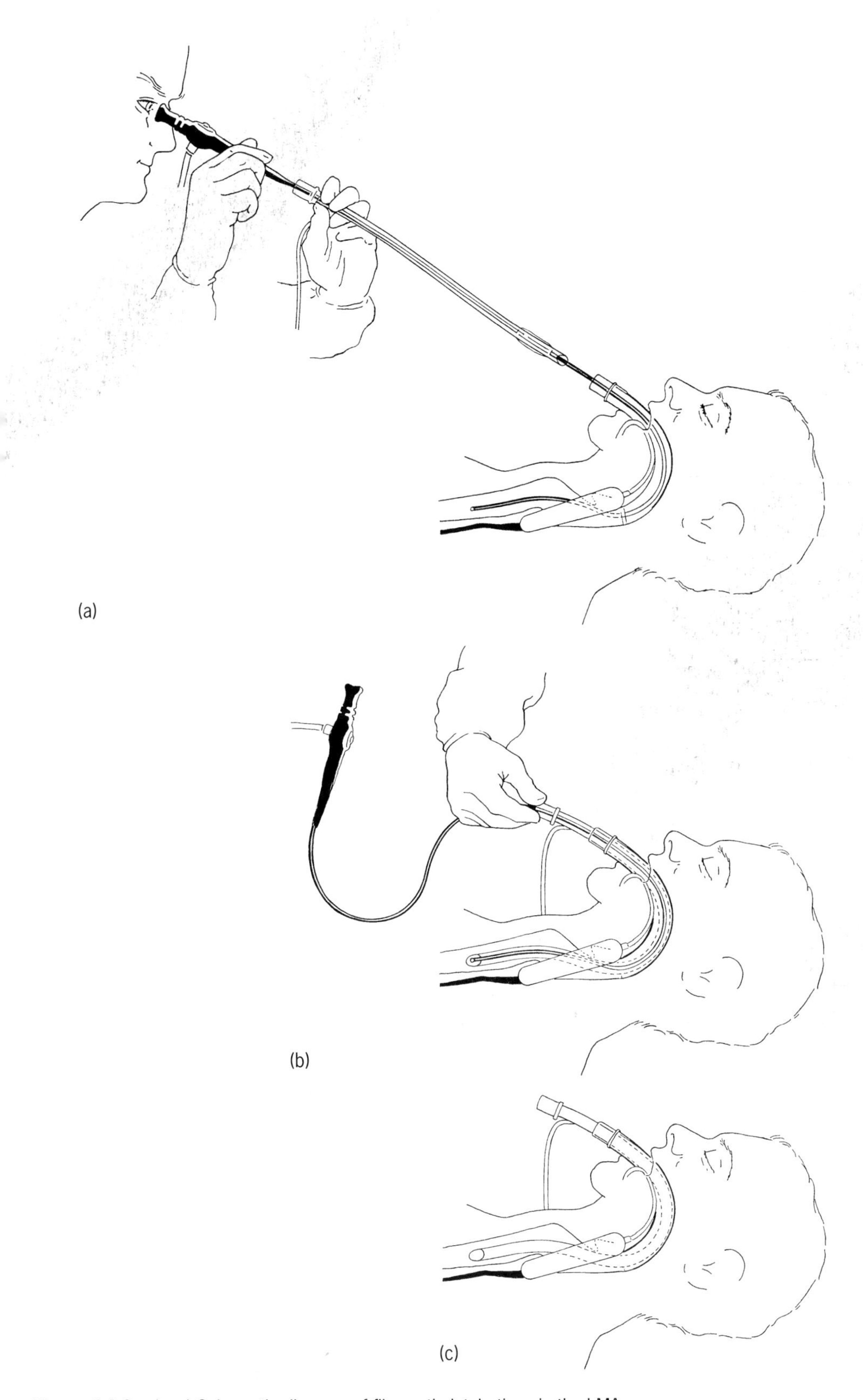

Figure 14.9 (a–c) Schematic diagram of fiberoptic intubation via the LMA.

There are numerous case reports of the successful use of a fiberoptic scope to aid intubation via the LMA in patients with abnormal airways[32,45]. Some of the equipment used to achieve tracheal intubation via the LMA is shown in Figure 14.8. The most common method is to prime the fiberoptic scope with a small well-lubricated tracheal tube which is railroaded into place once the scope is in the trachea[32,38,45,72,153,167,168] (Figure 14.9). Three small studies have investigated the use of the fiberoptic scope/tracheal tube (FOS/TT) combination in patients with abnormal airways. Kadota et al using a long PVC tube primed with the fiberoptic scope successfully intubated 5/5 adult patients, three of whom had severe rheumatoid arthritis, one a tongue malignancy and one ossification of the posterior longitudinal ligament[23]. In a more extensive study, Silk et al used the FOS/TT in 48 patients with anticipated intubation difficulty[25]. The technique was successful in 96% (46/48); the two failures resulted from one problem with LMA insertion and one failure to pass the tracheal tube. Langenstein reported the technique to be successful in 29/29 patients with known abnormal airways in whom the LMA had been successfully placed[64]. The fiberoptic scope may be used to guide a bougie[120] or wire[169,170] into the trachea in addition to direct passage of a tracheal tube. Atherton et al successfully intubated 24/24 paralyzed patients via the LMA using a fiberoptically guided exchange catheter[144].

It is important to practice the technique of fiberoptic laryngoscopy through the LMA to gain experience in orientation and manipulation of the scope. Initial valuable experience can be gained using an intubating mannequin. Fiberoptic techniques have been used in the emergency situation[142,171] but are time consuming, less available, and may be difficult to use where blood or secretions obscure the view.

The split LMA has been used as an aid to fiberoptic intubation following failed nasal and oral fiberoptic techniques which were hampered by blood and secretions[172]. Hornbein et al proposed using two elbow connectors to facilitate fiberoptic placement of a stylet while continuing to ventilate the patient[173]. This is a useful approach to instrumentation of the larynx and trachea, but the technique is limited by the increased resistance to gas flow secondary to the presence of both a stylet and a fiberoptic scope in the LMA tube. This may be particularly problematic in pediatric patients where the ratio of instrument size to tube internal diameter is high. Lopez-Gil et al have described a prototype LMA currently undergoing evaluation which offers similar advantages but overcomes the problems of gas flow[174] (see Chapter 17, *Double lumen LMA*).

Nasotracheal intubation

The LMA has been used to aid blind nasal intubation in a patient with severe micrognathia[47]. A size 12 FG catheter was passed into the trachea via the LMA and a size 10 FG inserted into the nostril and brought out through the mouth using Magill's forceps. The LMA was removed, the catheters sutured together and a 6.5 cuffed RAE nasal tube was railroaded into position[47]. This technique may be of interest if a fiberoptic scope is unavailable. Langenstein has described a similar technique using a reinforced stomach tube to substitute an uncuffed tracheal tube via the LMA with a nasotracheal tube[64]. The LMA has also been used to faciliate training for fiberoptic guided nasotracheal intubation by providing a clear airway during the attempt. Marjot et al[175] modified the LMA by (1) creating a window on the posterior distal tube, (2) splitting the cuff, and (3) removing the mask aperture bars. This allows passage of a fiberoptic scope into the trachea via the window and subsequent railroading of a nasotracheal tube. Alexander[176] pointed out that simply withdrawing the LMA into the oral cavity would suffice and would provide the operator with a more normal view of the laryngopharynx.

Predicted difficult airway

There is controversy over the use of the LMA in the known or strongly suspected difficult airway[15,137,177–183] and the American Task Force on Management of the Difficult Airway currently recommends awake intubation as the preferred option[89]. Reasons for avoiding LMA usage are that LMA placement may not always succeed and that face mask ventilation in the event of failure is not guaranteed. The counterargument is that to attempt intubation in someone in whom this is known to be difficult may itself represent an unnecessary risk. Asai and Morris consider that patients should not be paralyzed when using the LMA in this situation since placement may fail in up to 6% of patients with normal airways and subsequent success with the face mask is not guaranteed[137]. He also argues that the LMA may not always be replaced if it becomes dislodged and that subsequent replacement may not be easy since muscle relaxation decreases pharyngeal integrity[183]. Other authors argue that the LMA should not be used as a definitive airway in case the need for urgent intubation arises intraoperatively and that it may not function adequately in a substantial minority of patients[15,179]. However, there is no evidence that LMA insertion is affected by muscle relaxants[184] or that dislodgment is common. There are two clinical situations in which an adequately placed LMA might be exchanged for a tracheal tube: if high airway pressure ventilation is required or in the event of aspiration. Failure rates of 6% probably reflect inexperience and misuse of the device. Although Rose and Cohen[6] reported a failure rate of 4.7%, Verghese et al had a failure rate of 0.4% in 2359 patients[185], and the trial has been extended to over 11 000 patients with similar results[186]. The differences may also be explained by different criteria for failure of the technique. A further large series of over 9000 patients has shown an increased incidence of problems with the tracheal tube versus the LMA in terms of placement difficulties and laryngeal spasm in normal patients (0.9% versus 3.4%)[187]. There is evidence that placement of the LMA is safe in patients with normal airways, but who are coincidentally Mallampati III or IV[101]. Brimacombe reported no failed placement in 102 Mallampati grade III and 13 grade IV[101].

When the LMA is used in the anticipated difficult airway, the options are to insert the LMA either under general anesthesia or with the patient awake and the airway topicalized. The LMA may then be used either as a definitive airway or as an aid to oral intubation. If the LMA is used without intubation, then the operator should be prepared for urgent fiberoptic intubation or cricothyroid puncture should the need arise. Muscle relaxants should only be given when the airway is secured.

Unpredicted difficult airway

Background

The success of the LMA in rescuing patients from an unanticipated difficult airway situation depends on the nature of the airway problem and on the following factors: familiarity of the operator with the device in routine clinical practice, adherence to basic principles of failed intubation drills, the risk of aspiration and appreciation of the interaction between cricoid pressure and the LMA, and prior experience with intubation through the LMA. If tracheal intubation has failed, but face mask ventilation is adequate, there is no reason to substitute the face mask for the LMA. If patients are paralyzed and at low risk of aspiration, the LMA may be inserted and used as an aid to tracheal intubation. In deciding at what point in a failed intubation situation the LMA might be used, two essential points need to be considered: (1) although the LMA offers no protection against regurgitation, this may be made less likely by rapid relief of hypoxemia and upper airway obstruction; (2) hypoxic damage due to persistent attempts to intubate a cyanosed patient is the major problem in failed intubation, rather than acid aspiration[188].

There is scant data regarding the incidence of LMA usage in the unanticipated difficult airway. An audit survey revealed that there were three cases of failed tracheal intubation in approximately 25 000 patients in which the airway was secured with the LMA, giving an incidence of 1 : 8300 for airway rescue[186]. A 1995 British survey of 209 obstetric units with over 1000 deliveries a year showed that the LMA, available there since 1988, was now present in 91.4% of units, with 72% of anesthesiologists recommending its use following failed intubation and failed face mask ventilation and before cricothyrotomy[189]. There were 24 reports of the use of the LMA as an emergency airway; in eight of these it was considered to have been life saving. In three cases the LMA had not provided an adequate airway and face mask ventilation had just managed to maintain oxygenation. Hawthorne et al reported the successful use of the LMA for airway rescue in three patients, all of whom had laryngeal edema[93]. Cricoid pressure was maintained and spontaneous ventilation resumed. The LMA was unsuccessful in a fourth large woman with a short neck. More extensive data is being gathered in the USA regarding the incidence and success of LMA usage in these situations.

Algorithm for use of the LMA with cricoid pressure

The anatomical interaction between cricoid pressure and the LMA has been discussed in Chapter 2, *Cricoid pressure*. The incidence of aspiration with the LMA and the influence of cricoid pressure (CP) in patients considered 'at risk' of aspiration is unknown. When taking into account prospective trials and anecdotal reports of LMA insertion with CP applied, LMA insertion should probably be attempted before performing a cricothyroid puncture or cricothyrotomy, both of which require prolonged release of CP[190] and are associated with complication rates of up to 29%[191] and 14%[192] respectively. Published data would indicate that if a cricoid yoke or double handed CP is used, the safest method is to transiently release CP during LMA insertion. If single handed CP and probably also single handed CP with manual in-line traction is used, it would seem reasonable to initially attempt insertion with CP applied if the oxygen saturation is adequate (>95%). If failure of placement occurs, CP should be transiently and partially released for the second attempt. It is *essential* to faultlessly deflate the mask tip so that there is a smooth, thin leading edge before each attempt. If unsuccessful with CP applied the attempt will add an extra 20–30 s to the airway event.

If, however, oxygen saturation is low (<95%), the initial insertion attempt should probably be with CP transiently released as oxygenation is at maximum priority when compared with aspiration risk[193,194]. The risk of aspiration may be less than 10% without CP[195–197]. Vanner[198] has suggested that CP is released under direct vision and it may be appropriate to insert the LMA with the laryngoscope[199] to save time if the oxygen saturation is low or if the first blind insertion attempt fails. It is interesting to note the recent work of Pace et al which has shown that LMA placement is readily achieved following insertion of an esophageal tube[200]. This suggests that the LMA may be used to provide rapid and effective oxygenation if the tracheal tube is unintentionally placed in the esophagus. Drainage of regurgitated material may also be facilitated by passage of a tracheal tube into the upper esophagus following LMA placement.

Good preparation of the LMA and meticulous insertion technique are essential prerequisites to the use of the LMA for airway rescue in the presence of applied CP. An LMA deflation tool is now available and may be useful for paramedics and those involved in resuscitation as the LMA is maintained in a properly well-deflated shape in the device and is therefore ready for immediate use[201]. The LMA will not remain completely deflated even in the deflator tool, however; residual air should always be sucked out to a high vaccum immediately before use.

If the LMA has been successfully inserted without CP it would seem reasonable to apply CP. A further possible strategy may be to apply anterior neck pressure. This may have a further beneficial role in increasing leak pressure[202] and thus reducing the risk of gastric insufflation during manual ventilation through the LMA. If the application of CP impedes ventilation it should be released[203].

An algorithm has been proposed for the use of the LMA in a patient with a potentially full stomach in whom intubation has proved impossible[204] (Figure 14.10). The practicality of this algorithm has been questioned[198,205–208].

Emergency intubation via the LMA

Once the airway has been secured with the LMA consideration may be given to passing a suitable sized tracheal tube via the LMA, either blindly or fiberoptically. The results of blind intubation through the LMA are not dependable enough for the technique to

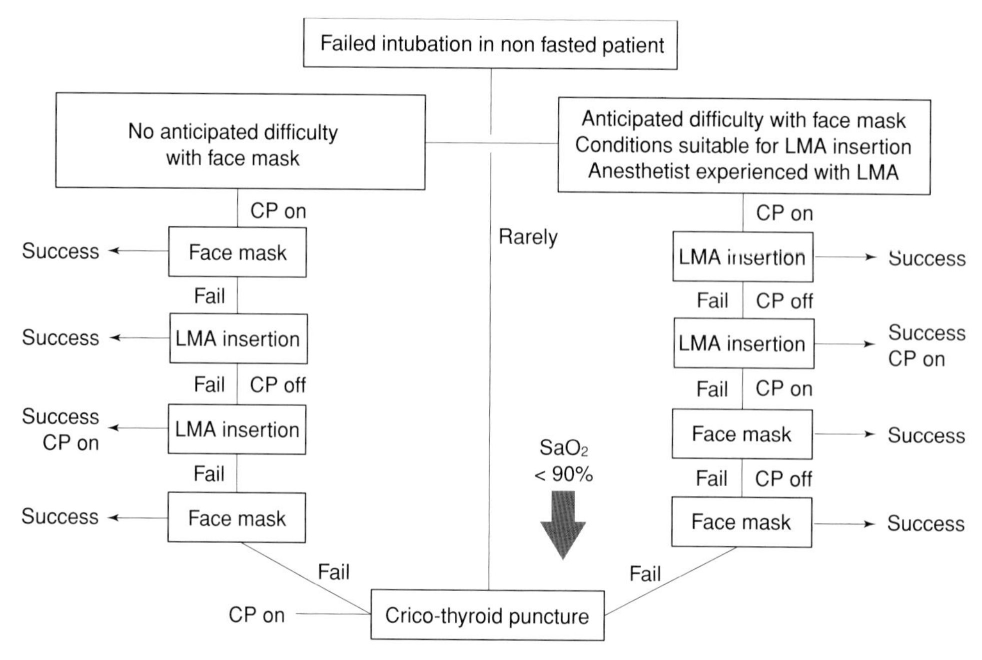

Figure 14.10 Proposed algorithm for LMA usage in the non-fasted patient. Reproduced with permission, *Anesthesiology Research Society.*

be considered a satisfactory option[209], although this has been successfully performed following failed intubation[142,210]. Gabbott and Sasada compared blind placement of a gum elastic bougie (with the angulated tip facing anteriorly) with applied CP and manual in-line stabilization[211]. The bougie entered the trachea in 22.5%, the esophagus in 52.5%, and either the vallecula, hypopharynx or arytenoid cartilages in the remainder. These results were similar to those obtained without CP and manual in-line stabilization. It is possible that, by tilting the cricoid cartilage cranially during the application of CP, this effect may be partially counteracted[212]. Fiberoptic intubation in patients with normal airways has a high first attempt success rate, but the presence of a downfolded epiglottis or the presence of CP may hinder the fiberoptic view. The authors consider that it is inappropriate to use the LMA as an aid to intubation if it is already functioning adequately with applied CP. A possible option is to view the glottis fiberoptically and for tracheal intubation to proceed only if there is good anatomical positioning and a high likelihood of success.

Comparison with other techniques

The place of the LMA when taken in the context of other techniques is unknown. Percutaneous transtracheal jet ventilation (TTJV) is extremely effective and well tested[7], but has been associated with a 29% complication rate in the emergency situation[213]. Benumof suggests that the low risk/benefit ratio associated with the LMA means that it may be a suitable alternative before TTJV is attempted in the difficult airway algorithm[214]. Experience with the esophageal tracheal combitube (ETC) and

TTJV during failed intubation is limited and neither device is used in routine anesthetic practice[214,215]. A study of use of the combitube in routine anesthetic practice where the patients had 'normal' airways gave a failure to ventilate in two attempts in a 'small number of cases' and there have been no studies on the use of the combitube in the abnormal airway[216]. Baraka and Salem have suggested that the ETC may be preferred to the LMA in the difficult intubation situation whenever the patient is considered to be at high risk of regurgitation and aspiration[217]. However, whilst the ETC probably offers increased airway protection, its value has not been proven in this clinical situation[218,219]. The LMA does not protect the trachea from regurgitated stomach contents but has been shown, by Baraka amongst others[37], to be life saving on occasions where tracheal intubation and face mask ventilation have both failed. The risk/benefit ratios of these two devices have not been assessed and it is premature to presume that one is superior to the other. Most authors agree that the LMA should be tried before attempting a cricothyroid puncture or cricothyrotomy, both of which require prolonged release of cricoid pressure[212,220–222]. Brimacombe and Berry have suggested that the rapidity with which the emergent airway can be secured with a LMA makes it a better option than the use of a face mask, and that it should be included in the failed intubation drill before a surgical airway is attempted[206].

Failed obstetric intubation

The incidence of failed intubation in the obstetric population is four times greater than in the general population[4,5] and hypoxia may occur rapidly due to reduced functional residual capacity[223]. Difficult or failed intubation was implicated in six out of eight anesthetic-related deaths in the 1985–1987 Report on Confidential Enquiries (RCE) into Maternal Deaths in England and Wales[220]. Vanner noted that the overall modern obstetric mortality rate is only marginally less than the mortality from aspiration pneumonitis when ether and a face mask were commonly used[195]. Rosen suggests that intubation should be limited to two attempts of 1 min each, separated by 30 s of ventilation[224]. Hasty surgical intervention during failed intubation (either tracheostomy or cricothyrotomy) is dangerous and time consuming[192,225–228], and three of the 10 anesthesia-related deaths in the 1982–1984 RCE were associated with failed tracheostomy[229].

Interestingly there have been two recent studies where the LMA was used for cesarean section. In a study of 48 patients undergoing elective cesarean section with the IPPV/LMA technique at peak airway pressures of 20 cm H_2O, Yang and Suh detected no episodes of aspiration[196]. Similarly, in a larger study of 224 patients undergoing elective and emergency cesarean section with the IPPV/LMA technique at peak airway pressures less than 15 cm H_2O, Liew and Chan-Liao detected no episodes of aspiration[197].

There is anecdotal evidence that the LMA may be useful in failed obstetric intubation[14,16–21,92,142,230,231], a view supported by several authorities in obstetric airway management[215,220,232,233]. There have been nine case reports of failed obstetric intubation in which the LMA was successfully used[14,16–18,20,21,92,142,230]. In seven of these reports CP was maintained during and after LMA insertion[14,16–18,20,142,230] and in one report CP was 'eased up' before insertion and then reapplied[21]. No specific problems were noted with LMA insertion. In a survey of 250 consultant obstetric anesthesiologists 24 reported using the LMA in obstetric anesthesia and on eight occasions it was considered life saving[189]. Christian et al reported functional failure of the LMA following insertion with CP applied which did not improve upon release of CP[19]. Dalmeida et al reported the failed placement of the LMA with applied CP and also subsequent failed transtracheal jet ventilation[92]. Fortunately, the LMA was successfully re-inserted without CP which was then reapplied. A formal tracheostomy was conducted at the end of surgery due to problems with laryngospasm during emergence. The authors considered the LMA to be a 'must in the obstetric suite'. Freeman et al have warned against the inappropriate use of the LMA during failed intubation and suggest that placement of the LMA when active reflexes are present may worsen the situation by causing aspiration[234]. To date there are no accounts of aspiration occurring in association with emergency LMA use in cases of failed intubation when patients have been at risk. It is also considered inappropriate to insert the LMA when an adequate airway has already been obtained with the face mask[16,235–238] or to use the LMA as an aid to intubation if the face mask is functioning adequately with applied cricoid pressure[142,209]. Reynolds has suggested that the LMA may be an option to consider as an alternative to awake tracheostomy in the obstetric patient with a known difficult airway in whom regional anesthesia was impossible or dangerous[239]. Gataure and Hughes suggest that the LMA has a role in obstetric anesthesia when tracheal intubation has failed and ventilation with a face mask proves to be impossible, and it should be inserted before attempting a cricothyrotomy[189]. The LMA has also been used as an aid to awake tracheal intubation in a morbidly obese patient with HELLP syndrome (hemolysis, elevated liver enzymes and low platelet count) requiring an urgent cesarean section for fetal distress[97].

Summary

Familiarity with the LMA should be obtained before using it in the management of the difficult airway and a full range of equipment and personnel should be available[240]. Most authors advocate the widespread availability of the LMA on the failed intubation carts[20,241–243]. Of some concern is the fact that only 87% of US trainees have practical experience of the LMA as a potential device for difficult airway management[244]. In view of the recommendations made by the American Society of Anesthetists Task Force of the Management of the Difficult Airway[89] and more recently by Benumof[86] it is essential that all trainees gain practical experience with the LMA.

Finally, many of the studies pertaining to the LMA and the difficult airway have included healthy paralyzed patients who would probably have been easy to intubate conventionally. The applicability of this data to the failed intubation scenario can only be inferred[245]. Further studies are needed to define the role of the LMA in these challenging circumstances. It is possible that a large multicenter US trial will be commenced in the near future collecting data about LMA usage in cases of failed intubation. This may allow further recommendations to be made regarding the exact role of the LMA.

References

1 Latto IP, Rosen M. Preface. In: *Difficulties in tracheal intubation*. London: Baillière Tindall, 1984;vii.

2 Rose DK, Cohen MM. The incidence of airway problems depends on the definition used. *Can J Anaesth* 1996;**43**:30–34.

3 Latto IP. Management of difficult intubation. In: Latto IP, Rosen M, eds. *Difficulties in tracheal intubation*. London: Baillière Tindall, 1987;99–141.

4 Davies JM, Weets S, Crone LA, Paulin E. Difficult intubation in the parturient. *Can J Anaesth* 1989;**36**:668–674.

5 Samsoon GLT, Young JRB. Difficult tracheal intubation: a retrospective study. *Anaesthesia* 1987;**42**:487–490.

6 Rose DK, Cohen MM. The airway: problems and predictions in 18,500 patients. *Can J Anaesth* 1994;**41**:372–383.

7 Benumof JL, Scheller MS. The importance of transtracheal jet ventilation in the management of the difficult airway. *Anesthesiology* 1989;**71**:769–778.

8 Oates JDL, MacLeod AD, Oates PD, Pearsall FJ, Howie JC, Murray GD. Comparison of two methods for predicting difficult intubation. *Br J Anaesth* 1991;**66**:305–309.

9 Frerk CM. Predicting difficult intubation. *Anaesthesia* 1991;**46**:1005–1008.

10 Benumof JL. Difficult laryngoscopy: obtaining the best view. *Can J Anaesth* 1994;**41**:361–365.

11 Tse JC, Rimm EB, Hussain A. Prediciting difficult endotracheal intubation in surgical patients scheduled for general anesthesia: a prospective blind study. *Anesth Analg* 1995;**81**:254–258.

12 Bainton CR. Difficult intubation – what's the best test? *Can J Anaesth* 1996;**43**:541–543.

13 Caplan RA, Posner KL, Ward RJ, Cheney FW. Adverse respiratory events in anesthesia: a closed claims analysis. *Anesthesiology* 1990;**72**:828–833.

14 McFarlane C. Failed intubation in an obese obstetric patient and the laryngeal mask. *Int J Obstet Anesth* 1993;**2**:183–184.

15 Todesco J, Dodd C, Tudor Williams R, Williams PJ, Bailey PM. Laryngeal mask airway: defining the limits. *Can J Anaesth* 1993;**40**:816–818.

16 Priscu V, Priscu L, Soroker D. Laryngeal mask for failed intubation in emergency Caesarean section. *Can J Anaesth* 1992;**39**:893.

17 Lim W, Wareham C, de Mello WF, Kocan M. The laryngeal mask in failed intubation. *Anaesthesia* 1990;**41**:689–690.

18 Chadwick LS, Vohra A. Anaesthesia for emergency Caesarean section using the Brain laryngeal mask airway. *Anaesthesia* 1989;**44**:261–262.

19 Christian AS, McClune S, Moore JA. Failed obstetric intubation. *Anaesthesia* 1990;**45**:995.

20 McClune S, Regan M, Moore J. Laryngeal mask airway for caesarean section. *Anaesthesia* 1990;**45**:227–228.

21 Storey J. The laryngeal mask for failed intubation at caesarean section. *Anaesth Intens Care* 1992;**20**:118–119.

22 Cork R, Monk JE. Management of a suspected and unsuspected difficult laryngoscopy with the laryngeal mask airway. *J Clin Anesth* 1992;**4**:230–234.

23 Kadota Y, Oda T, Yoshimura N. Application of a laryngeal mask to a fiberoptic bronchoscope-aided tracheal intubation. *J Clin Anesth* 1992;**4**:503–504.

24 Loken RG, Moir CL. The laryngeal mask airway as an aid to blind orotracheal intubation. *Can J Anaesth* 1992;**39**:518.

★ 25 Silk JM, Hill HM, Calder I. Difficult intubation and the laryngeal mask. *Eur J Anaesthesiol* 1991;**4**:47–51.
First series of LMA usage in the known difficult airway. Reported a success rate of 46/48 for fiberoptic guided intubation.

26 Calder I, Ordman AJ, Jackowski A, Crockard HA. The Brain laryngeal mask airway. An alternative to emergency tracheal intubation. *Anaesthesia* 1990;**45**:137–139.

27 Smith BL. Brain airway in anaesthesia for patients with juvenile chronic arthritis. *Anaesthesia* 1988;**43**:421.

28 Brain AI. Three cases of difficult intubation overcome by the laryngeal mask airway. *Anaesthesia* 1985;**40**:353–355.

29 Goldberg PL, Evans PF, Filshie J. Kinking of the laryngeal mask airway in two children. *Anaesthesia* 1990;**45**:487–488.

30 McCrirrick A, Pracilio JA. Awake intubation: a new technique. *Anaesthesia* 1991;**46**:661–663.
31 Higgins D, Astley BA, Berg S. Guided intubation via the laryngeal mask. *Anaesthesia* 1992;**47**:816.
32 Smith JE, Sherwood NA. Combined use of laryngeal mask airway and fibreoptic laryngoscope in difficult intubation. *Anaesth Intens Care* 1991;**19**:471–472.
33 Maroof M, Siddique MS, Khan RM. Modified laryngeal mask as an aid to fiberoptic endotracheal intubation. *Acta Anaesthesiol Scand* 1993;**37**:124.
34 Maroof M, Siddique M, Khan RM. Difficult diagnostic laryngoscopy and bronchoscopy aided by the laryngeal mask airway. *J Laryngol Otol* 1992;**106**:722.
35 Foster SJ, Clowes NW. Laryngeal mask airway for coronary artery bypass grafting. *Anaesthesia* 1991;**46**:701.
36 White A, Sinclair M, Pillai R. Laryngeal mask airway for coronary artery bypass grafting. *Anaesthesia* 1991;**46**:234.
37 Baraka A. Laryngeal mask airway in the cannot intubate, cannot ventilate situation. *Anesthesiology* 1993;**79**:1151.
38 Janssens M, Marechal J. The laryngeal mask – liege experience. *Acta Anaesthesiol Belg* 1991;**42**:199–206.
39 Sarna MC, Clapham MC, Watson CB. Failed tracheal intubation managed with laryngeal mask airway. *Anesthesiol News*, October 1989, p.36.
40 Chadd GD, Ackers JW, Bailey PM. Difficult intubation aided by the laryngeal mask airway. *Anaesthesia* 1989;**44**:1015.
41 Williams PJ, Bailey PM. Management of failed oral fibreoptic intubation with laryngeal mask airway insertion under topical anaesthesia. *Can J Anaesth* 1993;**40**:287.
42 Brain AIJ. The laryngeal mask – a new concept in airway management. *Br J Anaesth* 1983;**55**:801–805.
43 Russell R, Judkins KC. The laryngeal mask airway and facial burns. *Anaesthesia* 1990;**45**:894.
44 Thomson KD, Ordman AJ, Parkhouse N, Morgan BD. Use of the Brain laryngeal mask airway in anticipation of difficult tracheal intubation. *Br J Plast Surg* 1989;**42**:478–480.
45 Asai T. Fiberoptic tracheal intubation through the laryngeal mask airway in an awake patient with cervical spine instability. *Anesth Analg* 1993;**77**:404.
46 Logan A. Use of the laryngeal mask in a patient with an unstable fracture of the cervical spine. *Anaesthesia* 1991;**46**:987.
47 Thomson KD. A blind nasal intubation using a laryngeal mask airway. *Anaesthesia* 1993;**48**:785–787.
48 Owen G, Browning S, Davies CA, Saunders M, Thomas TA. Laryngeal mask. *Br Med J* 1993;**306**:580.
49 Dalrymple G, Lloyd E. Laryngeal mask: a more secure airway than intubation? *Anaesthesia* 1992;**47**:712–713.
50 Nanji GM, Maltby JR. Vomiting and aspiration pneumonitis with the laryngeal mask airway. *Can J Anaesth* 1992;**39**:69–70.
51 Tighe SQM, Greenslade D. The laryngeal mask airway and fibreoptic laryngoscopy. *Today's Anaesthetist* 1990;**5**:79.
52 Riley RH, Swan HD. Value of the laryngeal mask airway during thoracotomy. *Anesthesiology* 1992;**77**:1051.
53 Fuchs K, Kukule I, Knoch M, Wiegand W. Larynxmaske versus Intubation bei erschwerten Intubationsbedingungen beim Franceschetti–Zwahlen–Klein-Syndrom (Treacher–Collins-Syndrom). *Anaesthesiol Intensivmed Notfalmed Schmerzther* 1993;**28**:190–192.
54 Allen JG, Flower EA. The Brain laryngeal mask. An alternative to difficult intubation. *Br Dent J* 1990;**168**:202–204.
55 Lee JJ, Yau K, Barcroft J. LMA and respiratory arrest after anterior cervical fusion. *Can J Anaesth* 1993;**40**:395–396.
56 Thomson KD. Laryngeal mask airway for elective tracheostomy. *Anaesthesia* 1992;**47**:76.
57 Brimacombe J, Clarke G, Simons S. The laryngeal mask airway for endoscopic guided percutaneous tracheostomy. *Anaesthesia* 1994;**49**:358–359.
58 Dexter TJ. The laryngeal mask airway: a method to improve visualisation of the trachea and larynx during fibreoptic assisted percutaneous tracheostomy. *Anaesth Intens Care* 1994;**22**:35–39.
59 Brimacombe J, Berry A, van Duren P. Use of a size 2 laryngeal mask airway to relieve life threatening hypoxia in an adult with quinsy. *Anaesth Intens Care* 1993;**21**:475–476.
60 Brimacombe J. The laryngeal mask airway – use in the management of stridor. *Anaesth Intens Care* 1992;**20**:117–118.
61 Jun JH, Seung IS, Cho SY, Suh JK. Laryngeal mask airway – endotracheal intubation with laryngeal mask airway and fibreoptic bronchoscope. *J Kor Soc Anesthesiol* 1993;**26**:1029–1034.
62 Beahan PG. A aid to placing the laryngeal mask airway. *Anaesth Intens Care* 1996;**24**:511.
63 Watson CB. Changing the tracheal tube. *Anesthesiol News* 1995;13–19.
64 Langenstein H. Die Kehlkopfmaske bei schwieriger Intubation. *Anaesthetist* 1995;**44**:712–718.
65 Markakis DA, Sayson SC, Schreiner MS. Insertion of the laryngeal mask airway in awake infants with the Robin sequence. *Anesth Analg* 1992;**75**:822–824.
66 Cortes J, Franco A, Cid M, Vidal MI, Rabanal S. Uso de la mascarilla laringea para bronchoscopia fibroptica en un neonato con malformaciones faciales. *Revista Espanola* 1992;**39**:324–325.

67 Chadd GD, Crane DL, Phillips RM, Tunell WP. Extubation and reintubation guided by the laryngeal mask airway in a child with the Pierre-Robin syndrome. *Anesthesiology* 1992;**76**:640–641.

68 Zagnoev M, McCloskey J, Martin T. Fiberoptic intubation via the laryngeal mask airway. *Anesth Analg* 1994;**78**:813–814.

69 Denny NM, Desilva KD, Webber PA. Laryngeal mask airway for emergency tracheostomy in a neonate. *Anaesthesia* 1990;**45**:895.

70 Beveridge ME. Laryngeal mask anaesthesia for repair of cleft palate. *Anaesthesia* 1989;**44**:656–657.

71 Ebata T, Nishiki S, Masuda A, Amaha K. Anaesthesia for Treacher Collins syndrome using a laryngeal mask airway. *Can J Anaesth* 1991;**38**:1043–1045.

72 Goldie AS, Hudson I. Fibreoptic tracheal intubation through a modified laryngeal mask. *Paediatr Anaesth* 1992;**2**:344.

73 Nath G, Major V. The laryngeal mask airway in the management of a paediatric difficult airway. *Anaesth Intens Care* 1992;**20**:518–520.

74 Ravalia A, Goddard JM. The laryngeal mask and difficult tracheal intubation. *Anaesthesia* 1990;**45**:168.

75 Castresana MR, Stefansson S, Cancel AR, Hague KJ. Use of the laryngeal mask airway during thoracotomy in a pediatric patient with Cri-du-Chat syndrome. *Anesth Analg* 1994;**78**:817.

76 Johnson CM, Sims C. Awake fibreoptic intubation via a laryngeal mask in an infant with Goldenhar's syndrome. *Anaesth Intens Care* 1994;**22**:194–197.

77 Bailey C, Chung R. Use of the laryngeal mask airway in a patient with Edward's syndrome. *Anaesthesia* 1992;**47**:713.

78 Lawson R, Lloyd-Thomas AR. Three diagnostic conundrums solved using the laryngeal mask airway. *Anaesthesia* 1993;**48**:790–791.

79 Theroux MC, Kettrick RG, Khine HH. Laryngeal mask airway and fiberoptic endoscopy in an infant with Schwartz–Jampel syndrome. *Anesthesiology* 1995;**82**:605.

80 Brimacombe J, Gandini D. Paediatric airway management. *Br J Hosp Med* 1995;**53**:175.

81 Brimacombe J, De Maio B. Emergency use of the laryngeal mask airway during helicopter transfer of a neonate. *J Clin Anesth* 1995;**7**:689–690.

82 Lee SK, Lee JR. A case of general anaesthesia with the laryngeal mask airway in a patient with Pierre Robin syndrome. *J Kor Soc Anesthesiol* 1994;**27**:95–96.

83 Rabb MF, Minkowitz HS, Haberg CA. Blind intubation through the laryngeal mask airway for management of the difficult airway in children. *Anesthesiology* 1996;**84**:1510–1511.

84 Brimacombe J, Berry A, Brain A. The laryngeal mask airway. In: Sandler AN, Doyle DJ, eds. *The difficult airway I*. Philadelphia: WB Saunders, 1995;411–437.

85 Bogetz MS. The laryngeal mask airway – role in managing the difficult airway. *Int Anesthesiol Clin* 1994;**32**:109–117.

★ 86 Benumof J. The laryngeal mask airway and the ASA difficult airway algorithm. *Anesthesiology* 1996;**84**:686–699.
A scholarly analysis of LMA usage in the difficult airway. Discusses the role of the device in the ASA algorithm and suggests five situations where the device would be useful. After Brain's original description this is probably the most important reference in the LMA literature.

87 Galdi L, Grossi P, Di Lizia A. L'intubazione difficile mediante maschera laringea. *Minerva Anestesiol* 1995;**61**:33–38.

88 Brimacombe J, Dunbar-Reid K. The effect of introducing fibreoptic bronchoscopes on gas flow in laryngeal masks and tracheal tubes. *Anaesthesia* 1996;**51**:923–928.

89 Practice Guidelines for Management of the Difficult Airway – a Report by the American Society of Anesthesiologists Task Force on Management of the Difficult Airway. *Anesthesiology* 1993;**78**:597–602.

90 Judkins KC. When the chips are down – the laryngeal mask in anger. *Anaesthesia* 1993;**48**:353.

91 Lee C, Yang H. Case of difficult intubation overcome by the laryngeal mask airway. *J Kor Med Sci* 1993;**8**:290–292.

92 Dalmeida RE, Mayhew J, Gallagher T, Herring LE. The laryngeal mask airway: a must in the obstetric suite. *J Clin Anesth* (in press).

93 Hawthorne L, Wilson R, Lyons G, Dresner M. Failed intubation revisited: 17-yr experience in a teaching maternity unit. *Br J Anaesth* 1996;**76**:680–684.

94 Adejumo SWA, Davies MW. The laryngeal mask airway – another trick. *Anaesthesia* 1996;**51**:604.

95 Maltby JR, Loken RG, Beriault MT, Archer DP. Laryngeal mask airway with mouth opening less than 20 mm. *Can J Anaesth* 1995;**42**:1140–1142.

96 Aye T, Milne B. Use of the laryngeal mask prior to definitive intubation in a difficult airway: a case report. *J Emerg Med* 1995;**13**:711–714.

97 Godley M, Ramachandra AR. Use of LMA for awake intubation for Caesarean section. *Can J Anaesth* 1996;**43**:299–302.

98 Greene MK, Roden R, Hinchley G. The laryngeal mask airway. Two cases of prehospital trauma care. *Anaesthesia* 1992;**47**:688–689.

99 Sher M, Brimacombe J, Laing D. Anaesthesia for laser pharyngoplasty – a comparison of the tracheal tube versus reinforced laryngeal mask airway. *Anaesth Intens Care* 1995;**23**:149–154.

100 Brimacombe J, Berry A. Mallampatti classification and laryngeal mask insertion. *Anaesthesia* 1993;**48**:347.

101 Brimacombe J. Analysis of 1500 laryngeal mask uses by one anaesthetist in adults undergoing routine anaesthesia. *Anaesthesia* 1996;**51**:76–80.

102 Mahiou P, Narchi P, Veyrac P, Germond M, Gory G, Bazin G. Is laryngeal mask easy to use in case of difficult intubation? *Anesthesiology* 1992;**77**:A1228 (Abstract).

103 McCrory CR, Moriarty DC. Laryngeal mask airway positioning is related to Mallampati grading in adults. *Anesth Analg* 1995;**81**:1001–1004.

104 Brimacombe J, Berry A. Mallampati grade and laryngeal mask placement. *Anesth Analg* 1996;**82**:1112–1113.

105 McCrory C, Moriarty D. Mallampati grade and laryngeal mask placement. *Anesth Analg* 1996;**82**:1112–1113.

106 Asai T. The view of the glottis at laryngoscopy after unexpectedly difficult placement of the laryngeal mask. *Anaesthesia* 1996;**51**:1063–1065.

107 Voyagis G, Doka P, Papakalou E, Kaklis S, Kontopoulou S, Roussaki-Danoe E. Comparison of laryngeal mask with endotracheal tube for airway control. Is the laryngeal mask easy to use in case of difficult intubation? *Acta Anaesth Hell* 1994;**28**:260–266.

108 Brimacombe J. Positive pressure ventilation with the size 5 LMA. *J Clin Anesth* (in press).

109 Brain AIJ. Modification of laryngeal mask insertion technique in children. *Anesth Analg* 1995;**81**:212.

110 Mallampati SR, Gatt SP, Gugino LD, et al. A clinical sign to predict difficult tracheal intubation: a prospective study. *Can J Anaesth* 1985;**32**:429–434.

111 Mason DG, Bingham RM. The laryngeal mask airway in children. *Anaesthesia* 1990;**45**:760–763.

112 Collier C. A hazard with the laryngeal mask airway. *Anaesth Intens Care* 1991;**19**:301.

113 Russell SH, Hirsch NP. Simultaneous use of two laryngoscopes. *Anaesthesia* 1993;**48**:918.

114 Ishimura H, Minami K, Sata T, Shigematsu A, Kadoya T. Impossible insertion of the laryngeal mask airway and oropharyngeal axes. *Anesthesiology* 1995;**83**:867–869.

115 Sheppard IM, Sheppard FM. Maximal incisal opening: a diagnostic index. *J Dent Med* 1965;**20**:13–15.

116 Monso E, Carreras A, Bassons J, Gonzalez Tadeo M. Fibreoptic laryngoscopy as a method of assessing the risk of airway obstruction following laryngeal mask airway insertion. *Anaesthesia* 1992;**47**:631–632.

117 Brimacombe J. Assessing the risk of airway obstruction following laryngeal mask insertion. *Anaesthesia* 1993;**48**:79.

118 Brain AIJ. The development of the laryngeal mask – a brief history of the invention, early clinical studies and experimental work from which the laryngeal mask evolved. *Eur J Anaesthesiol* 1991;**4**:5–17.

119 Brain AIJ. The laryngeal mask airway – a possible new solution to airway problems in the emergency situation. *Arch Emerg Med* 1984;**1**:229–232.

120 Allison A, McCrory J. Tracheal placement of a gum elastic bougie using the laryngeal mask airway. *Anaesthesia* 1990;**45**:419–420.

121 Brimacombe J, Johns K. Modified Intavent LMA. *Anaesth Intens Care* 1991;**19**:607.

122 Smigovec E, Sakic K, Tripkovic B. [The laryngeal mask – news in orthopedic anesthesia]. *Lijec Vjesn* 1993;**115**:166–169.

123 Myles PS, Venema HR, Lindholm DE. Trauma patient managed with the laryngeal mask airway and percutaneous tracheostomy after failed intubation. *Med J Aust* 1994;**161**:640.

124 Fawcett WJ, Ravilia A, Radford P. The laryngeal mask airway in children. *Can J Anaesth* 1991;**38**:685–686.

125 Benumof JL. Intubation and extubation of the patient with Pierre–Robin syndrome. *Anesthesiology* 1992;**77**:401.

126 Denman WT, Goudsouzian NG, Chadd GD, Crane DL. Position of the laryngeal mask airway. *Anesthesiology* 1992;**77**:401–402.

127 Wheatley RS, Stainthorp SF. Intubation of a one-day-old baby with the Pierre–Robin syndrome via a laryngeal mask. *Anaesthesia* 1994;**49**:733.

128 Robichon J. Utilite du masque larynge en cas d'intubation difficile. *Cahiers d'Anesthesiologie* 1993;**41**:525–527.

129 Mecklem D, Brimacombe J, Yarker J. Glossopexy in Pierre Robin sequence using the laryngeal mask airway. *J Clin Anesth* 1995;**7**:267–269.

130 De Mattos AL, Lauretti GR, Garcia LV, Dos Reis MP. Mascara laringea em artrogripose multiplex congenita. Relato de um caso. *Rev Brasil Anestesiol* 1994;**44**:CBA 141.

131 Haxby EJ, Liban JB. Fibreoptic intubation via a laryngeal mask in an infant with Goldenhar syndrome. *Anaesth Intens Care* 1995;**23**:753.

132 Pennant JH, Gajraj NM, Griffith K. Puncture of the laryngeal mask airway cuff. *Anaesthesia* 1994;**49**:448.

133 Goldik Z, Mecz Y, Bornstein J, Heifetz M. LMA insertion after accidental extubation. *Can J Anaesth* 1995;**42**:1065.

134 Brimacombe J, Berry A. Insertion of the laryngeal mask airway – a prospective study of four techniques. *Anaesth Intens Care* 1993;**21**:89–92.

135 Charters P. Digital exploration and the laryngeal mask. *Anaesthesia* 1996;**51**:990.

136 Dasey N, Mansour N. Coughing and laryngospasm with the laryngeal mask. *Anaesthesia* 1989;**44**:865.

137 Asai T, Morris S. Elective use of the laryngeal mask in patients with difficult airways. *Can J Anaesth* 1993;**40**:1221–1222.

138 Carey MF, Smith J, Cooney CM. Laryngeal mask to aid tracheal intubation. *Anaesthesia* 1991;**46**:1083.

139 Knoll W, Wafai Y, Salem MR, Joseph NJ. Facilitation of blind intubation through the laryngeal mask airway by the use of the self-inflating bulb. *Mid-west Anesthesiology Resident's Conference, Cleveland, Ohio, 26–27 March 1994* (Abstract).

140 Brimacombe J, Berry A. Placement of the Cook Airway Exchange Catheter via the laryngeal mask airway. *Anaesthesia* 1993;**48**:351–352.

141 Vickers R, Springer A, Hindmarsh J. Problem with the laryngeal mask airway. *Anaesthesia* 1992;**47**:639.

142 Hasham FM, Andrews PJD, Juneja MM, Ackermann III WE. The laryngeal mask airway facilitates intubation at cesarean section. A case report of difficult intubation. *Int J Obstet Anesth* 1993;**2**:181–182.

143 Hasham F, Kumar CM, Lawler PG. The use of the laryngeal mask airway to assist fibreoptic orotracheal intubation. *Anaesthesia* 1991;**46**:891.

144 Atherton DPL, O'Sullivan E, Charters P. A fibreoptically guided exchange bougie. *Br J Anaesth* 1996;**73**:288P–289P (Abstract).

145 Brimacombe J, Berry A. Preliminary experience with the size 5 laryngeal mask airway. *Anaesth Intens Care* 1993;**21**:888–889.

146 Kapila A, Addy EV, Verghese C, Brain AIJ. Intubating laryngeal mask airway: a preliminary assessment of performance. *Br J Anaesth* 1995;**75**:228P–229P (Abstract).

★ 147 Asai T, Latto IP, Vaughan RS. The distance between the grille of the laryngeal mask airway and the cords. Is conventional intubation through the laryngeal mask safe? *Anaesthesia* 1993;**48**:667–669.
Study of 60 patients showing that the tracheal tube must protrude beyond the end of the mask aperture bars by 9.5 cm to ensure that the cuff inflates distal to the vocal cords.

148 Pennant JH, Joshi GP. Intubation through the laryngeal mask airway. *Anesthesiology* 1995;**83**:891–892.

149 Asai T. Tracheal intubation through the laryngeal mask. *Anesthesiology* 1996;**85**:439.

150 Brimacombe J, Berry A. Laryngeal mask airway for difficult intubation and head and neck surgery in children. *Paediatr Anaesth* 1993;**3**:320–321.

151 Breen PH. Simple technique to remove laryngeal mask airway 'guide' after endotracheal intubation. *Anesth Analg* 1996;**82**:1302.

152 Chadd GD, Walford AJ, Crane DL. The 3.5/4.5 modification for fiberscope-guided tracheal intubation using the laryngeal mask airway. *Anesth Analg* 1992;**75**:307–308.

153 Reynolds PI, O'Kelly SW. Fiberoptic intubation and the laryngeal mask airway. *Anesthesiology* 1993;**79**:1144.

154 Crichlow A, Locken R, Todesco J. The laryngeal mask airway and fibreoptic laryngoscopy. *Can J Anaesth* 1992;**39**:742–743.

155 Asai T, Morris S. The laryngeal mask airway: its features, effects and role. *Can J Anaesth* 1994;**41**:930–960.

156 Brimacombe J. Split laryngeal mask airway. *Anaesthesia* 1993;**48**:639.

157 Catala JC, Garcia-Pedrajas F, Carrera J, Monedero P. Placement of an endotracheal device via the laryngeal mask airway in a patient with tracheal stenosis. *Anesthesiology* 1996;**84**:239–240.

158 Nakano A, Aoyagi M. Blind tracheal intubation through the LM. *J Clin Anesth (Rinsho-Masui)* 1992;**16**:657–658.

★ 159 Heath ML, Allagain J. Intubation through the laryngeal mask – a technique for unexpected difficult intubation. *Anaesthesia* 1991;**46**:545–548.
Early study of 100 patients reporting a 90% success rate for blind intubation via the LMA, decreasing to 56% with cricoid pressure. These success rates probably represent the highest achievable with the standard LMA.

★ 160 Lim SL, Tay DHB, Thomas E. A comparison of three types of tracheal tube for use in laryngeal mask assisted blind orotracheal intubation. *Anaesthesia* 1994;**49**:255–257.
Study of 90 normal patients determining success rates for blind intubation using a variety of tracheal tubes and maneuvers. Success rates ranged from 30 to 93% within three attempts.

161 White AP, Billingham IM. Laryngeal mask guided tracheal intubation in paediatric anaesthesia. *Paediatr Anaesth* 1992;**2**:265.

162 Inada T, Fujise K, Tachibana K, Shingu K. Orotracheal intubation through the laryngeal mask airway in paediatric patients with Treacher Collins syndrome. *Paediatr Anaesth* 1995;**5**:129–132.

163 Brain AIJ. Orotracheal intubation through the laryngeal mask in paediatric patients with Treacher Collins syndrome. *Paediatr Anaesth* 1995;**5**:342.

164 Dean VS, Jurai SA, Bethelmy L. Gum elastic bougies and the laryngeal mask. *Anaesthesia* 1996;**51**:1078.

165 Wafai Y, Knoll W, Salem MR. Facilitation of blind intubation through the laryngeal mask airway. *Anesthesiology* 1995;**83**:A19 (Abstract).

166 Witton TH. An introduction to the fiberoptic scope. *Can Anaesth Soc J* 1981;**28**:475–478.
167 Ezri T, Priscu V, Szmuk P, Soroker D. Laryngeal mask and pulmonary edema. *Anesthesiology* 1993;**78**:219.
168 Thomas DI. Another approach with the laryngeal mask airway. *Anesth Analg* 1992;**75**:156.
169 Miyawaki H. LM-aided tracheal intubation. *J Clin Anesth (Rinsho-Masui)* 1992;**16**:1588–1589.
170 Heard CMB, Caldicott LD, Fletcher JE, Selsby DS. Fiberoptic guided endotracheal intubation via the laryngeal mask airway in paediatric patients. A report of a series of cases. *Anesth Analg* 1996;**82**:1287–1289.
171 Swayne P, Greenslade GL. Emergency intubation through the laryngeal mask airway. The effective application of cricoid pressure. *Anaesthesia* 1994;**49**:696–697.
172 Maroof M, Khan RM, Bonsu A, Raza HS. A new solution to fibreoptic intubation in the presence of blood and secretions. *Can J Anaesth* 1995;**42**:177.
173 Hornbein TF, Turnquist K, Freund P. Another way through a laryngeal mask airway. *Anesthesiology* 1995;**83**:880.
174 Lopez-Gil M, Brimacombe J, Brain AIJ, Wenck D, Wilkins H. The double-lumen LMA. *Anesthesiology* 1996;**84**:1263–1264.
175 Marjot R, Cook TM, Baylis R. Teaching fibreoptic nasotracheal intubation via the laryngeal mask airway. *Anaesthesia* 1996;**51**:511–512.
176 Alexander R. Modifying the laryngeal mask for nasotracheal intubation. *Anaesthesia* 1996;**51**:7.
177 Fisher JA, Ananthanarayan C, Edelist G. Role of the laryngeal mask in airway management. *Can J Anaesth* 1992;**39**:1–3.
178 Maltby JR, Neil SG. Laryngeal mask airway and difficult intubation. *Anesthesiology* 1993;**78**:994–995.
179 Benumof JL. Laryngeal mask airway and difficult intubation. *Anesthesiology* 1993;**78**:995.
180 Brimacombe J, Berry A. The laryngeal mask airway in elective difficult intubation. *J Clin Anesth* 1994;**6**:450–451.
181 Brimacombe J, Shorney N. The role of the LMA? *Can J Anaesth* 1993;**40**:394.
182 Fisher JA, Ananthanarayan C, Edelist G. The role of the LMA? *Can J Anaesth* 1993;**40**:394–395.
183 Nandi PR, Charlesworth CH, Taylor SJ, Nunn JF, Dore CJ. Effect of general anaesthesia on the pharynx. *Br J Anaesth* 1991;**66**:157–162.
184 Brimacombe J, Berry A, Yaddanapudi LN, Kashyap L. Neuromuscular blockade and insertion of the laryngeal mask airway. *Br J Anaesth* 1993;**71**:166–167.
185 Verghese C, Smith TGC, Young E. Prospective survey of the use of the laryngeal mask airway in 2359 patients. *Anaesthesia* 1993;**48**:58–60.
186 Verghese C, Brimacombe J. Survey of laryngeal mask usage in 11 910 patients – safety and efficacy for conventional and nonconventional usage. *Anesth Analg* 1996;**82**:129–133.
187 Haden RM, Pinnock CA, Campbell RL. The laryngeal mask for intraocular surgery. *Br J Anaesth* 1993;**71**:772.
188 Bailey PM. Failed intubation: the problems faced and strategies for coping. *Clin Risk* 1995;**1**:136–138.
189 Gataure PS, Hughes JA. The laryngeal mask airway in obstetrical anaesthesia. *Can J Anaesth* 1995;**42**:130–133.
190 Brimacombe J, Berry A. The laryngeal mask airway – an alternative to emergency cricothyrotomy when conventional airway management fails in the field. *J Trauma* (in press).
191 Smith WB, Schaer WB, Pfaeffle J. Percutaneous transtracheal ventilation for anaesthesia and resuscitation: a review and report of complications. *Can Anaesth Soc J* 1975;**22**:607.
192 Toye FJ, Weinstein JD. Clinical experience with percutaneous tracheostomy and cricothyrotomy in 100 patients. *J Trauma* 1986;**26**:1034–1040.
193 Morrison AG, O'Donnell NG. Laryngeal mask insertion, cricoid pressure and manual in-line stabilisation. *Anaesthesia* 1996;**51**:285–286.
194 Gabbott DA, Sasada MP. Laryngeal mask insertion, cricoid pressure and manual in-line stabilisation. *Anaesthesia* 1996;**51**:285–286.
195 Vanner RG. Mechanisms of regurgitation and its prevention with cricoid pressure. *Int J Obstet Anesth* 1993;**3**:207–215.
196 Yang H, Suh B. Laryngeal mask airway in cesarean section. *11th World Congress of Anesthesiology, Sydney, 14–20 April 1996, Abstract Handbook* p.439.
197 Liew E, Chan-Liao M. Experience of using laryngeal mask anesthesia for caesarean section. *11th World Congress of Anesthesiology, Sydney, 14–20 April 1996, Abstract Handbook* p.439.
198 Vanner RG. The role of the laryngeal mask in the failed intubation drill. *Int J Obstet Anesth* 1995;**4**:191–192.
199 Jenkins J. The laryngoscope and the laryngeal mask airway. *Anaesthesia* 1993;**48**:735.
200 Pace NA, Gajraj NM, Pennant JH, Victory RA, Johnson ER, White PF. Use of the laryngeal mask airway after oesophageal intubation. *Br J Anaesth* 1994;**73**:688–689.
201 Brimacombe J, Brain AIJ, Branagan H, Spry M, Schofield J. Optimal shape of the laryngeal mask cuff: the influence of three deflation techniques. *Anaesthesia* 1996;**51**:673–676.
202 Brimacombe J, Berry A. Leak reduction with the laryngeal mask airway – the application of external neck pressure. *Can J Anaesth* 1996;**43**:537.

203 Asai T, Barclay K, McBeth C, Vaughan RS. Cricoid pressure applied after placement of the laryngeal mask prevents gastric insufflation but inhibits ventilation. *Br J Anaesth* 1996;**76**:772–776.

204 Brimacombe J, Berry A, White A. An algorithm for use of the laryngeal mask airway during failed intubation in the patient with a full stomach. *Anesth Analg* 1993;**77**:398–399.

205 Asai T, Morris S. The role of the laryngeal mask for failed tracheal intubation in the patient with a 'full stomach'. *Anesth Analg* 1994;**78**:817–818.

206 Brimacombe J, Berry A. The role of the laryngeal mask airway for failed tracheal intubation in the patient with a 'Full Stomach'. *Anesth Analg* 1994;**78**:818–819.

207 Asai T, Barkley K, Power I, Vaughan RS. The role of the laryngeal mask in obstetric anaesthesia. *Int J Obstet Anesth* 1995;**4**:190–191.

208 Brimacombe J, Berry A. The role of the laryngeal mask in obstetric anaesthesia. *Int J Obstet Anesth* 1995;**4**:192–194.

209 Brimacombe J, Berry A. Failed obstetric intubation – use of the laryngeal mask airway as an airway intubator? *Int J Obstet Anesth* 1994;**3**:120–121.

210 Kokkinis K. The use of the laryngeal mask airway in CPR. *Resuscitation* 1994;**27**:9–12.

211 Gabbott DA, Sasada MP. Tracheal intubation through the laryngeal mask using a gum elastic bougie in the presence of cricoid pressure and manual in line stabilisation of the neck. *Anaesthesia* 1996;**51**:389–390.

212 Salem MR, Heyman HJ, Mahdi M. Facilitation of tracheal intubation by cephalad displacement of the larynx – rediscovered. *J Clin Anesth* 1994;**6**:167–168.

213 Smith RB, Babinski M, Klain M, Pfaaffle H. Percutaneous transtracheal ventilation. *J Am Coll Emerg Phys* 1976;**5**:765–770.

214 Benumof JL. Management of the difficult adult airway – with special emphasis on awake tracheal intubation. *Anesthesiology* 1991;**75**:1087–1110.

215 Lawlor M, Johnson C, Weiner M. Airway management in obstetric anesthesia. *Int J Obstet Anesth* 1993;**3**:225–232.

216 Green KS, Beger TH. Proper use of the combitube. *Anesthesiology* 1994;**81**:513–514.

217 Baraka A, Salem R. The combitube oesophageal–tracheal double lumen airway for difficult intubation. *Can J Anaesth* 1993;**40**:1222–1223.

218 Brimacombe J, Berry A. The oesophageal tracheal combitube for difficult intubation. *Can J Anaesth* 1994;**41**:656–657.

219 Baraka A. The oesophageal tracheal combitube for difficult intubation. *Can J Anaesth* 1994;**41**:657.

220 Department of Health. *Report on confidential enquiries into maternal death in England and Wales 1985–1987.* London: HMSO, 1991.

221 McCrirrick A, Ramage DT, Pracilio JA, Hickman JA. Experience with the laryngeal mask airway in two hundred patients. *Anaesth Intens Care* 1991;**19**:256–260.

222 O'Sullivan G, Stoddart PA. Failed tracheal intubation. *Br J Anaesth* 1991;**67**:225.

223 Byrne F, Oduro-Dominah A, Kipling R. The effect of pregnancy on pulmonary nitrogen washout. A study of pre-oxygenation. *Anaesthesia* 1987;**42**:148–150.

224 Rosen M. Difficult and failed intubation in obstetrics. In: Latto IP, Rosen M, eds. *Difficulties in tracheal intubation.* London: Baillière Tindall, 1984;152–155.

225 King TA, Adams AP. Failed tracheal intubation. *Br J Anaesth* 1990;**65**:409–410.

226 Griggs WM, Worthley LIG, Gilligan JE, Thomas PD, Myburg JA. A simple percutaneous tracheostomy technique. *Surg Gynecol Obstet* 1990;**170**:543–545.

227 Silk JM, Marsh AM. Pneumothorax caused by a minitracheostomy. *Anaesthesia* 1989;**44**:663–664.

228 Wain JC, Wilson DJ, Mathisen DJ. Clinical experience with minitracheostomy. *Ann Thorac Surg* 1990;**49**:881–886.

229 Department of Health. *Report on confidential enquiries into maternal deaths in England and Wales 1982–1984.* London: HMSO, 1987.

230 Brimacombe J. Emergency airway management in rural practice: use of the laryngeal mask airway. *Aust J Rural Hlth* 1995;**3**:10–19.

231 de Mello WF, Restall J. Difficult intubation. *Can J Anaesth* 1990;**37**:486.

232 Tunstall ME. Failed intubation in the parturient. *Can J Anaesth* 1989;**36**:611–613.

233 Castelletti I, Gollo E, Martello A. Uso della maschera laringea in ginecologia ed ostetricia. *Minerva Anestesiol* 1995;**61**:39–41.

234 Freeman R, Baxendale B, McClune S, Moore JA. Laryngeal mask airway for caesarean section. *Anaesthesia* 1990;**45**:1094–1095.

235 Brimacombe J, Berry A. The laryngeal mask airway for failed intubation (3). *Can J Anaesth* 1993;**40**:802–803.

236 Levy DM. LMA for failed intubation (1). *Can J Anaesth* 1993;**40**:801–802.

237 Asai T, Appadurai I. LMA for failed intubation (2). *Can J Anaesth* 1993;**40**:802.

238 Priscu V, Priscu L, Soroker D. LMA in failed intubation (reply). *Can J Anaesth* 1993;**40**:803.

239 Reynolds F. Tracheostomy in obstetric practice – how about the laryngeal mask airway. *Anaesthesia* 1989;**44**:870.

240 Pennant JH, White PF. The laryngeal mask airway. Its uses in anesthesiology. *Anesthesiology* 1993;**79**:144–163.
241 de Mello WF. Management of failed endotracheal intubation at caesarean section. *Anaesth Intens Care* 1991;**19**:303–304.
242 Pennant JH, Walker MB. Comparison of the endotracheal tube and laryngeal mask in airway management by paramedical personnel. *Anesth Analg* 1992;**74**:531–534.
243 Brimacombe J, Shorney N. The laryngeal mask airway. *Br J Hosp Med* 1992;**47**:252–256.
244 Koppel JN, Reed AP. Formal instruction in difficult airway management. A survey of anesthesiology residency programs. *Anesthesiology* 1995;**83**:1343–1346.
245 Frerk CM, Heath ML, Allagain J. Intubation through the laryngeal mask. *Anaesthesia* 1991;**46**:985–986.

15 Nonanesthetic uses

Training

It has been suggested that the LMA is included in the curriculum of any airway management training program and that all nonanesthetic personnel involved in airway management should receive some training in LMA usage[1]. The precise nature of initial and continued training has yet to be determined. However, a standardized training course has been established in several major centers in the UK and is proving popular with nursing staff. For example, over 50% of nurses at the Conquest Hospital in Hastings, UK, are LMA trained for resuscitation. Recent data from this hospital show: (1) those trained in Hastings chose the LMA in 95% of arrests; (2) of the 382 arrests between January 1994 and August 1995, 203 were managed with the LMA; (3) observed regurgitations during airway use in these patients were 28% for the bag and mask and 1.5% for the LMA; (4) of the three regurgitations with the LMA, all had prior management with the face mask.

Emergency medicine

There is a high risk of gastric insufflation and pulmonary aspiration occurring during cardiopulmonary resuscitation (CPR)[2,3]. The incidence of pulmonary aspiration is between 9 and 29%, being higher in nonsurvivors. Tracheal intubation is therefore the most suitable method of securing the airway during CPR, but it is not a simple skill to acquire or maintain and may occasionally be inappropriate or impossible. Early management of the airway during CPR is commonly with a face mask, is performed by nonanesthesiologists and is frequently unsuccessful. Other airway devices have been used for CPR. The esophageal obturator airway (EOA) device has been widely used, but ventilation is impossible if the EOA is inserted into the trachea[4,5]. Ventilation may also fail due to difficulty in placement or an inadequate seal with the face mask. Major trauma to the esophagus, stomach and trachea have been reported. The esophageal tracheal combitube (ETC)[6] has also been recommended for CPR and has advantages over the EOA in that neck movement is not required for placement and ventilation is possible if the ETC is inserted into the trachea or esophagus[7]. The ETC is currently only available in one size and cannot be used in patients with an intact gag reflex or patients less than 1.5 m tall. It may also be difficult to determine if the ETC is correctly placed and this may result in hypoxia. As with all airway devices, successful placement of the ETC is not guaranteed[8–11]. A comparison of different emergency airway equipment is given in Table 15.1.

Use of the LMA in emergency medicine was first described by Brain in 1984[12], but an LMA prototype was first used to resuscitate a patient who suffered a cardiac arrest by a nurse in the Intensive Therapy Unit of St Andrews Hospital in London in 1983. The advantages of the LMA for first responders are that it is relatively easy to insert, and the risks of esophageal and right main bronchus intubation are avoided. However, the risks of aspiration and inability to achieve high pressure ventilation are relatively undefined in this patient population. These limitations imply that it should be regarded as a device providing temporary airway support, but not as a replacement for a tracheal tube.

Three hospital studies have demonstrated that unskilled personnel insert the LMA more rapidly and reliably than the tracheal tube[13–15] and two studies indicated that it provides better ventilation than a bag and mask[16,17]. Pennant and Walker showed that success rates (mean time to achieve adequate ventilation) were 94% (38 s) with the LMA and 69% (88 s) with the tracheal tube[13]. Interestingly, Reinhart and Simmons found that health care providers who already had a small amount of tracheal tube experience placed an LMA and achieved effective ventilation faster and more reliably than with a tracheal tube in the same anesthetized and paralyzed patients[18]. Hayes and McCarroll showed that nonanesthetic personnel had an 80% first time placement rate within 25 s and that the LMA was superior to the bag and mask and similar to mouth to mask ventilation[17]. Tolley et al found that the bag and mask was superior for inexperienced personnel[19], but this study has been criticized as the LMA training program was inadequate[20]. By comparison, studies on successful tracheal

Table 15.1 Comparisons of emergency airway equipment

Description	*LMA*	*TT*	*FM*	*ETC*	*EOA*
Ease of use	+++	+	++	+	+
Protection against aspiration*	+	+++	0	++	++
Safe drainage of gastric contents	0	+++	0	++	++
Functions when blindly passed into trachea	NA	Yes	NA	Yes	No
Functions when blindly passed into esophagus	NA	No	NA	Yes	Yes
Requires effective face mask fit	No	No	Yes	No	Yes
Pediatric sizes available	Yes	Yes	Yes	No	No
Cardiorespiratory stability	+++	+	+++	+	+
Aid to intubation	Yes	NA	No	No	No
Ease of ventilation	++	+++	+	++	+
Potential for trauma	+	++	+	++	++

*Both gastric contents and oropharyngeal contamination.

Key: LMA = laryngeal mask airway; TT = tracheal tube; FM = face mask; ETC = esophageal tracheal combitube; EOA = esophageal obturator airway; NA = not applicable.

intubation by trained paramedics report 90% successful intubation rates[21,22], but Stewart et al reported that only 50–60% of these were at the first attempt[22]. Most complications were related to prolonged attempts at intubation and esophageal intubation which suggests that the LMA may be a useful alternative airway for paramedics and ambulance staff.

The degree to which these studies are applicable to the clinical circumstances of emergency airway management where patients are at risk of aspiration and often have pulmonary pathology has been questioned[23], but there is prospective evidence from field studies that the LMA has a role during CPR, albeit undefined. Grantham et al trained 30 ambulance officers in the use of the LMA and 233 insertions were attempted in the field over a 12-month period[24–28]. The LMA provided an effective airway in 90% of patients sufficiently comatose to compromise airway care and soiling occurred in 10 patients. A large multicenter trial showed that, after a training program, ward nurses obtained satisfactory chest expansion with the LMA in 86% of cases during CPR[29]. In 7% of these subsequent intubation by an anesthesiologist proved difficult and ventilation was continued through the LMA. There was one case of aspiration which may well have occurred at the time of the arrest. The interval between cardiac arrest and LMA insertion was 2.4 min. Kokkinis reported 49/50 successful LMA placements during in-hospital CPR by junior anesthesiologists with very good blood gases for both survivors and nonsurvivors and no instances of aspiration[30]. Pellanda et al reported the successful use of the LMA in 28/32 patients requiring CPR[31]. Verghese et al surveyed the success of airway management by nonanesthesiologists in a 407 bed hospital over a 2-year period and found that survival improved after the introduction of the LMA[32]. A follow-up survey confirmed this finding[33]. The LMA training program included five successful placements in a mannequin and five in anesthetized patients. Finally, LMA trained neonatologists were able to initially resuscitate 21/21 neonates with the LMA and in all cases insertion was successful at the first attempt[34].

The Japanese Ministry of Health and Welfare approved the use of the LMA by paramedics during CPR in February 1992 and the world's first symposium on the LMA in prehospital care was held in Japan in May 1993. In 1996, the LMA was included in the guidelines of the European Resuscitation Council for the advanced management of the airway and ventilation during resuscitation[35]. A UK-wide trial will shortly commence on its use in the field. Until the results of such trials are available, the role of the LMA in the emergency situation will remain unproven. In assessing the potential role of the LMA outside the operating room, the risks of a less secure airway must be balanced against the benefits of ease of training, possible wider availability than tracheal intubation, skills maintenance and speed of insertion[24]. In addition consideration must be given to those difficult airway situations where the face mask or tracheal tube fail to secure the airway. Myles et al recently reported failed intubation in a trauma patient in whom LMA insertion was life saving and facilitated subsequent percutaneous tracheostomy[36]. Aye and Milne reported successful use of the LMA to provide temporary airway support in the emergency department in an obese trauma patient with micrognathia, a short bull neck and nasopharyngeal bleeding[37]. Most authors consider that the LMA would be a preferable option to emergency cricothyrotomy[36–39], which is a technically difficult and occasionally time consuming procedure and is associated with a survival rate of less than 50%[40,41]. Blind passage of a cannula into the trachea via the LMA for the purposes of drug administration during resuscitation is not recommended due to the high failure rate (82%)[42]. In Australia and Japan the LMA is already in regular use in some regions by ambulance personnel for pre-hospital care[43]. It is possible that the LMA will find a role in emergency room management of suspected cervical spine injury as it may be inserted with the head maintained in the neutral position[44–49].

Lessons learnt from the multicenter trial[29,50,51] are:

1. nurses can easily be trained to insert the LMA and become very enthusiastic;
2. it is essential to set up an organized training program;
3. personnel who have not been correctly trained must not be permitted to use the device;
4. significant time can be saved in starting effective ventilation when the LMA is used by nurses on the ward;
5. the LMA is a face mask substitute, not a tracheal tube substitute, and as soon as an intubation competent person becomes available the decision to intubate or continue with the LMA must be made by them; and
6. the frequency of intubation difficulty is higher after cardiac arrest than in the operating theater.

It was also considered that the risk of regurgitation/aspiration was greater in (a) the semiconscious patient when muscle tone was present, (b) if previous face mask ventilation was performed and was difficult, and (c) if airway reflexes were not present when the LMA was removed. Warwick et al have suggested that basic life support training for nursing staff should incorporate early use of the LMA[52]. Curry suggests that situations where it may be appropriate to use the LMA include:

1. an unconscious but breathing patient when it is not reasonable (without the presence of an anesthesiologist) to paralyze the patient to allow intubation and when blind nasal intubation is not an appropriate alternative;
2. where attempts at tracheal intubation have failed – a failure rate of 30–40% would not be unusual for paramedics;
3. in situations where access to the patient is limited and appropriate positioning for tracheal intubation is impossible;
4. where facial damage causes disturbance of the anatomy such that successful intubation is precluded[53].

Patient transportation

It has been proposed that the LMA should be available for aeromedical evacuation teams[54]. Loss of airway control during transportation may present enormous management difficulties, even in the presence of experienced personnel. Even an intubated patient may occasionally suffer a tracheal tube-related incident and urgently require another form of airway control[55,56]. Restricted access, constant movement and noise may make re-intubation and face mask ventilation not just difficult, but impossible. The appropriate sized LMA should be immediately available on the difficult airway tray during transport of critically ill patients both within and between hospitals. The successful use of the LMA during helicopter transfer of a neonate has been reported[54].

Intensive care

The ideal requirements for any airway device used in this setting are reliability in terms of airway patency and fixation stability, effective protection against aspiration of gastric contents or other secretions, low airflow resistance, lack of trauma when used over a period of days or weeks, ease of insertion and replacement in case of accidental dislodgment, good patient acceptance, preservation of an effective cough reflex, and absence of infection transmission risk. Clearly no existing device can claim to fulfill all these criteria.

There are several anecdotal reports[46,57–63] and four small series[64–67] where the LMA has been used in the intensive care unit (ICU) for airway rescue, percutaneous tracheostomy and for minimally invasive airway control. Most authors consider it to have a role in the management of the difficult airway in ICU[60,68–70] and this is supported by a number of case reports where the LMA may have been life saving[46,71]. For instance, it was used in a patient who developed severe acute upper airway obstruction 48 h after an anterior cervical fusion[46]. Manual ventilation by face mask, and laryngoscopy and intubation were impossible owing to the nature of the surgery and halo jacket. More specialized uses, however, have been proposed.

The LMA is better tolerated than the tracheal tube and may be useful in selected patients where weaning with a tracheal tube may require sedation to a degree that compromises adequate spontaneous ventilation[63] or where intubation is unnecessary, but airway support required[57,62]. It may be useful where a noninterventionist decision has been made not to intubate the patient[58] or where the hemodynamic stress response to intubation would be harmful, such as in acute cerebrovascular disease[64]. It may also be useful for short-term assistance during weaning since it can be used to provide continuous positive airway pressure[62] or inspiratory pressure support[72,73]. Its use, however, would depend on the patient having an empty stomach, and in theory chest physiotherapy may be difficult since turning and suctioning might precipitate laryngeal spasm and regurgitation. Blind suction of the upper airway but not easily of the lower would be possible; this restricts its usefulness for chest physiotherapy to those patients with an active cough reflex. However, in this context an important advantage of the LMA is that it permits effective coughing, theoretically reducing the need for physiotherapy with the LMA in place.

Other potential applications would be as an aid to awake bronchoscopy and conventional tracheostomy when it avoids the risk of tracheal tube cuff rupture and the need to withdraw the airway during surgery[74]. Endoscopic guided percutaneous tracheostomy performed on the ICU is now a common technique in the UK and Australia, in which a guidewire is inserted through the cricothyroid membrane and dilators used prior to inserting a tracheostomy tube[75]. It can also be performed with fiberoptic guidance via the LMA in fasted patients with normal lung compliance and no glottic edema[76,77]. The advantages over the tracheal tube are that the LMA allows better views of the trachea without interfering with the surgical field so that misplacement of the wire is avoided[61,65]. The LMA has also been used for the bronchoscopic removal of a sputum plug[60] and for diagnostic fiberoptic bronchoscopy in patients with respiratory failure[67]. In the latter study lung function returned to preoperative status within 1 h. Aoyagi has reported a series of 30 patients using the LMA in combination with a minitracheostomy for overnight management of patients with poor respiratory function as a means of avoiding intubation and ventilation[66]. It has also been used in ICU for the management of pneumothorax, including a 63-year-old woman 3 weeks post multitrauma who had a large bulla[78], where PPV was considered undesirable. The LMA has been used in the ICU to provide respiratory support for 10–24 h with no apparent problems[62,66]. Costa e Silva reported use of the LMA as an airway intubator in a patient with an acute subarachnoid hemorrhage in whom the LMA remained in situ with a partially deflated cuff for 8 days (L Costa e Silva, personal communication, 1996). This resulted in a small area of pharyngeal necrosis and meant that accidental tracheal extubation went unnoticed. Interestingly, on two occasions following LMA removal the patient required urgent airway control and on neither occasion was the LMA available. On the second occasion an emergency tracheostomy was required. It was suggested that the LMA should be removed within 24 h (see Chapter 14, *Technical considerations*) of its use as an airway intubator and that prior to this the cuff should be deflated. Where the LMA has been required for airway rescue one should be immediately available in case of further problems.

Careful consideration must be given to the risk/benefit ratio of any intervention in each individual. It should be noted that the relationship between length of fasting and gastric volume is unpredictable in a critically ill patient. The introduction of the LMA into the ICU as an emergency airway device would seem appropriate for those situations where the trachea cannot be intubated and face mask ventilation is ineffective. The safe and effective use of the LMA in ICU requires that potential users acquire basic skills and a full understanding of the limitations of the device. In this respect communication between anesthetists and intensivists is critical. Prototypes are currently being assessed which may be more appropriate for ICU use, having both an improved seal and the ability to separate the gastrointestinal and respiratory tracts, potentially reducing the risk of aspiration[79] (see Chapter 17, *Future designs*).

References

1 Brimacombe J, Berry A. The laryngeal mask airway. *Br Med J* 1993;**306**:580.
2 Nagel EL, Fine EG, Krischer JP, Davis JH. Complications of CPR. *Crit Care Med* 1981;**9**:424.
3 Lawes EG, Baskett PJF. Pulmonary aspiration during unsuccessful cardiopulmonary resuscitation. *Intens Care Med* 1987;**13**:379–382.
4 Don Michael TA, Gordon AS. The oesophageal obturator airway: a new device in emergency cardiopulmonary resuscitation. *Br Med J* 1980;**281**:1531–1534.
5 Tunstall ME, Geddes C. 'Failed intubation' in obstetric anaesthesia. An indication for use of the 'Esophageal Gastric Tube Airway'. *Br J Anaesth* 1984;**56**:659–661.
6 Frass M, Frezner R, Zdrahal F, Hoflehner G, Porges P, Lackner F. The esophageal tracheal combitube: preliminary results with a new airway for cardiopulmonary resuscitation. *Ann Emerg Med* 1987;**16**:768–772.
7 Wissler RN. The esophageal–tracheal combitube. *Anaesth Rev* 1993;**20**:147–152.
8 Brimacombe J, Berry A. The oesophageal tracheal combitube for difficult intubation. *Can J Anaesth* 1994;**41**:656–657.

9 Baraka A. The oesophageal tracheal combitube for difficult intubation. *Can J Anaesth* 1994;**41**:657.

10 Green KS, Beger TH. Proper use of the combitube. *Anesthesiology* 1994;**81**:513–514.

11 Kline JS. Proper use of the combitube (a reply). *Anesthesiology* 1994;**81**:514.

12 Brain AIJ. The laryngeal mask airway – a possible new solution to airway problems in the emergency situation. *Arch Emerg Med* 1984;**1**:229–232.

★ 13 Pennant JH, Walker MB. Comparison of the endotracheal tube and laryngeal mask in airway management by paramedical personnel. *Anesth Analg* 1992;**74**:531–534.
Prospective study comparing the performance of paramedics with the LMA and tracheal tube in normal anesthetized patients. Placement of the LMA was more rapid and successful than that of the tracheal tube.

14 Davies PRF, Tighe SQ, Greenslade GL, Evans GH. Laryngeal mask airway and tracheal tube insertion by unskilled personnel. *Lancet* 1990;**336**:977–979.

15 Reinhart DJ. Laryngeal mask airway (LMA) vs endotracheal tube (ETT) placement by paramedics, respiratory therapists and registered nurses. *Anesthesiology* 1993;**79**:A1058 (Abstract).

16 Martin PD, Cyna AM, Hunter WAH, Henry J, Pamayya GP. Training nursing staff in airway management for resuscitation – a clinical comparison of the facemask and laryngeal mask. *Anaesthesia* 1993;**48**:33–37.

17 Hayes A, McCarrol SM. Airway management in unskilled personnel – a comparison of laryngeal mask airway, pocket mask and bag-valve-mask techniques. *Anesthesiology* 1995;**83**:A223 (Abstract).

18 Reinhart DJ, Simmons G. Comparison of placement of the laryngeal mask airway with endotracheal tube by paramedics and respiratory therapists. *Ann Emerg Med* 1994;**24**:260–263.

19 Tolley PM, Watts DJ, Hickman JA. Comparison of the use of the laryngeal mask and face mask by inexperienced personnel. *Br J Anaesth* 1992;**69**:320–321.

20 Walker MB, Goodwin APL, Verghese C, et al. Use of the laryngeal mask and face mask by inexperienced personnel. *Br J Anaesth* 1993;**70**:114–115.

21 Vertesi L. The paramedic ambulance: a Canadian experience. *Can Med Assoc J* 1978;**119**:25.

22 Stewart RD, Paris PM, Pelton GH, Cannon GM. Field endotracheal intubation by paramedical personnel. *Chest* 1984;**85**:341.

23 Devitt JH. Mask lung ventilation by ambulance personnel. *Can J Anaesth* 1994;**41**:872–873.

24 Grantham H, Phillips G, Gilligan JE. The laryngeal mask in pre-hospital emergency care. *Emerg Med* 1994;**6**:193–197.

25 Brimacombe J. The laryngeal mask airway in pre-hospital emergency care. *Emerg Med* 1994;**6**:351–352.

26 Grantham H. The laryngeal mask in pre-hospital emergency care. *Emerg Med* 1994;**6**:352–353.

27 Oxer HF. The laryngeal mask in pre-hospital emergency care. *Emerg Med* 1995;**7**:56–57.

28 Grantham H, Phillips G, Gilligan JE. The laryngeal mask in pre-hospital emergency care. *Emergency Medicine* 1995;**7**:57.

★ 29 Stone BJ, Leach AB, Alexander CA, et al. The use of the laryngeal mask airway by nurses during cardiopulmonary resuscitation – results of a multicentre trial. *Anaesthesia* 1994;**49**:3–7.
Multicenter trial looking at use of the LMA for resuscitation for paramedics and nurses. Showed a high success rate. Notable features were the short time between arrest and gaining control of the airway and the low incidence of LMA-related aspiration.

30 Kokkinis K. The use of the laryngeal mask airway in CPR. *Resuscitation* 1994;**27**:9–12.

31 Pellanda A, Ruffini C, Conti L, Fagnoni L, Avanzi GL. Utilita e limiti dell masschera laringea nella rianimazione extraospedaliera. *Minerva Anestesiol* 1995;**61**:51–52.

32 Verghese C, Prior-Willeard PFS, Baskett PJF. Immediate management of the airway during cardopulmonary resuscitation in a hospital without a resident anaesthesiologist. *Eur J Emerg Med* 1994;**1**:123–125.

33 Verghese C, Eastwick-Field PFS, Barnes IL. Management of the immediate airway during cardio-pulmonary resuscitation with the laryngeal mask airway. *Third Scientific Congress of the European Resuscitation Council, Seville, Spain, 6–8 June 1996.*

34 Paterson SJ, Byrne PJ, Molesky MG, Seal RF, Finucane BT. Neonatal resuscitation using the laryngeal mask airway. *Anesthesiology* 1994;**80**:1248–1253.

35 Baskett PJF, Bossaert L, Carli P, et al. Guidelines for the advanced management of the airway and ventilation during resuscitation. *Resuscitation* 1996;**31**:201–230.

36 Myles PS, Venema HR, Lindholm DE. Trauma patient managed with the laryngeal mask airway and percutaneous tracheostomy after failed intubation. *Med J Aust* 1994;**161**:640.

37 Aye T, Milne B. Use of the laryngeal mask prior to definitive intubation in a difficult airway: a case report. *J Emerg Med* 1995;**13**:711–714.

38 Brimacombe J, Berry A. The laryngeal mask airway – an alternative to emergency cricothyrotomy when conventional airway management fails in the field. *J Trauma* (in press).

39 Coluccia R, Grossi P. La maschera laringea in urgenza ed emergenza. *Minerva Anestesiol* 1995;**61**:13–15.

40 Miklus RM, Elliott C, Snow N. Surgical cricothyrotomy in the field: experience of a helicopter transport team. *J Trauma* 1989;**29**:506–508.

41 Xeropotamos NS, Coats TJ, Wilson AW. Prehospital surgical airway management: 1 year's experience from the Helicopter Emergency Medical Service. *Injury* 1993;**24**:222–224.
42 Alexander R, Smith G. Laryngeal mask airway (LMA) and tracheal route for drug administration in resuscitation. *Third Scientific Congress of the European Resuscitation Council, Seville, Spain, 6–8 June 1996*, p.56 (Abstract).
43 Brimacombe J. Does the laryngeal mask airway have a role outside the operating theatre? *Can J Anaesth* 1995;**42**:258–259.
44 Calder I, Ordman AJ, Jackowski A, Crockard HA. The Brain laryngeal mask airway. An alternative to emergency tracheal intubation. *Anaesthesia* 1990;**45**:137–139.
45 Logan A. Use of the laryngeal mask in a patient with an unstable fracture of the cervical spine. *Anaesthesia* 1991;**46**:987.
46 Lee JJ, Yau K, Barcroft J. LMA and respiratory arrest after anterior cervical fusion. *Can J Anaesth* 1993;**40**:395–396.
47 Asai T. Fiberoptic tracheal intubation through the laryngeal mask airway in an awake patient with cervical spine instability. *Anesth Analg* 1993;**77**:404.
48 Pennant JH, Pace NA, Gajraj NM. Role of the laryngeal mask airway in the immobile cervical spine. *J Clin Anesth* 1993;**5**:226–230.
49 Gabbott DA, Sasada MP. Laryngeal mask airway insertion using cricoid pressure and manual in-line neck stabilisation. *Anaesthesia* 1995;**50**:674–676.
50 Brain AIJ. Use of the laryngeal mask airway as a face-mask substitute in cardio-pulmonary resuscitation. *Minerva Anestesiol* 1995;**61**:7–8.
51 Baskett PJF. The laryngeal mask in resuscitation. *11th World Congress of Anesthesiology, Sydney, 14–20 April 1996, Abstract Handbook*, p.530 (Abstract).
52 Warwick JP, Mackie K, Spencer I. Towards early defibrillation – a nurse training programme in the use of automated external defibrillators. *Resuscitation* 1995;**30**:231–235.
53 Curry P. The laryngeal mask in pre-hospital care. *J Br Assoc Immediate Care* 1994;**17**:55–57.
54 Brimacombe J, De Maio B. Emergency use of the laryngeal mask airway during helicopter transfer of a neonate. *J Clin Anesth* 1995;**7**:689–690.
55 Guidelines for the transfer of critically ill patients. Guidelines Committee of the American College of Critical Care Medicine; Society of Critical Care Medicine and American Association of Critical Care Nurses Transfer Guidelines Task Force. *Crit Care Med* 1993;**21**:931–937.
56 Kanter RK, Tompkins JM. Adverse events during interhospital transport: physiologic deterioration associated with pretransport severity of illness. *Pediatrics* 1989;**84**:43–48.
57 Salib YM. The use of the laryngeal mask airway in intensive care. *Today's Anaesthetist* 1989;**4**:268.
58 Lim W. Yet another use for the laryngeal mask. *Anaesthesia* 1992;**47**:175–176.
59 Fullekrug B, Pothmann W, Druge G. Unkonventioneller Einsatz der Kehlikopfmaske zur Therapie einer postoperativen, atelektasenbedingten Ateminsuffizienz. *Anaesthesiol Intensivmed Notfallmed Schmerzther* 1993;**28**:187–189.
60 Mabuchi N. Laryngeal mask airway in the ICU. *J Clin Exp Med* 1992;**162,12,9**:876–878.
61 Brimacombe J, Clarke G, Simons S. The laryngeal mask airway for endoscopic guided percutaneous tracheostomy. *Anaesthesia* 1994;**49**:358–359.
62 Arosio EM, Conci F. Use of the laryngeal mask airway for respiratory distress in the intensive care unit. *Anaesthesia* 1995;**50**:635–636.
63 Taylor JC, Bell GT. An asthmatic weaned from a ventilator using a laryngeal mask. *Anaesthesia* 1995;**50**:454–455.
64 Ito N, Aikawa N, Hori S, et al. Laryngeal mask airway in acute cerebrovascular disease. *Lancet* 1992;**339**:69.
★ 65 Dexter TJ. The laryngeal mask airway: a method to improve visualisation of the trachea and larynx during fibreoptic assisted percutaneous tracheostomy. *Anaesth Intens Care* 1994;**22**:35–39.
Paper describing the use of the LMA for fiberoptic guided percutaneous tracheostomy in nine ICU patients. Suggested that the technique may be useful in selected patients.
66 Aoyagi M. Application of the laryngeal mask airway in ICU. *40th Meeting of the Japanese Society of Anesthesiology, Iwate Prefectual Hall, Japan, 22 April 1993*, pp.6–7 (Abstract).
67 Buzzetti V, Cigada M, Solca M, Iapichino G. Use of the laryngeal mask airway during fibreoptic bronchoscopy. *Intens Care World* 1996;**13**:72–74.
68 Brimacombe J, Berry A, Verghese C. The laryngeal mask airway in critical care medicine. *Intens Care Med* 1995;**21**:361–364.
69 Brimacombe J. The role of the laryngeal mask airway (LMA) in the intensive care unit. *19th Australian and New Zealand Scientific Meeting on Intensive Care, Darling Harbour, Sydney, 20–23 October 1994, Conference Handbook*, p.172 (Abstract).
70 Brimacombe J, Berry A. The laryngeal mask airway in emergency and intensive care medicine. *Intens Care World* 1994;**11**:26–27.
71 Brimacombe J, Gandini D. Paediatric airway management. *Br J Hosp Med* 1995;**53**:175.

72 Groudine SB, Lumb PD, Sandison MR. Pressure support ventilation with the laryngeal mask airway: a method to manage severe reactive airway disease postoperatively. *Can J Anaesth* 1995;**42**:341–343.

73 Capdevila X, Biboulet P, Vallee M, Drissi S, D'Athis F. Pressure support ventilation with a laryngeal mask during general anesthesia. *Anesthesiology* 1995;**83**:A1226 (Abstract).

74 Thomson KD. Laryngeal mask airway for elective tracheostomy. *Anaesthesia* 1992;**47**:76.

75 Miyasaka K. Laryngeal mask airway in pediatric anesthesia. *J Clin Exp Med* 1992;**162**:872–875.

76 Dexter TJ. Laryngeal oedema, a marker of an 'at risk' airway. *Anaesthesia* 1994;**49**:826.

77 Ip-Yam C, Shaw S. The laryngeal mask airway and endoscopic guided percutaneous tracheostomy. *Anaesthesia* 1994;**49**:733–734.

78 Yamauchi M. Use of the LM in patients with pneumothorax. *J Clin Anesth (Rinsho-Masui)* 1993;**17**:239–240.

79 Brain AIJ, Verghese C, Strube P, Brimacombe J. A new laryngeal mask prototype – preliminary evaluation of seal pressures and glottic isolation. *Anaesthesia* 1995;**50**:42–48.

16 Pediatrics and neonatal resuscitation

Introduction

The LMA has been widely used in the pediatric population and its use in children is supported by a large number of studies[1–35] and case reports[36–72]. The size 1 LMA is suitable for neonates up to 5 kg babies; the recently developed size 1.5 is suitable for babies from 5 to 10 kg; size 2 is suitable for babies from 10 to 20 kg; size 2.5 is suitable for children between 20 and 30 kg; and size 3 should be used for children over 30 kg (see Table 5.7). The size 1 LMA has been used for resuscitation of premature neonates weighing 1–1.5 kg[73] and for low birth weight infants with bronchopulmonary dysplasia undergoing cryopexy[74,75], but its routine use in very small infants cannot be recommended without further study.

Some authors consider that experience with the LMA in adults is essential before attempting its use in children because difficulties are encountered more commonly[76], but provided there is adequate supervision such precautions are unnecessary, at least for older children. It has been suggested that the complication rate increases with decreasing LMA size[20,77]. This may be related to the increased anesthetic requirement of children[78,79] or to a smaller error margin for accurate placement. Much of it is probably related to the well-known difficulties of anesthetizing small children[80]. One study has shown that the complication rates occurring between the size 1 and size 2 LMA were similar[9]. There have been no controlled studies comparing the problems in adults and children, but a large prospective survey failed to show an increased incidence of problems compared with adults[81]. LMA usage in pediatric anesthesia has been reviewed by Haynes and Morton[82] and Miyasaka[83] and has been the subject of an editorial by Wilson[84].

Anatomy and physiology

Anatomy

The LMA was designed for use in adults, but a scaled down version was found empirically to work equally effectively in children in spite of the differences in the infant larynx. Anatomical studies subsequently showed the pharyngeal sac to be substantially the same in children as in adults[55]. The incidence of anatomical misplacement is considered to be higher in children than in adults[2,9,84,85], but the incidence of functional success is similar. Goudsouzian et al examined the radiological localization of the LMA in infants and children using magnetic resonance imaging or CT scans[7]. In 86% the epiglottis was deflected down by 90 degrees or more, but this had no effect on ventilatory parameters. Gurpinar et al in a fiberoptic study of 100 children using the standard insertion technique found that the epiglottis was within the bowl in 38%, but that function was unaffected[31].

Physiology

Reignier et al have shown that in children aged 6–24 months anesthetized with halothane there is less paradoxic inspiratory movement breathing through the LMA than the tracheal tube[22]. Watcha et al have shown that following induction with halothane LMA placement produces less hemodynamic stress response and lower intraocular pressure than tracheal intubation[5]. Demiralp et al showed that intraocular pressure rises were similar when comparing the tracheal tube (thiopentone–fentanyl–atracurium) with the LMA (either thiopentone–fentanyl or halothane), but heart rate was higher in the tracheal tube group[32]. Gonzalez-Zarco et al showed that there were minimal hemodynamic changes to LMA insertion and removal in 225 children[27]. This has been confirmed in a further study of 200 patients by Mora et al[68]. Jung et al have shown that placement with a laryngoscope produces a more exaggerated hemodynamic stress response than the standard technique[86]. There were no differences in blood pressure or pulse rate following LMA insertion with propofol 2.5 versus 3.5 mg kg^{-1}[87]. Ferrari and Goudsouzian have shown that the LMA is suitable for children with bronchopulmonary dysplasia[88].

Safety and efficacy

Braun and Fritz reported LMA use in 3000 children with a 0.1% incidence of serious complications[17]. Lopez-Gil et al undertook a survey of LMA usage in 1400 pediatric patients by 10 trainee anesthesiologists to provide information about insertion and complication rates using the standard insertion technique[20]. The overall problem rate was 11.5%, but oxygen saturation briefly fell below 90% on 23 occasions (1.7%). The incidence of problems was unrelated to the mode of ventilation, or whether isoflurane or total intravenous anesthesia with propofol was used for maintenance. Watcha et al showed that there were fewer hypoxic episodes with the LMA compared with the face mask for myringotomy[89]. One study failed to demonstrate any outcome differences between the face mask and tracheal tube for peripheral orthopedic procedures[90].

Anesthesia

The insertion technique is the same as in adults, but a greater degree of gentleness and deftness of touch is required and occasional pediatric anesthetists should first gain experience in adults. Preoxygenation is recommended where possible[79]. It is likely that the standard technique is also superior in pediatric patients[20,21,84], although some authors have recommended semi-inflation[91] or use of the Guedel airway technique[92], or a laryngoscope[78,93]. First time insertion rates in children vary between 67 and 90%, depending on the level of experience[3,4,26,29,77]; this improves considerably with increased experience to around 98%[3,21]. In a study of 1400 pediatric LMA insertions using the standard technique, placement was successful in 90% at the first attempt, 8% at the second attempt and 2% required an alternative technique[20]. Alternative techniques are not generally recommended unless the standard technique fails (see Chapter 6, *Alternative insertion techniques*). The inventor has consistently found when teaching that those who recommend the inflated technique have failed to understand one or more details of the standard technique.

Gaseous induction with halothane provides excellent conditions for insertion. Isoflurane is not generally considered a suitable gaseous induction agent in children[94]. However, Rungreungvanich et al detected no difference in problem rates in 88 children undergoing inhalational induction with halothane or isoflurane, and conditions for LMA insertion were similar[95]. Enflurane is less irritant and may be suitable in those undergoing repeat anesthesia. Sevoflurane is reported to be an excellent induction agent when the LMA is used in children[16]. Desflurane is an unsuitable agent for inhalational induction due to airway irritability[80,94], but may be utilized following intravenous induction and facilitates a rapid emergence[96]. Ketamine has been used successfully in combination with halothane-enriched air, but has not been adequately investigated[97]. Mizikov et al reported a 10% incidence of laryngospasm following induction with ketamine, midazolam and fentanyl[33]. Taguchi et al have shown that the minimum alveolar concentration for LMA insertion is lower than for the tracheal tube in children[16]. Larger doses of propofol (3.5–5.0 mg kg^{-1})[78,79,87,98] are required than in adults and safe placement is aided by preoxygenation[79]. Martlew et al determined the dose–response curves for LMA insertion with propofol in premedicated and unpremedicated children[99]. The doses required for satisfactory LMA insertion in 50% and 90% of unpremedicated patients (95% confidence interval) were 3.4–4.2 mg kg^{-1} and 4.7–6.8 mg kg^{-1}, respectively; those for premedicated patients were 2.2–2.8 and 3.2–4.3 mg kg^{-1}, respectively. The authors considered that, both rate of injection and timing of insertion are important factors in lowering propofol requirements. Thiopentone has the same disadvantages as in adults and insertion should be delayed until reflex response has been abolished by inhalational anesthesia. Inhalational induction or high dose propofol is the preferred method.

Spontaneous ventilation is an acceptable technique in children even though it commonly leads to moderate hypercapnea[100]. Controlled ventilation may be readily achieved in children and is considered relatively safe and effective provided certain precautions are adhered to[24,101,102]. Epstein et al showed that the initial mean leak pressure in children was 25.9 cm H_2O with less than 3% having leak pressures less than 10 cm H_2O and 7% greater than 34 cm H_2O [24] (see Chapter 6, *Positive pressure ventilation*). Precautions include using moderate tidal volumes, minimal peak inspiratory pressures and continual monitoring of airway integrity, gas leak and abdominal distension[101]. Where gastric insufflation is a concern it is preferable to insert a nasogastric tube prior to LMA insertion.

Infants

Sorba et al conducted a prospective study of 37 infants (<6.5 kg) undergoing 42 surgical procedures[19]. Induction was with halothane and LMA insertion was successful in 80.9% at the first attempt and a good airway obtained in 93%. Orfei et al reported the successul use of the LMA in 50 infants aged approximately 100 (2–400) days undergoing a variety of general surgical procedures (n = 15) or for airway management prior to tracheal intubation (n = 35)[103]. In the latter group oxygen saturation was greater than 95% in all patients. The most frequent cause of insertion failure was insufficient depth of anesthesia. Insertion in infants even at adequate levels of anesthesia often causes temporary interference with normal ventilation, noisy breathing due to mild laryngeal spasm or vocalization being typical. Experience will tell the anesthesiologist whether such sounds represent transient reaction to insertion or true obstruction. With correct insertion technique the latter will be rare. As the airway is so small, even slight reaction to surgical stimulus may cause reversible obstruction at the laryngeal level. Gentle application of continuous positive airway pressure (CPAP) often suffices to overcome the obstruction, but the key to success is to achieve adequate anesthetic depth.

Emergence and postoperative aspects

There is conflicting evidence as to whether the LMA should be removed deep or awake in children[19,104]. Varughesa et al showed that there were fewer complications if the LMA was removed deep[104], but Sorba et al recommended late removal[19]. In infants recovery is probably best carried out in the operating room with the infant in the lateral position. The advantages of the LMA in terms of sore throat have not been adequately demonstrated in children[105]. Fung et al have shown that emergence times are reduced with the LMA compared with the tracheal tube in children undergoing hepatic angiography prior to liver transplant surgery[35]. The inventor recommends awake removal provided: (1) cuff pressure is not excessive (60 cm H_2O); (2) adequate pain relief has been given; (3) the device is correctly positioned and secured in place; (4) an appropriate bite block is in place; and (5) removal is not attempted before complete return of protective reflexes. Laryngeal spasm associated with secretions is best managed with CPAP.

Pediatric difficult airway

The LMA has been used for a wide variety of pediatric airway problems, many associated with congenital syndromes[38,41,45,50–52,61–63,66,67,69,70,72,106–113] (Table 16.1). There are no studies correlating ease of insertion of the LMA and factors known to predict or score difficult intubation in children. Mallampati scoring is not a good predictor of difficult intubation in children[114]. The vocal cords are visible from the mask aperture bars in approximately 75% of children[2,9,84,85]. Blind intubation through the LMA is possible in children[115] and infants[116], but, as in adults, direct fiberoptic techniques are safer and more reliable[117]. Heard et al assessed a technique of using the LMA to facilitate the use of a fiberoptic scope to position a guidewire for directing the placement of a tracheal tube in 15 normal children undergoing dental surgery[23]. The authors demonstrated that the technique was 100% successful and was without undesirable cardiovascular or respiratory side effects. Experience of the LMA as an airway intubator in infants is limited, but blind and fiberoptic techniques have been performed in both awake and anesthetized infants[38,41,62,107,108,111,113,118]. Inada et al reported two patients with Treacher Collins syndrome in whom intubation was accomplished via the LMA with a FOS/TT combination following failure with the blind passage of a bougie[119]. The LMA has been used to secure the airway of a 13-year-old girl with a laryngeal fracture and soft tissue swelling following gaseous induction[120]. The safety of such an approach is questionable. Rabb et al reported successful blind intubation via the LMA in two infants (weight 7 and 5 kg) in whom conventional intubation was impossible[116]. The role of the LMA in the pediatric difficult airway has been discussed by Vener and Lerman[121].

Table 16.1 Pediatric airway problems managed successfully with the LMA

Airway rescue (helicopter transfer)[122]	Hurler's syndrome*[51]*
Airway rescue (special care baby unit)[123]	Kenny–Caffey syndrome[124]
Arthrogryphosis multiplex congenita[45,67,69]	Neck contracture[54,50]
Cervical spine anomaly*[117]*	Obstructed hydrocephalus[116]
Cri du chat[61]	Pierre Robin sequence[38,56,109,*118*,*41*,52,70,110,*125*,112]
Diagnostic laryngobronchoscopy[63]	Schwartz–Jampel syndrome*[111]*
Down's syndrome*[72]*	Tongue tumor[45]
Edwards' syndrome[50]	Tracheostomy[41]
Freeman–Sheldon syndrome[116]	Treacher Collins syndrome*[51,126]*
Goldenhar's syndrome*[62,113]*	

Reference numbers in italic indicate that the LMA was also used as airway intubator.

Neonatal resuscitation

It is well known that neonatal airway management is difficult, even for those with advanced airway control skills. In theory, the LMA offers several advantages over the face mask during neonatal resuscitation. It avoids the necessity to form a seal on a slippery surface and manipulation of the head, neck and jaw is not required. It avoids pressure to the eyes and it may free the operator to perform other tasks such as CPR or administer drugs. The advantages over the tracheal tube include avoidance of laryngoscopy and its associated adverse effects, less invasion of the respiratory tract, and avoidance of the risks of endobronchial or esophageal intubation. An attenuated hemodynamic stress response to LMA insertion is likely and this may be important in preventing intraventicular hemorrhage. Furthermore, placement is probably independent of factors governing ease of intubation, making the LMA particularly useful in the 'cannot intubate, cannot ventilate' situation in neonates. Tracheal intubation may also cause laryngeal edema and in the newborn 1 mm of edema reduces the cross-sectional area of the larynx by 65%[127]. It is worth pointing out that other emergency airway management options such as cricothyrotomy puncture, the esophageal tracheal combitube and transtracheal jet ventilation may not be applicable to the neonate. However, potential limitations of the LMA are that it may not be suitable for removal of meconium aspirate and may be inadequate for neonates who require high airway pressures – in these situations it is not a substitute for a tracheal tube.

A large proportion of neonatal resuscitation is performed by nonmedical personnel[128] who are infrequently exposed to advanced resuscitation techniques and may have difficulty in maintaining proficiency[129]. Tests on neonatal intubation training models have shown that midwives and junior doctors can obtain a clear airway more rapidly with the LMA than the tracheal tube and with fewer failures[130], a similar finding to adults[131]. In a prospective pilot study of neonates born with apnea or heart rate <110 min^{-1}, experienced LMA users were able to resuscitate 20/20 neonates with the LMA at the first attempt[1]. Mean time for LMA insertion was <9 s and peak circuit pressure was 37 cm H_2O. Oxygenation and restoration of heart rate occurred in most neonates within 30 s. Other groups have also reported a rapid increase in oxygen saturation for neonates resuscitated with the LMA[132] or a rapid improvement in Apgar score[103]. Our experience is similar and extends to 39/40 successful resuscitations[133]. Three of these neonates weighed 1–1.5 kg[73]. Margaria et al randomly allocated 100 neonates requiring resuscitation to receive either the face mask or LMA and found that the rate of rise in oxygen saturation was more rapid with the LMA[134]. Denny et al used an LMA to successfully resuscitate a 2.75 kg neonate with Pierre Robin syndrome in whom intubation and face mask ventilation had failed[41]. A similar case has been reported by Baraka[112].

It has been suggested that the LMA should be available wherever resuscitation is performed[131]. We consider that the LMA warrants consideration for inclusion in the neonatal resuscitation algorithm[135] for use when other forms of airway management fail, as it has been in difficult airway algorithms in adults[136–139], although this has been contested[133,140,141]. The LMA may have a significant future role in the routine management of neonatal resuscitation as the initial airway of choice where tracheal intubation is not essential. Further randomized prospective studies comparing the LMA with the face mask are currently underway.

References

★ 1 Paterson SJ, Byrne PJ, Molesky MG, Seal RF, Finucane BT. Neonatal resuscitation using the laryngeal mask airway. *Anesthesiology* 1994;**80**:1248–1253.
Prospective study showing the potential value of the LMA for neonatal resuscitation.

2 Rowbottom SJ, Simpson DL, Grubb D. The laryngeal mask airway in children. A fibreoptic assessment of positioning. *Anaesthesia* 1991;**46**:489–491.

3 Johnston DF, Wrigley SR, Robb PJ, Jones HE. The laryngeal mask airway in paediatric anaesthesia. *Anaesthesia* 1990;**45**:924–927.

4 Mason DG, Bingham RM. The laryngeal mask airway in children. *Anaesthesia* 1990;**45**:760–763.

★ 5 Watcha MF, White PF, Tychsen L, Steven JL. Comparative effects of laryngeal mask airway and endotracheal tube insertion on intraocular pressure in children. *Anesth Analg* 1992;**75**:355–360.
Comparative study of 41 children looking at cardiovascular and intraocular reponses to the LMA and tracheal tube. Showed that the LMA was less stimulating.

6 Bailie R, Barnett MB, Fraser JF. The Brain laryngeal mask – a comparative study with the nasal mask in paediatric dental outpatients. *Anaesthesia* 1991;**46**:358–360.

★ 7 Goudsouzian NG, Denman W, Cleveland R, Shorten G. Radiologic localisation of the laryngeal mask airway in children. *Anesthesiology* 1992;**77**:1085–1089.
The first CT and NMR study of the position of the LMA in children. Fifty children were investigated and there was little correlation between position and function. In 46/50 patients the cuff was in the pharynx and covered the laryngeal opening.

8 Williams PJ, Bailey PM. Comparison of the reinforced laryngeal mask airway and tracheal intubation for adenotonsillectomy. *Br J Anaesth* 1993;**70**:30–33.

9 Dubreuil M, Laffon M, Plaud B, Penon C, Ecoffey C. Complications and fiberoptic assessment of size 1 laryngeal mask airway. *Anesth Analg* 1993;**76**:527–529.

10 Webster AC, Morley-Forster PK, Dain S, et al. Anaesthesia for adenotonsillectomy: a comparison between tracheal intubation and the armoured laryngeal mask airway. *Can J Anaesth* 1993;**40**:1171–1177.

11 Spahr-Schopfer IA, Bissonnette B, Hartley EJ. Capnometry and the paediatric laryngeal mask airway. *Can J Anaesth* 1993;**40**:1038–1043.

12 Epstein RH, Halmi BH. Oxygen leakage around the laryngeal mask airway during laser treatment of port-wine stains in children. *Anesth Analg* 1994;**78**:486–489.

13 St Claire Logan A, Morris P. Complications following use of the laryngeal mask airway in children. *Paediatr Anaesth* 1993;**3**:297–300.

14 McGinn G, Haynes SR, Morton NS. An evaluation of the laryngeal mask airway during routine paediatric anaesthesia. *Paediatr Anaesth* 1993;**3**:23–28.

15 Miyasaka K, Suzuki Y, Kondo Y, Nakagawa S, Asahara S. The use of the laryngeal mask airway in paediatric anaesthesia. *J Anaesth* 1991;**5**:160–165.

16 Taguchi M, Watanabe S, Asakura N, Inomata S. End-tidal sevoflurane concentrations for laryngeal mask airway insertion and for tracheal intubation in children. *Anesthesiology* 1994;**81**:628–631.

★ 17 Braun U, Fritz U. Die Kehlopfmaske in der Kinderanasthesie. *Anaesthesiol Intensivmed Notfalmed Schmerzther* 1994;**29**:286–288.
Reports the use of the LMA in 3000 pediatric patients with a high success rate and a 0.1% major complication rate. One patient aspirated with no adverse outcome.

18 Efrat R, Kadari A, Katz S. The laryngeal mask airway in pediatric anesthesia: experience with 120 patients undergoing elective groin surgery. *J Pediatr Surg* 1994;**29**:206–208.

19 Sorba F, Courreges P, Lecoutre D, Bayard-Gary R. Evaulation du Masque Larynge. *Cahiers d'Anesthesiol* 1994;**42**:567–570.

★ 20 Lopez-Gil M, Brimacombe J, Alvarez M. Safety and efficacy of the laryngeal mask airway – a prospective survey of 1400 paediatric patients. *Anaesthesia* 1996;**51**:969–972.
Prospective survey of 1400 LMA uses in pediatrics. Presents data about the frequency of problems during induction, maintenance and emergence. The overall problem rate was 11.5% and the oxygen saturation fell briefly below 90% in 1.7%.

21 Lopez-Gil M, Brimacombe J, Cebrian J, Arranz J. The laryngeal mask airway in pediatric practice – a prospective study of skill acquisition by resident anesthesiologists. *Anesthesiology* 1996;**84**:807–811.

22 Reignier J, Ameur MB, Ecoffey C. Spontaneous ventilation with halothane in children. A comparison between endotracheal tube and laryngeal mask airway. *Anesthesiology* 1995;**83**:674–678.

23 Heard CMB, Caldicott LD, Fletcher JE, Selsby DS. Fiberoptic guided endotracheal intubation via the laryngeal mask airway in paediatric patients. A report of a series of cases. *Anesth Analg* 1996;**82**:1287–1289.

24 Epstein RH, Ferouz F, Jenkins MA. Airway sealing pressures of the laryngeal mask airway in pediatric patients. *J Clin Anesth* 1996;**8**:93–98.

25 Prosperi M, Heinen M, Fantini G. La maschera laringea nell'anestesia ambulatoriale pediatrica. *Minerva Anestesiol* 1995;**61**:53–55.

26 Lopez Gil T, Pazos JC, Zarco LMG. Aplicacion de la mascarilla laringea en anestesia pediatrica. *Rev Esp Anestesiol Reanim* 1995;**42**:332–335.

27 Gonzalez-Zarco L, Mateos M, Lopez-Gil T, Cebrian J. Respuesta hemodinamica de la utilizacion de la mascarilla laringea en anestesia pediatrica. *Rev Esp Anestesiol Reanim* 1993;**40**:64 (Abstract).

28 Mateos M, Gonzalez-Zarco L, Cebrian J, Lopez-Gil T. Problemas de mantenimiento asociados al uso de la mascarilla laringea en anestesia pediatrica. *Rev Esp Anestesiol Reanim* 1993;**40**:64 (Abstract).

29 Mateos M, Gonzalez-Zarco L, Cebrian J, Lopez-Gil T. Utilizacion de la mascarilla laringea en anestesia pediatrica por personal sin experiencia previa. *Rev Esp Anestesiol Reanim* 1993;**40**:65 (Abstract).

30 Lacroix O, Billard V, Bourgain JL, Debaene B. Prevention of postoperative sore throat during use of the laryngeal mask airway. *European Society of Anaesthesiologists Annual Congress, London, 1–5 June 1996;* A51 (Abstract).

31 Gurpinar A, Yavascaoglu B, Korfali G, Dogruyol H. Fibreoptic assessment of positioning of the laryngeal mask airway in children. *European Society of Anaesthesiologists Annual Congress, London, 1–5 June 1996;* A306 (Abstract).

32 Demiralp S, Ates Y, Yorukoglu D, Basar H, Alanoglu Z. Laryngeal mask airway does not increase intraocular pressure regardless of the induction method. *European Society of Anaesthesiologists Annual Congress, London, 1–5 June 1996;* A307 (Abstract).

33 Mizikov V, Variuschina T, Esakov I. The laryngeal mask in paediatric anaesthesia: the first experience in Russia. *11th World Congress of Anesthesiology, Sydney, 14–20 April 1996, Abstract Handbook*, p.465 (Abstract).

34 George JM, Sanders GM. The reinforced laryngeal mask in paediatric outpatient dental surgery. *11th World Congress of Anesthesiology, Sydney, 14–20 April 1996, Abstract Handbook*, p.477 (Abstract).

35 Fung ST, Cheung HK, Jawan B, Tsai PS, Chen CC, Lee JH. Use of the laryngeal mask in off-floor anesthesia for hepatic angiography in pediatric liver transplant candidates. *Transplant Proc* 1996;**28**:1723–1724.

36 Langton JA, Wilson I, Fell D. Use of the laryngeal mask airway during magnetic resonance imaging. *Anaesthesia* 1992;**47**:532.

37 Ngan Kee WD. Laryngeal mask airway for radiotherapy in the prone position. *Anaesthesia* 1992;**47**:446–447.

38 Chadd GD, Crane DL, Phillips RM, Tunell WP. Extubation and reintubation guided by the laryngeal mask airway in a child with the Pierre–Robin syndrome. *Anesthesiology* 1992;**76**:640–641.

39 Molloy AR. Unexpected position of the laryngeal mask airway. *Anaesthesia* 1991;**46**:592.

40 Marjot R. Trauma to the posterior pharyngeal wall caused by a laryngeal mask airway. *Anaesthesia* 1991;**46**:589–590.

41 Denny NM, Desilva KD, Webber PA. Laryngeal mask airway for emergency tracheostomy in a neonate. *Anaesthesia* 1990;**45**:895.

42 Waite K, Filshie J. The use of a laryngeal mask airway for CT radiotherapy planning and daily radiotherapy. *Anaesthesia* 1990;**45**:894.

43 Rowbottom SJ, Simpson DL. Partial obstruction of the laryngeal mask airway. *Anaesthesia* 1990;**45**:892.

44 Smith BL. Brain airway in anaesthesia for patients with juvenile chronic arthritis. *Anaesthesia* 1988;**43**:421.

45 Ravalia A, Goddard JM. The laryngeal mask and difficult tracheal intubation. *Anaesthesia* 1990;**45**:168.

46 Goldberg PL, Evans PF, Filshie J. Kinking of the laryngeal mask airway in two children. *Anaesthesia* 1990;**45**:487–488.

47 Taylor DH, Child CSB. The laryngeal mask for radiotherapy in children. *Anaesthesia* 1990;**45**:690.

48 Maekawa H, Mikawa K, Tanaka O, Goto R, Obara H. The laryngeal mask may be a useful device for fiberoptic airway endoscopy in pediatric anesthesia. *Anesthesiology* 1991;**75**:169–170.

49 Wilson IG, Eastley R. A modification of the laryngeal mask airway. *Anesthesiology* 1991;**74**:1157 (Abstract).

50 Bailey C, Chung R. Use of the laryngeal mask airway in a patient with Edward's syndrome. *Anaesthesia* 1992;**47**:713.

51 Goldie AS, Hudson I. Fibreoptic tracheal intubation through a modified laryngeal mask. *Paediatr Anaesth* 1992;**2**:344.

52 Beveridge ME. Laryngeal mask anaesthesia for repair of cleft palate. *Anaesthesia* 1989;**44**:656–657.

53 Smith TGC, Whittet H, Heyworth T. Laryngomalacia – a specific indication for the laryngeal mask. *Anaesthesia* 1992;**47**:910.

54 Nath G, Major V. The laryngeal mask airway in the management of a paediatric difficult airway. *Anaesth Intens Care* 1992;**20**:518–520.

55 Brain AIJ. The development of the laryngeal mask – a brief history of the invention, early clinical studies and experimental work from which the laryngeal mask evolved. *Eur J Anaesthesiol* 1991;**4**:5–17.

56 Cortes J, Franco A, Cid M, Vidal MI, Rabanal S. Uso de la mascarilla laringea para bronchoscopia fibroptica en un neonato con malformaciones faciales. *Revista Espanola* 1992;**39**:324–325.

57 Stott SA. Use of the laryngeal mask airway in the developing world. *Anaesthesia* 1993;**48**:450.
58 Tatsumi K, Furuya H, Nagahata T, et al. [Removal of a bronchial foreign body in a child using the laryngeal mask]. *Masui* 1993;**42**:441–444.
59 Steib A, Beller JP, Lleu JC, Otteni JC. Intubation difficile reglée par un masque larynge et un fibroscope. *Ann Fr Anesth Reanim* 1992;**11**:601–603.
60 Alexander R, Arrowsmith JE, Frossard RJ. The laryngeal mask airway: safe in the X-ray department. *Anaesthesia* 1993;**48**:734.
61 Castresana MR, Stefansson S, Cancel AR, Hague KJ. Use of the laryngeal mask airway during thoracotomy in a pediatric patient with Cri-du-Chat syndrome. *Anesth Analg* 1994;**78**:817.
62 Johnson CM, Sims C. Awake fibreoptic intubation via a laryngeal mask in an infant with Goldenhar's syndrome. *Anaesth Intens Care* 1994;**22**:194–197.
63 Lawson R, Lloyd-Thomas AR. Three diagnostic conundrums solved using the laryngeal mask airway. *Anaesthesia* 1993;**48**:790–791.
64 Tham LCH. Children and size of laryngeal masks. *Can J Anaesth* 1994;**41**:354.
65 Ravalia D, Kumar N. Rotation of reinforced laryngeal mask airway. *Anaesthesia* 1994;**49**:541–542.
66 Wheatley RS, Stainthorp SF. Intubation of a one-day-old baby with the Pierre–Robin syndrome via a laryngeal mask. *Anaesthesia* 1994;**49**:733.
67 Robichon J. Utilité du masque larynge en cas d'intubation difficile. *Cahiers d'Anesthesiol* 1993;**41**:525–527.
68 Mora J, Lopez Gil MT, Blanco T, et al. Aplicacion de la mascarilla laringea en cirugia pediatrica. *Cir Pediatr* 1995;**8**:55–57.
69 De Mattos AL, Lauretti GR, Garcia LV, Dos Reis MP. Mascara laringea em artrogripose multiplex congenita. Relato de um caso. *Rev Brasil Anestesiol* 1994;**44**:CBA 141.
70 Lee SK, Lee JR. A case of general anaesthesia with the laryngeal mask airway in a patient with Pierre Robin syndrome. *J Kor Soc Anesthesiol* 1994;**27**:95–96.
71 Ismail-Zade IA, Vanner RG. Regurgitation and aspiration of gastric contents in a child during general anaesthesia using the laryngeal mask airway. *Paediatr Anaesth* 1996;**6**:325–328.
72 Gronert BJ. Laryngeal mask airway for management of a difficult airway and extracorporeal shock wave lithotripsy. *Paediatr Anaesth* 1996;**6**:147–150.
73 Brimacombe J. The use of the laryngeal mask airway in very small neonates. *Anesthesiology* 1994;**81**:1302.
74 Webster AC, Reid WD, Siebert LF, Taylor MD. Laryngeal mask airway for anaesthesia for cryopexy in low birth weight infants. *Can J Anaesth* 1995;**42**:361–362.
75 Lonnqvist PA. Successful use of laryngeal mask airway in low-weight expremature infants with bronchopulmonary dysplasia undergoing cryotherapy for retinopathy of the premature. *Anesthesiology* 1995;**83**:422–424.
76 Maroof M, Khan RM, Siddique MS. Intraoperative aspiration pneumonitis and the laryngeal mask airway. *Anesth Analg* 1993;**77**:409–410.
77 McLeod DH, Narang VPS. Functional and anatomical assessment of the laryngeal mask airway in infants and children. *Anaesth Intens Care* 1992;**20**:109 (Abstract).
78 Robinson DN, Shaikh L, Best CJ. Laryngeal mask airway placement in paediatric patients: a comparison of two general anaesthetic techniques. *Paediatr Anaesth* 1995;**4**:371–374.
79 Logan A, Ashford P, Gosling AJ. Arterial oxygen saturation during induction of anaesthesia and laryngeal mask insertion in children: prospective evaluation of two techniques. *Br J Anaesth* 1994;**73**:718P–719P. (Abstract).
80 Zwass MS, Fisher DM, Welborn LG, et al. Induction and maintenance characteristics of anesthesia with desflurane and nitrous oxide in infants and children. *Anesthesiology* 1992;**76**:373–378.
81 Verghese C, Brimacombe J. Survey of laryngeal mask usage in 11 910 patients – safety and efficacy for conventional and nonconventional usage. *Anesth Analg* 1996;**82**:129–133.
82 Haynes SR, Morton NS. The laryngeal mask airway: a review of its use in paediatric anaesthesia. *Paediatr Anaesth* 1993;**3**:65–73.
83 Miyasaka K. Laryngeal mask airway in pediatric anesthesia. *J Clin Exp Med* 1992;**162**:872–875.
84 Wilson IG. The laryngeal mask airway in paediatric practice. *Br J Anaesth* 1993;**70**:124–125.
85 Mizushima A, Wardall GJ, Simpson DL. The laryngeal mask airway in infants. *Anaesthesia* 1992;**47**:849–851.
86 Jung K, Cho C, Yang H. Clinical investigation of the laryngeal mask airway in children. *J Kor Soc Anesthesiol* 1993;**26**:763–769.
87 Allsop E, Innes P, Jackson M, Cunliffe M. Dose of propofol required to insert the laryngeal mask airway in children. *Paediatr Anaesth* 1995;**5**:47–51.
88 Ferrari LR, Goudsouzian NG. The use of the laryngeal mask airway in children with bronchopulmonary dysplasia. *Anesth Analg* 1995;**81**:310–313.
89 Watcha MF, Garner FT, White PF, Lusk R. Laryngeal mask airway vs face mask and Guedel airway during pediatric myringotomy. *Arch Otolaryngol Head Neck Surg* 1994;**120**:877–880.
90 Watcha MF, Tan TSH, Safavi F, Payne CT, Teufel AE. Comparison of outcome with the use of the laryngeal mask, face mask–oral airway and endotracheal tube in children. *Anesth Analg* 1994;**78**:S471 (Abstract).

91 O'Neill B, Caramico L, Templeton JJ, Schreiner MS. Inflated vs deflated insertion of the laryngeal mask airway in infants and children. *Anesthesiology* 1993;**79**:A1188 (Abstract).

92 McNicol LR. Insertion of the laryngeal mask airway in children. *Anaesthesia* 1991;**46**:330.

93 Elwood T, Cox RG. Laryngeal mask insertion with a laryngoscope in paediatric patients. *Can J Anaesth* 1996;**43**:435–437.

94 Phillips J, Brimacombe J, Simpson D. Anaesthetic induction with isoflurane or halothane. Oxygen saturation during induction with isoflurane or halothane in unpremedicated children. *Anaesthesia* 1988;**43**:927–929.

95 Rungreungvanich M, Sriswasdi S, Soranastaporn C. Comparison of halothane and isoflurane for laryngeal mask insertion in pediatric patients. *11th World Congress of Anesthesiology, Sydney, 14–20 April 1996, Abstract Handbook* p.395 (Abstract).

96 Ghouri AF, Bodner M, White PF. Recovery profile after desflurane–nitrous oxide versus isoflurane–nitrous oxide in outpatients. *Anesthesiology* 1991;**74**:419–424.

97 Prasiko D, Shrestha BM. Laryngeal mask airway in pediatric burn contractures in Nepal. *11th World Congress of Anesthesiology, Sydney, 14–20 April 1996, Abstract Handbook* p.119 (Abstract).

98 Dain SL, Webster AC, Morley-Forster P, Ruby R, Weberpals J, Cook MJ. Propofol for insertion of the laryngeal mask airway for short ENT procedures in children. *Anesth Analg* 1996;**82**:S83 (Abstract).

99 Martlew RA, Meakin G, Wadsworth R, Sharples A, Baker RD. Dose of propofol for laryngeal mask insertion in children: effect of premedication with midazolam. *Br J Anaesth* 1996;**76**:308–309.

100 Recio A, Jacobson K, Gronert B, Motoyama E. The use of the LMA in children under halothane anesthesia: is spontaneous ventilation acceptable? *Anesthesiology* 1995;**83**:A1153 (Abstract).

101 Gursoy F, Algren JT, Skjonsby BS. Positive pressure ventilation with the laryngeal mask airway in children. *Anesth Analg* 1996;**82**:33–38.

102 Burnett YL, Brennan MP, Salem MR. Controlled ventilation and the laryngeal mask airway: effect on $ETCO_2$, O_2, PIP and gastric secretions in pediatric patients. *Anesthesiology* 1994;**81**:A1320 (Abstract).

103 Orfei P, Misiti FR, Pinto G, Aragona P. The laryngeal mask airway in paediatric anaesthesia and in neonatal resuscitation. *International Symposium on Perinatal Medicine and Human Reproduction, Rome, 26–29 June 1995*, pp.421–425 (Abstract).

104 Varughesa A, McCulloch D, Lewis M, Stokes M. Removal of the laryngeal mask airway (LMA) in children: awake or deep? *Anesthesiology* 1994;**81**:A1321 (Abstract).

105 Splinter WM, Smallman B, Rhine EJ, Komocar L. Postoperative sore throat in children and the laryngeal mask airway. *Can J Anaesth* 1994;**41**:1081–1083.

106 Fawcett WJ, Ravilia A, Radford P. The laryngeal mask airway in children. *Can J Anaesth* 1991;**38**:685–686.

107 Benumof JL. Intubation and extubation of the patient with Pierre–Robin syndrome. *Anesthesiology* 1992;**77**:401.

108 Denman WT, Goudsouzian NG, Chadd GD, Crane DL. Position of the laryngeal mask airway. *Anesthesiology* 1992;**77**:401–402.

109 Markakis DA, Sayson SC, Schreiner MS. Insertion of the laryngeal mask airway in awake infants with the Pierre Robin sequence. *Anesth Analg* 1992;**75**:822–824.

110 Mecklem D, Brimacombe J, Yarker J. Glossopexy in Pierre Robin sequence using the laryngeal mask airway. *J Clin Anesth* 1995;**7**:267–269.

111 Theroux MC, Kettrick RG, Khine HH. Laryngeal mask airway and fiberoptic endoscopy in an infant with Schwartz–Jampel syndrome. *Anesthesiology* 1995;**82**:605.

112 Baraka A. Laryngeal mask airway for resuscitation of a newborn with Pierre Robin syndrome. *Anesthesiology* 1995;**83**:645–646.

113 Haxby EJ, Liban JB. Fibreoptic intubation via a laryngeal mask in an infant with Goldenhar syndrome. *Anaesth Intens Care* 1995;**23**:753.

114 Kopp VJ, Bailey A, Valley RD, et al. Utility of the Mallampati classification for predicting difficult intubation in pediatric patients. *Anesthesiology* 1995;**83**:A1147 (Abstract).

115 White AP, Billingham IM. Laryngeal mask guided tracheal intubation in paediatric anaesthesia. *Paediatr Anaesth* 1992;**2**:265.

116 Rabb MF, Minkowitz HS, Haberg CA. Blind intubation through the laryngeal mask airway for management of the difficult airway in children. *Anesthesiology* 1996;**84**:1510–1511.

117 Silk JM, Hill HM, Calder I. Difficult intubation and the laryngeal mask. *Eur J Anaesthesiol* 1991;**4**:47–51.

118 Zagnoev M, McCloskey J, Martin T. Fiberoptic intubation via the laryngeal mask airway. *Anesth Analg* 1994;**78**:813–814.

119 Inada T, Fujise K, Tachibana K, Shingu K. Orotracheal intubation through the laryngeal mask airway in paediatric patients with Treacher Collins syndrome. *Paediatr Anaesth* 1995;**5**:129–132.

120 O'Kelly SW, Reynolds PI, Collito M. The use of fibreoptic endoscopy and laryngeal mask airway in securing the traumatized airway in the paediatric patient. *Am J Anesthesiol* 1995;**22**:152–153.

121 Vener DF, Lerman J. The pediatric airway and associated syndromes. In: Doyle DJ, Sandler AN, eds. *The difficult airway II*. Philadelphia: WB Saunders, 1995;585–614.

122 Brimacombe J, De Maio B. Emergency use of the laryngeal mask airway during helicopter transfer of a neonate. *J Clin Anesth* 1995;**7**:689–690.

123 Brimacombe J, Gandini D. Paediatric airway management. *Br J Hosp Med* 1995;**53**:175.

124 Janke EL, Fletcher JE, Lewis IH. Anaesthetic management of the Kenny–Caffey syndrome using the laryngeal mask. *Paediatr Anaesth* 1996;**6**:235–238.

125 Andrews PJ, Marchant RB. A new technique for difficult intubation in babies. *Technic* 1995;**143**:12–14.

126 Ebata T, Nishiki S, Masuda A, Amaha K. Anaesthesia for Treacher Collins syndrome using a laryngeal mask airway. *Can J Anaesth* 1991;**38**:1043–1045.

127 Holinger P, Johnston K. Factors responsible for laryngeal obstruction in infants. *J Am Med Assoc* 1950;**143**:1229.

128 Standards and guidelines for cardiopulmonary resuscitation (CPR) and emergency cardiac care (ECC). Part VI. Neonatal advanced life support. *J Am Med Assoc* 1986;**255**:2969–2973.

129 Gibbs CP, Krischer J, Peckham BM, Sharp H, Kirschbaum TH. Obstetric anesthesia: a national survey. *Anesthesiology* 1986;**65**:298–306.

130 Lavies NG. Use of the laryngeal mask airway in neonatal resuscitation. *Anaesthesia* 1993;**48**:352.

131 Pennant JH, Walker MB. Comparison of the endotracheal tube and laryngeal mask in airway management by paramedical personnel. *Anesth Analg* 1992;**74**:531–534.

132 Gollo E, Mutani C, Reilia P, Margaria E. Primary resuscitation of the newborn. In: *Abstracts of the 2nd World Congress of Perinatal Medicine, Rome, 19–24 September 1993*, p.102 (Abstract).

133 Brimacombe J, Gandini D. Resuscitation of neonates with the laryngeal mask – a caution. *Pediatrics* 1995;**95**:453–454.

134 Margaria E, Mutani C, Treves S. La maschera laringea nella rianmazione primaria del neonato. *Minerva Anestesiol* 1995;**61**:43–44.

135 Brimacombe J, Berry A. The laryngeal mask airway – a consideration for the NRP guidelines? *Can J Anaesth* 1995;**42**:88–89.

136 Practice Guidelines for Management of the Difficult Airway – a Report by the American Society of Anesthesiologists Task Force on Management of the Difficult Airway. *Anesthesiology* 1993;**78**:597–602.

137 Williamson JA, Webb RK, Szekely S, Gillies ERN. Difficult intubation: an analysis of 2000 incident reports. *Anaesth Intens Care* 1993;**21**:602–607.

138 Brimacombe J. Neonatal resuscitation and the laryngeal mask airway. *Anaesthesia* 1995;**50**:1003.

139 Benumof J. The laryngeal mask airway and the ASA difficult airway algorithm. *Anesthesiology* 1996;**84**:686–699.

140 Williams RK. Resuscitation of neonates with the laryngeal mask – a caution. *Pediatrics* 1995;**95**:454.

141 Thomas EO. Neonatal resuscitation and the laryngeal mask airway. *Anaesthesia* 1995;**50**:569–570.

17 Future directions

Clinical research

A considerable amount of work is yet needed to identify the merits and demerits of the LMA in many areas of advanced and nonanesthetic use. Anecdotal reports, where possible, should be followed up by prospective research. It is particularly important that the LMA is used correctly during future studies and that rigorous criteria for successful placement are defined[1] to help differentiate between user and device related problems. For example, a fiberoptic scoring system has been devised to standardize the position of the LMA (Table 17.1)[2], although this is not infallible[3]. There is also a need for a very large controlled study (>10 000 patients) comparing the LMA, face mask and tracheal tube and a reporting system established for life threatening or rare complications.

Table 17.1 Fiberoptic scoring system to standardize the position of the LMA

Score	Description
Score 4	Only cords
Score 3	Cords plus posterior epiglottis
Score 2	Cords plus anterior epiglottis
Score 1	Cords not seen, but function adequate
Score 0	Failure to insert or to function

Physiology research

Interest in the anatomy and physiology of the upper airway has increased in recent years, stimulated by clinical disorders such as dysphagia and sleep apnea. The physiological implications of the LMA are relatively unexplored but, by occupying a space at the intersection of the respiratory and gastrointestinal tracts, the LMA may provide new insights into their physiological interaction. Use of the LMA as a research tool may be enhanced by modifications to the basic design (see *Future modifications*). In addition, the glottis and tracheobronchial tree may be synchronously observed by passing a fiberoptic scope via the lumen of the LMA[4]. Also, the cuff may be expanded to variable volumes and the intracuff pressure can vary from a low range, in which the surrounding anatomy dictates the shape of the cuff (low trauma risk), to a high range, in which the cuff dictates the shape of the anatomy (high trauma risk). Devices such as sleeve manometers and pH probes may be readily passed behind the device into the esophagus, for example to investigate the effects of the device on the sphincter at different intracuff pressures. There is a need for animal studies to clarify the present uncertainty concerning possible effects of the LMA on esophageal sphincters and gastroenterologists would make useful allies in this field. The LMA can be used in the cat[5] and dog[6], which are accepted models for assessment of pharyngo–upper esophageal reflexes[7].

Future modifications

Many modifications to the standard device are possible. Some that have been suggested include:

1. making the pilot tube integral with the main tube[8];
2. provision of an additional tube for CO_2 sampling[9];
3. increasing the resistance to lasers[10];
4. using nonferromagnetic wires in the FLMA for MRI[11];
5. strengthening the wires of the FLMA to prevent collapse[12];
6. manufacturing a size 0.5 for premature neonates[13]; and
7. producing a range of LMAs with pre-inflated cuffs[14] (unlikely to be of benefit[15,16]).

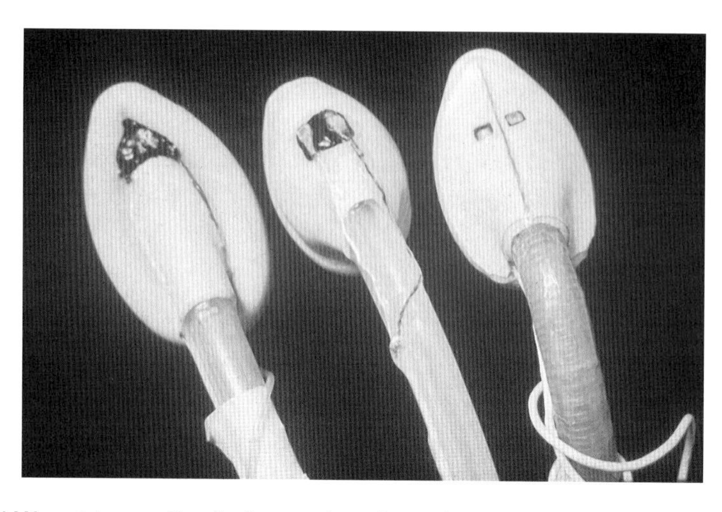

Figure 17.1 LMA prototypes with reflectance pulse oximeter incorporated.

Miura has suggested adding markers to the side of the LMA tube to give a better idea of depth[17]. Patent protection has been sought for a number of potentially useful clinical modifications. It is possible to incorporate an electromyograph (AM Berry, personal communication, 1994), pulse oximeter, temperature probe, pH probe and pressure transducer into the LMA cuff (Figure 17.1). There is also theoretical utility in mounting stimulating electrodes on the LMA cuff. It has been shown in animals that the upper esophageal sphincter tone can be influenced by weak electrical stimulation applied to the sphincter mucosa from electrodes placed in the extremity of the mask. A study in progress is examining the possible value of stimulating specific laryngeal muscles such as the posterior cricoarytenoid. Another possibility is the use of the mask as one of the electrodes in cardiac defibrillation. A considerable amount of work still needs to be done to define the usefulness of these modifications for research and clinical practice.

Future designs

General

Twenty-seven different kinds of LMA of potential utility have been patented, built and tested by the inventor and remain to be exploited commercially. The only variation to become commercially available to date is the flexible (reinforced – UK) LMA which was first described by Alexander in 1990[18] (see Chapter 4, *The flexible laryngeal mask airway*). The intubating LMA and disposable LMA are scheduled for release in 1997. An LMA with a shortened tube is also available in the UK (see Chapter 4, *Modifications*). Two modifications have been described which are not produced by the manufacturer: the split LMA to overcome the problems of size limitation when using the LMA as a conduit for intubation and to facilitate device removal after intubation[19–27], and a partially flexible LMA with a nonkinkable corrugated upper shaft to provide some of the benefits of the FLMA[28]. A nasal LMA with a detachable tube and flanged cuff has been designed and tested, but may be too impractical for common clinical use[6]. The disposable LMA may be more appropriate for resuscitation use and has been produced for assessment in this situation (Figure 17.2).

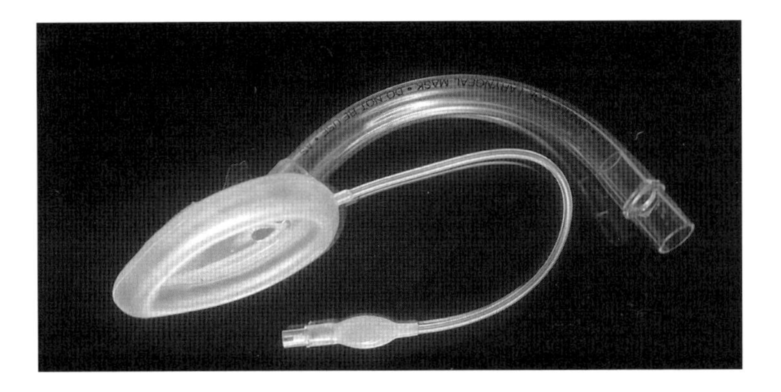

Figure 17.2 Disposable LMA.

In 1994 Akhtar described the esophageal vent-laryngeal mask airway which attempted to provide protection against regurgitation by adding a tracheal tube fused to the dorsal surface of the LMA which rested in the upper esophagus[29]. A similar device was investigated by Brain almost a decade before, but discarded since it was difficult to place, invasive, and thought likely to provoke reflux or impact with the glottis[6,30]. These objections have been reiterated by Asai[31], Sorooshian[32] and Gajraj et al[33]. Akhtar has emphasized that the presence of the LMA anteriorly forces the tracheal tube along the posterior pharyngeal wall, making impaction with the glottis unlikely[34]. Brain, however, has suggested that placement of a tracheal tube in the esophagus is best conducted once the LMA is placed since it can act as a shield protecting the glottis from trauma[30]. Cheam has recently pointed out that the presence of a tracheal tube in the upper esophagus does not prevent reflux[35].

Double lumen LMA

The double lumen laryngeal mask airway comprises a standard LMA with an additional tube fused onto the posterolateral aspect of the main tube just proximal to the cuff. In effect this increases the bore of the LMA tubing and allows ventilation and airway instrumentation to take place in separate tubes[36]. It may be useful for bronchoscopy in small children where the fiberoptic scope may occupy most of the LMA tubing. Insertion is similar to the standard device. When utilizing it for diagnostic laryngobronchoscopy the fiberoptic scope is passed down the main tube and the additional tube is connected to the circuit. When utilizing it as an airway intubator the fiberoptic scope and circuit are connected to the additional tube and the airway instruments are passed via the main tube. It has been shown that flow resistance is lower than with the standard LMA[36] (see Chapter 14, *Fiberoptic techniques*). This device is not currently available commercially. A similar tube arrangement is shown in Figure 17.7.

Intubating LMA

The first intubating LMA prototype (ILM) (see Figure 14.2) was used in three cases of difficult intubation in 1983[37]. It differed from other prototypes in having a wider, shorter and stiffer tube and a raised area in the bowl of the mask to direct the tracheal tube anteriorly. The 12 mm ID tube accepted a 9 mm tracheal tube whose cuff could be passed distal to the vocal cords and was stiff enough to permit a degree of control over LMA cuff position during tracheal tube insertion attempts. Although shown to work effectively, the idea was set aside pending completion of development of the standard device, which took a further 5 years. However, ILM development was resumed in 1993. In 1995, Kapila et al used a prototype ILM with a wide bore tube and guiding handle mounted on a conventional mask for elective intubation of 78 patients[38] (see Figure 14.7). They found that the device was successfully placed in 72 patients and that intubation was possible in 80% at the first attempt and 12% at the second attempt. Following this trial the ILM was further modified and the final device (due for release in 1997) comprises a curved stainless steel airway tube of ID 13 mm sheathed in silicone and formed into a 15 mm connector at its outer end which is fixed permanently to a laryngeal mask of conventional general shape (Figure 17.3). Attached to the metal tube near the connector end is a handle to guide the mask into place and to steady the device while an endotracheal tube is being passed through it. The mask aperture is partly covered by a moveable flap firmly fixed to the upper rim of the mask. This is called the epiglottic elevating bar (EEB), which describes its function. Within the aperture behind the bar the floor of the channel is formed into a V-shaped ramp to centralize and direct the tracheal tube towards the glottis.

The ILM may be inserted with the patient awake after pharyngeal topicalization or under general anesthesia. The insertion sequence and technique for intubation via the ILM is shown in Figure 17.4. It is not necessary to insert the finger into the patient's mouth and the head and neck should be in the neutral position with the head supported on a pillow. The ILM may be either used as an airway by itself or as an aid to intubation after paralysis, using up to an 8.0 mm cuffed tracheal tube. The manufacturer recommends the use of a dedicated straight 8 mm cuffed silicone tube for intubation through the device for the best results. Once inserted in the patient with the cuff inflated, the patient may be ventilated using the ILM alone by connecting the outer end to the anesthesia circuit. This permits oxygenation prior to and during intubation attempts. The device may be left in place or removed after intubation has been accomplished and may be re-inserted behind the tracheal tube to provide an immediate airway if deep extubation is planned or extubation is thought to be hazardous.

The intubation procedure may be carried out blindly or using a fiberscope (see Figure 17.4 and accompanying text). An unpublished pilot study of 66 patients conducted by the inventor has shown that the success rate for blind intubation with or without two device manipulations is 98.5% using a special tube designed for use with the device. The success rate may be higher with fiberoptic guidance. The ILM has a potential role in difficult intubation, paramedic use, suspected injury to the cervical spine, bronchoscopy and one-lung anesthesia. Ten cases of either known previous difficult intubation, Mallampati 3/4 or Cormack and Lehane grade 3 have all been successfully intubated

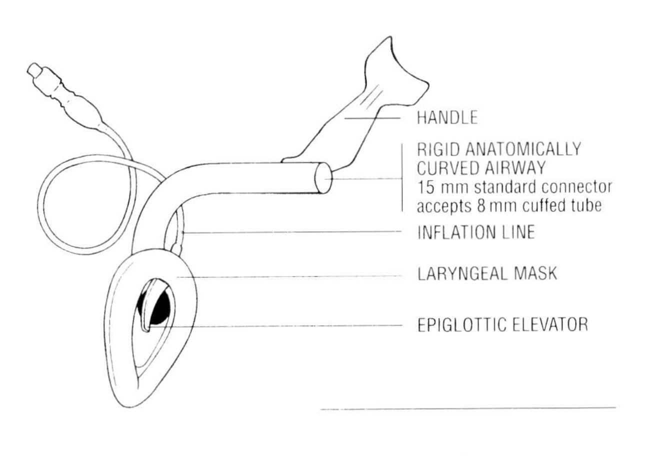

Figure 17.3 Intubating LMA.

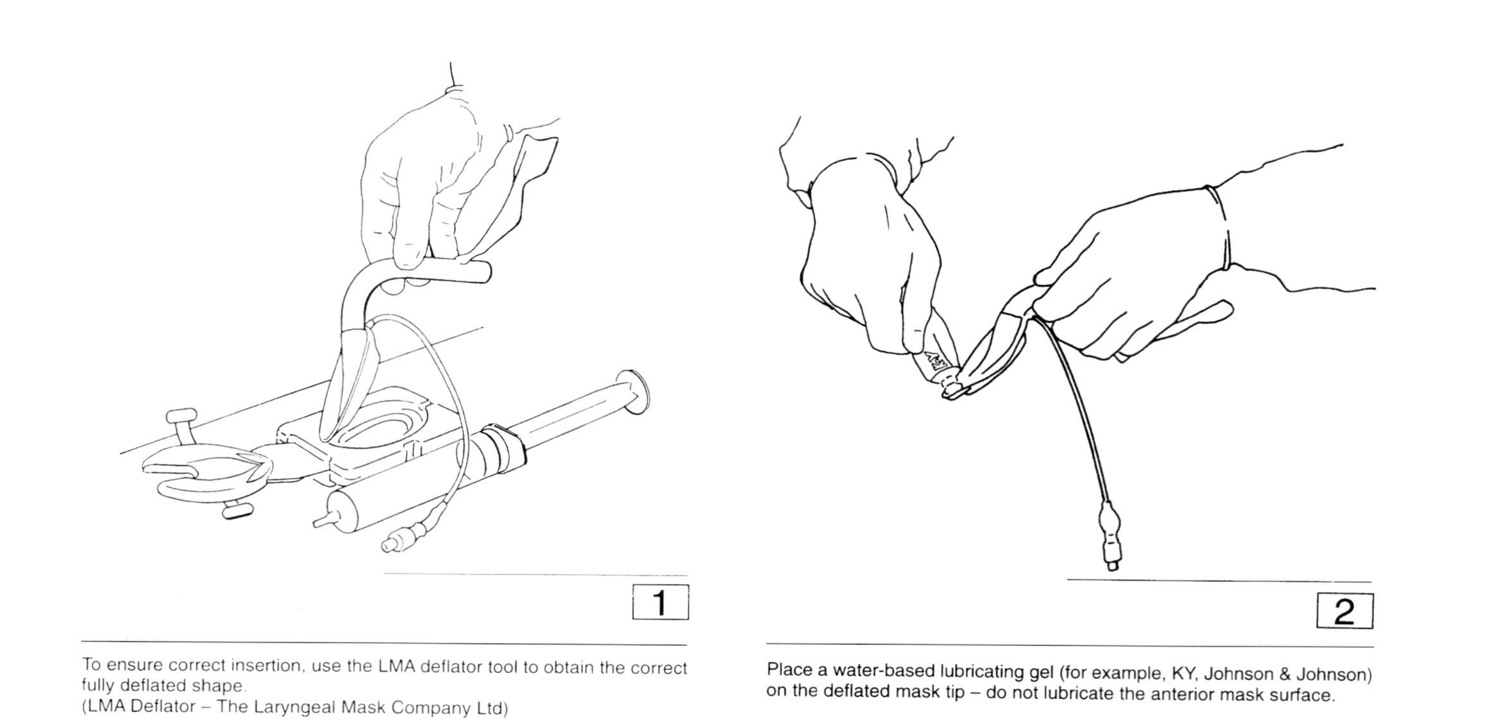

Figure 17.4 How to use the ILM. (1)–(6) inserting the device, (7)–(21) inserting the TT through it.

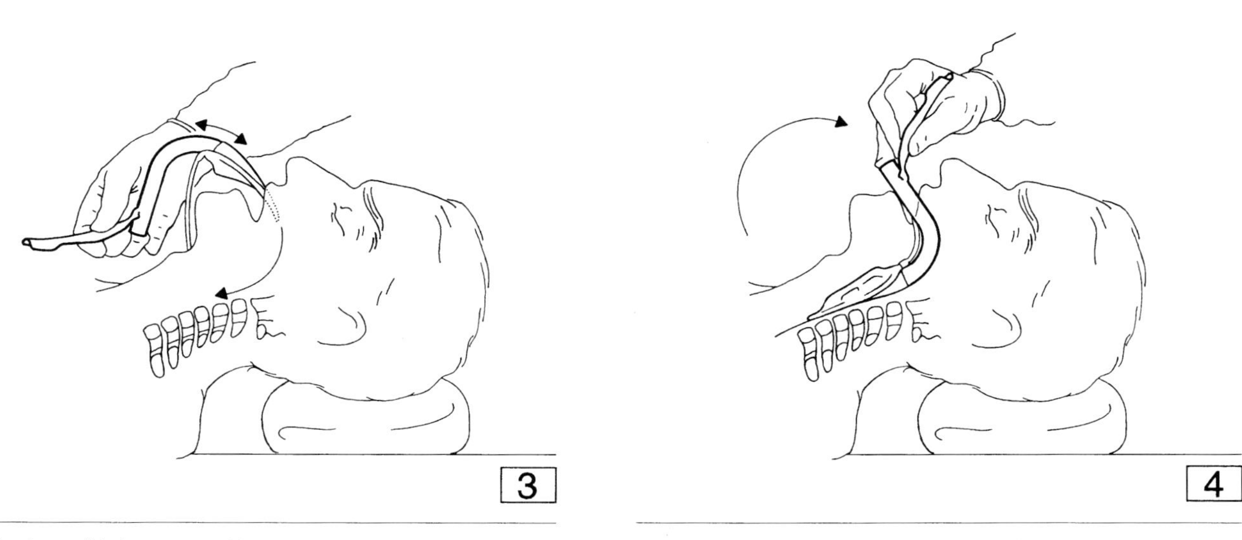

Insertion is possible from any position – no head or neck manipulation is required but rub the lubricant over the anterior hard palate with the device exactly in the position shown here.

The mask is swung into place in a single circular movement ensuring pressure is maintained against palate and posterior pharynx.

Figure 17.4 *(continued)*.

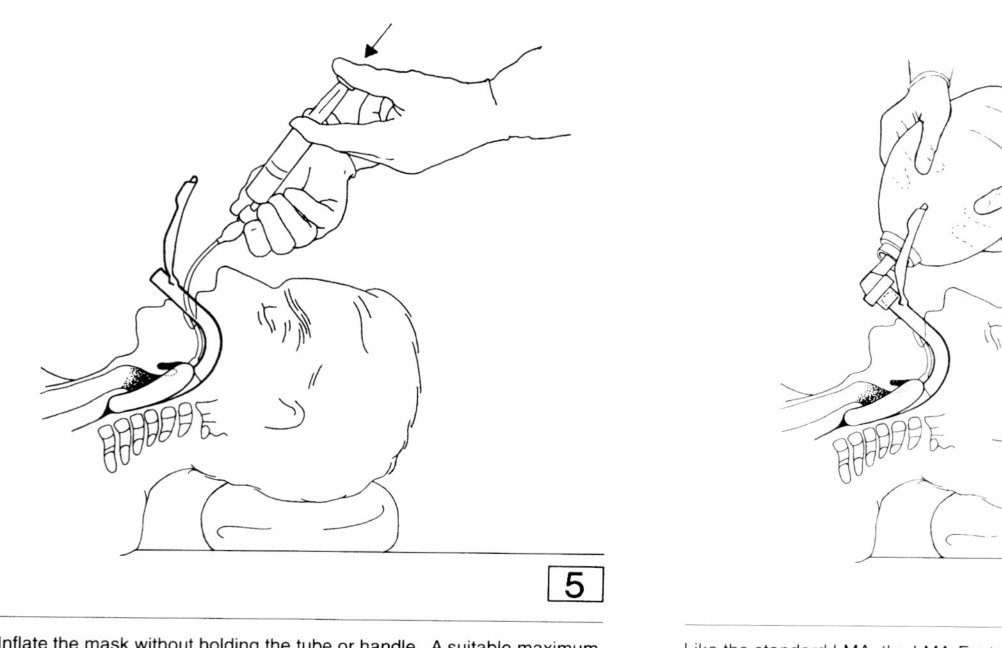

Inflate the mask without holding the tube or handle. A suitable maximum mask inflation pressure would be 60–80 cm H_2O. Before any further step is taken, oxygenate the patient using gentle positive pressure ventiation.

Like the standard LMA, the LMA-Fastrach™ can be used to ventilate the patient on its own. Take care not to dislodge the tube from the midline.

Figure 17.4 *(continued)*.

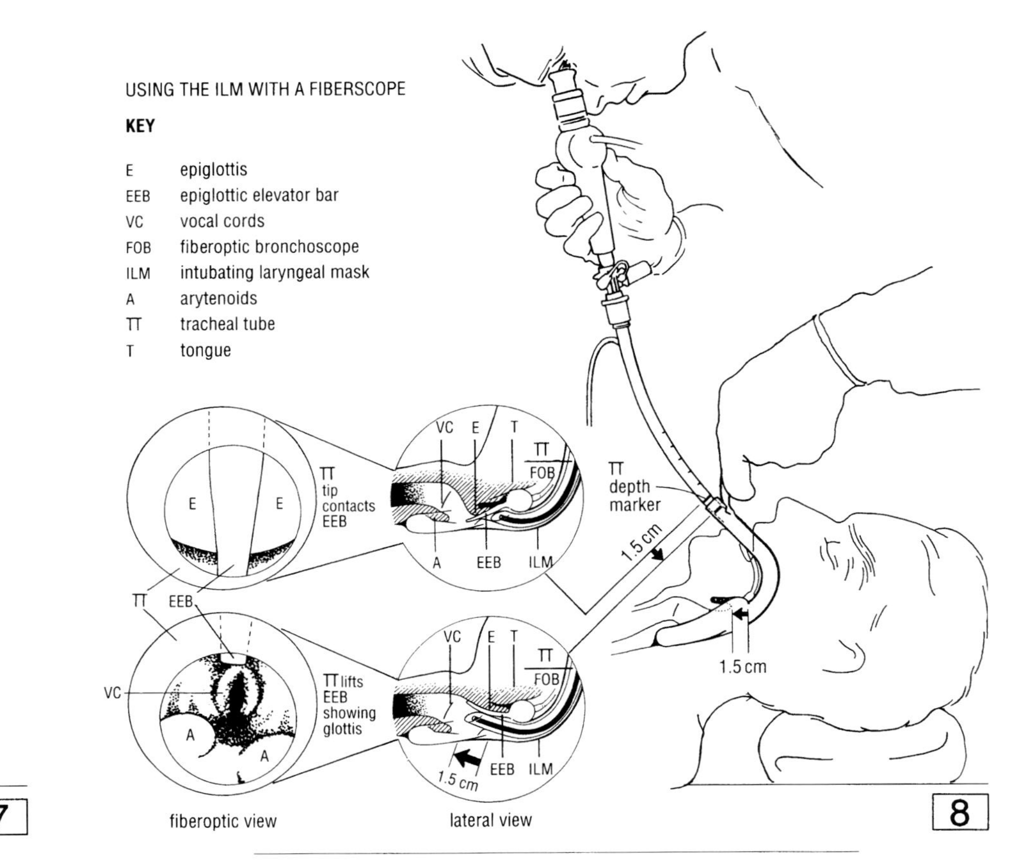

BLIND INTUBATION – NO FIBERSCOPE AVAILABLE

Grasp the handle firmly to steady the device while passing the lubricated tracheal tube up and down to lubricate the metal tube. Do not yet pass the tracheal tube beyond the depth marker indicating tube entry through the mask aperture.

Now the tube is carefully advanced about 2 cm. A fiberscope may be used when available. If the device is the correct size, intubation should be possible without resistance. Do not use force.

Figure 17.4 *(continued)*.

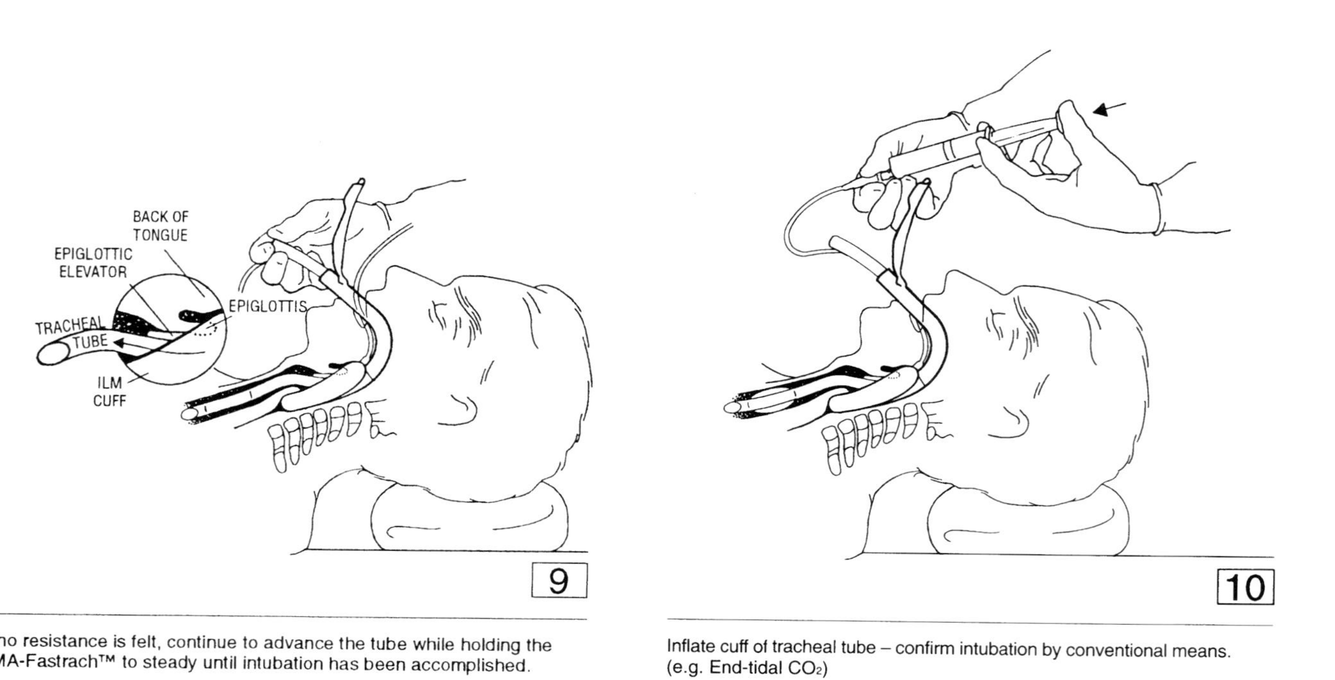

Figure 17.4 *(continued)*.

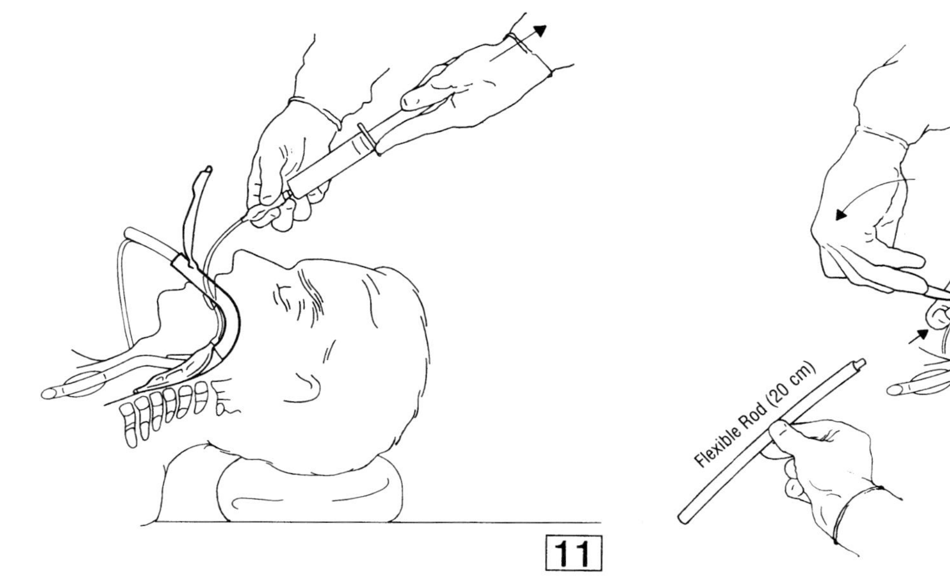

After achieving intubation, the LMA-Fastrach™ may be left in place or removed. If left in place it should be deflated to a pressure of 20–30 cm H_2O.

Removal of LMA-Fastrach™:-

1. Ensure patient well oxygenated.
2. Remove tracheal tube connector.
3. Deflate mask cuff (keep TT cuff inflated).

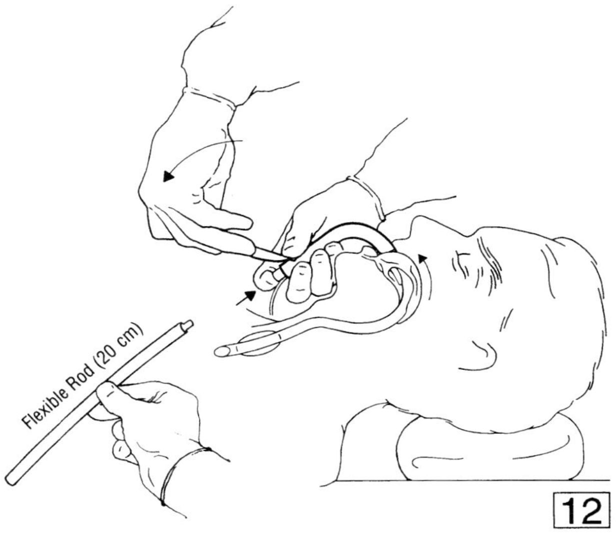

Swing mask out of pharynx into oral cavity applying counter-pressure to tracheal tube with finger as shown, prior to insertion of 20 cm flexible rod. The LMA-Fastrach™ can be eased out by tapping or swinging the handle around the chin as shown. The rod can be conveniently used to measure how far the tracheal tube protrudes from the mouth before device removal to ensure it is correctly repositioned afterwards.

Figure 17.4 *(continued)*.

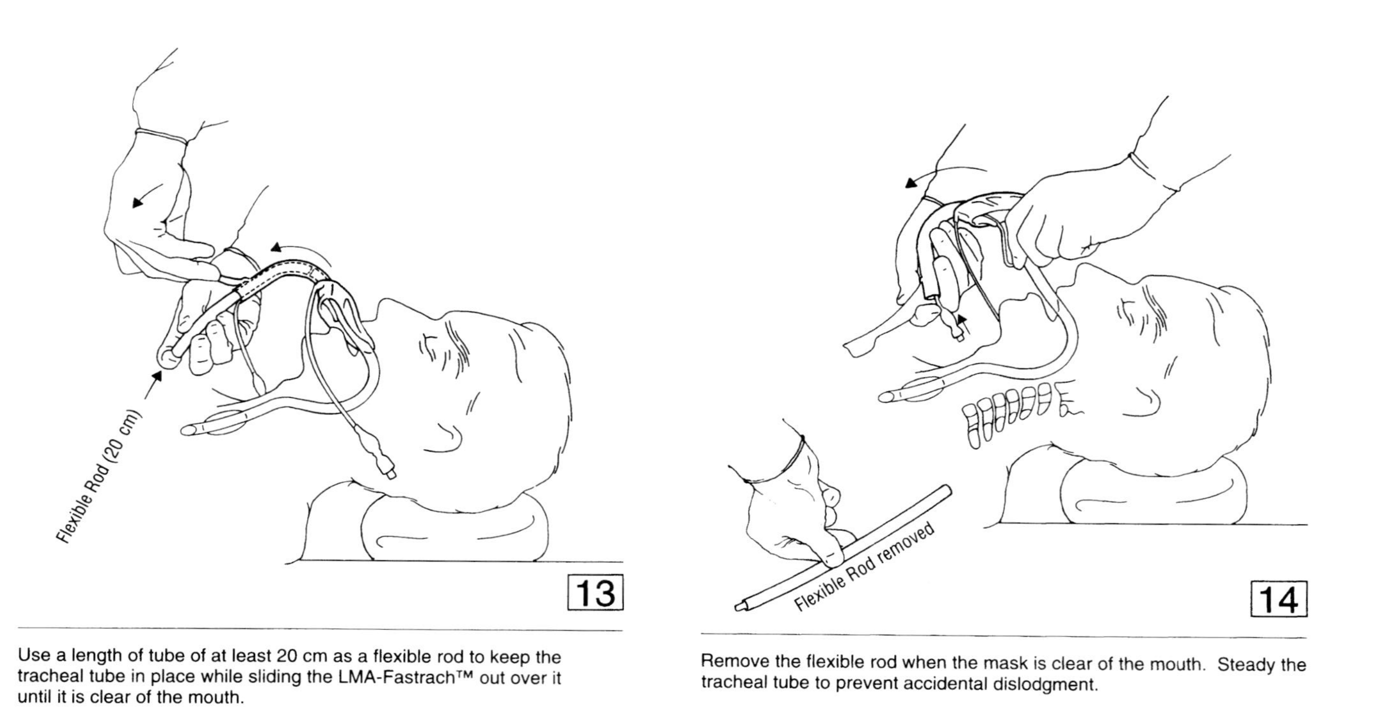

Use a length of tube of at least 20 cm as a flexible rod to keep the tracheal tube in place while sliding the LMA-Fastrach™ out over it until it is clear of the mouth.

Remove the flexible rod when the mask is clear of the mouth. Steady the tracheal tube to prevent accidental dislodgment.

Figure 17.4 *(continued)*.

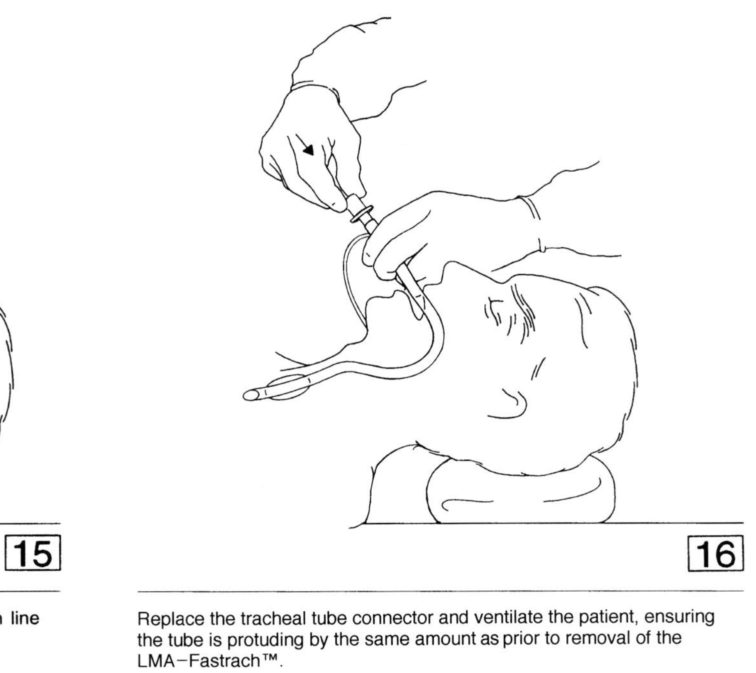

Grasp the tracheal tube firmly while gently unthreading its inflation line and pilot balloon from the LMA-Fastrach™ tube.

Replace the tracheal tube connector and ventilate the patient, ensuring the tube is protuding by the same amount as prior to removal of the LMA–Fastrach™.

Figure 17.4 *(continued)*.

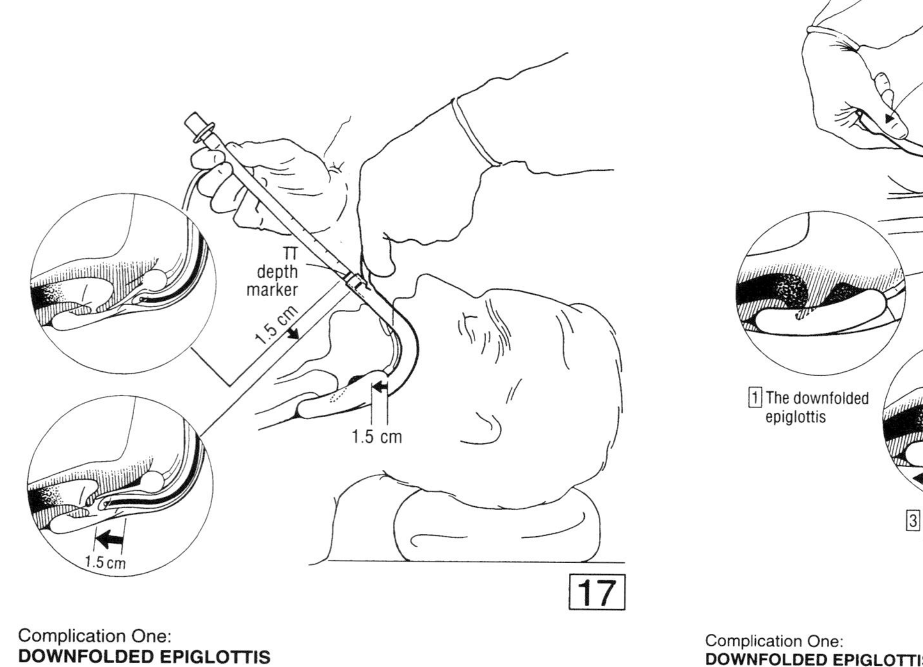

Complication One:
DOWNFOLDED EPIGLOTTIS

If the epiglottis is downfolded, resistance is often felt about 1.5 cm beyond the depth marker on the tracheal tube.

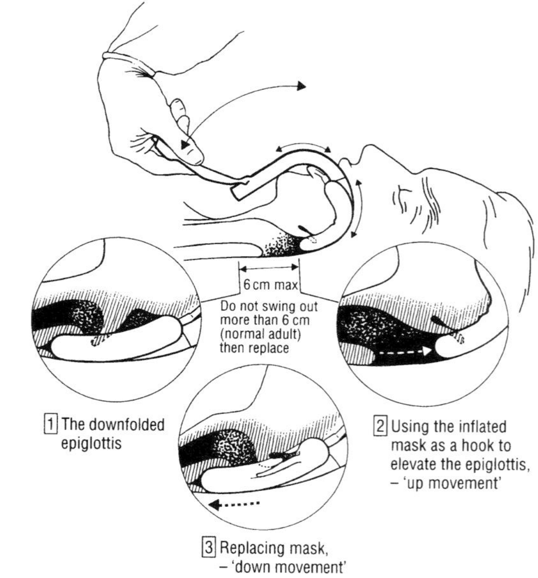

Complication One:
DOWNFOLDED EPIGLOTTIS

How to overcome using the 'up-down' movement
Swing the device back outwards no more than 6 cm; then replace.
Do this without deflating the cuff of the mask.

Figure 17.4 *(continued).*

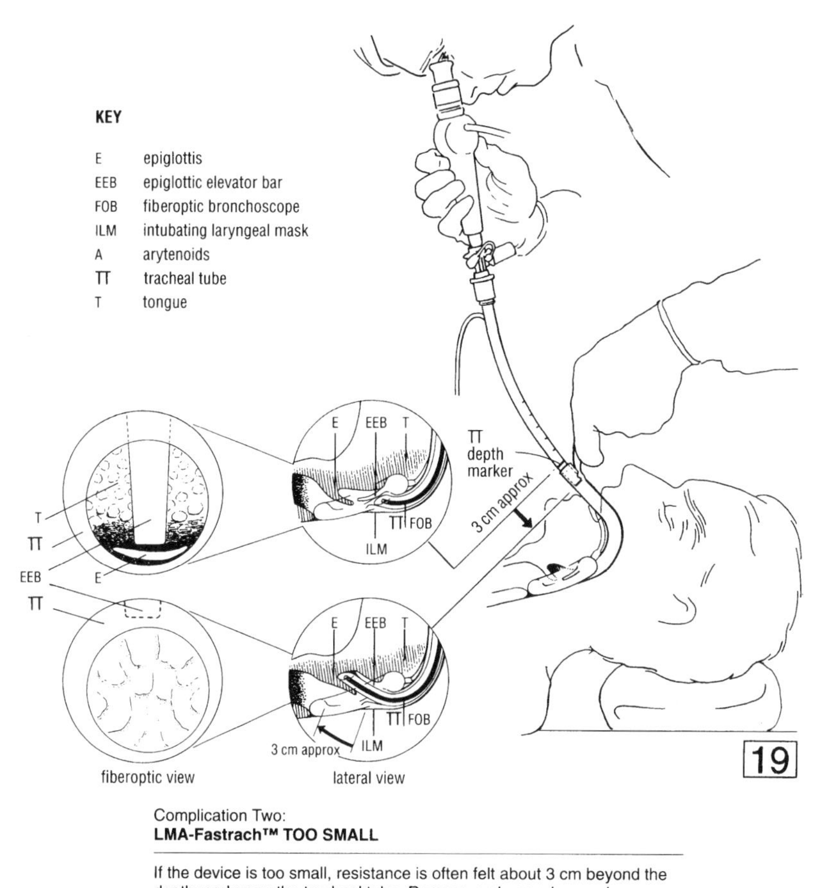

Figure 17.4 (*continued on Page 242*).

through the ILM. The disadvantages are that the ILM tube cannot be inserted through less than a 20 mm interdental gap, the rigid tube cannot adapt to changing neck position, so loss of cuff seal may occur if the head is tilted, and the fixed curve and relatively shorter tube means that the mask may not always reach the base of the hypopharynx. However, evidence is still lacking that these disadvantages are important clinically. Longer tubes are currently being developed to complete the adult range of sizes.

Double cuff LMA

Like the ILM, the double cuff LMA has a wide and short tube (ID 13 mm), permitting low flow resistance and easy insertion of suction equipment, appropriate sized tracheal tubes or fiberscopes (Figure 17.5). A posteriorly placed cuff communicates with the main cuff so that both inflate together, giving a higher seal pressure than the standard LMA. In addition, the curvature of the tube is more anatomical than that of the LMA tube, so little pressure is exerted by the tube on the posterior pharyngeal wall. This may be important in long cases. It does not have an esophageal vent,

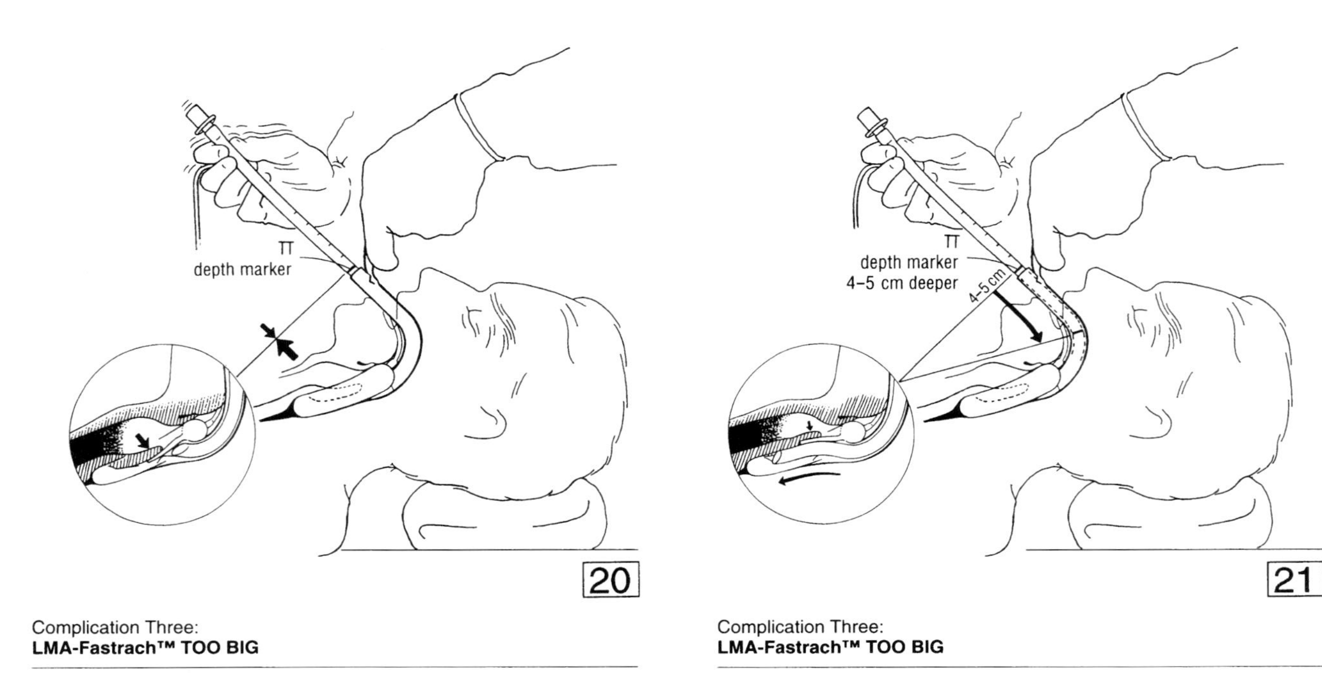

Complication Three:
LMA-Fastrach™ TOO BIG

(A) Resistance may be felt with depth marker still visible / a few millimeters into metal tube = EEB trapped behind arytenoids (normal/thin necked subject)

Complication Three:
LMA-Fastrach™ TOO BIG

(B) Slight resistance felt at 4–5 cm beyond depth marker = TT wedged between inflated mask tip and arytenoid area (more likely in wide, short-necked subject)

Figure 17.4 *(continued)*.

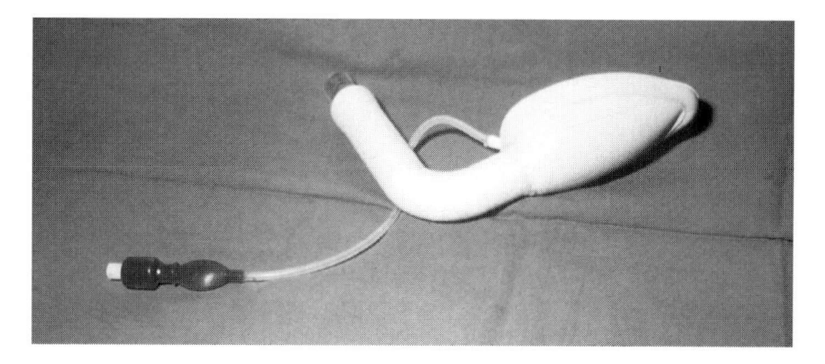

Figure 17.5 Double cuff LMA[231].

unlike the gastrolaryngeal mask (GLM) or LMA II. Formal studies in large numbers of patients have not yet been carried out but preliminary work shows it is easy to insert and appears well tolerated with excellent recovery. The disadvantages of the device are:

1. the higher seal pressures obtained may introduce the risk of barotrauma (if the lungs are accidentally overinflated – normally a risk factor associated with tracheal intubation and not the standard LMA) or esophageal trauma (if vomiting occurs with the device in place);
2. the shorter tube length compared with the LMA does not reduce dead space (25 ml as opposed to 15 ml); and
3. the moulded tube resists rotation when the head is turned to the side, causing the mask to tilt towards the same side. This increases the pressure of the cuff against the contralateral pyriform fossa and possibly reduces overall seal efficacy.

However, the double cuff LMA may be a more effective device than the LMA for prolonged surgery and the higher pressure seal may reduce the risk of aspiration by more effective isolation of the glottis from the upper esophagus.

Gastrolaryngeal mask

A prototype GLM which provides direct access to the esophagus and a higher seal pressure has been recently described by Brain et al[39] (Figure 17.6). This design incorporates a second mask to isolate the upper esophagus and a second dorsal cuff to increase the seal against the glottis. The prototype GLM can be regarded in principle as a double mask forming two end-to-end junctions, one sealing around the opening into the entrance to the respiratory tract, the other sealing around and opening into the entrance to the digestive tract. A within-patient comparison of seal pressures between this prototype and standard LMA showed that leak pressure was significantly higher for the prototype and equalled or exceeded 5.0 kPa in all patients. The prototype GLM also provided functional isolation of the respiratory tract from the gastrointestinal tract as judged by leak and placement of a gastric tube via the esophageal mask. It was concluded that the prototype GLM, while lacking the simplicity and ease of insertion of the standard device, exhibited potentially useful new features which justify further evaluation and development.

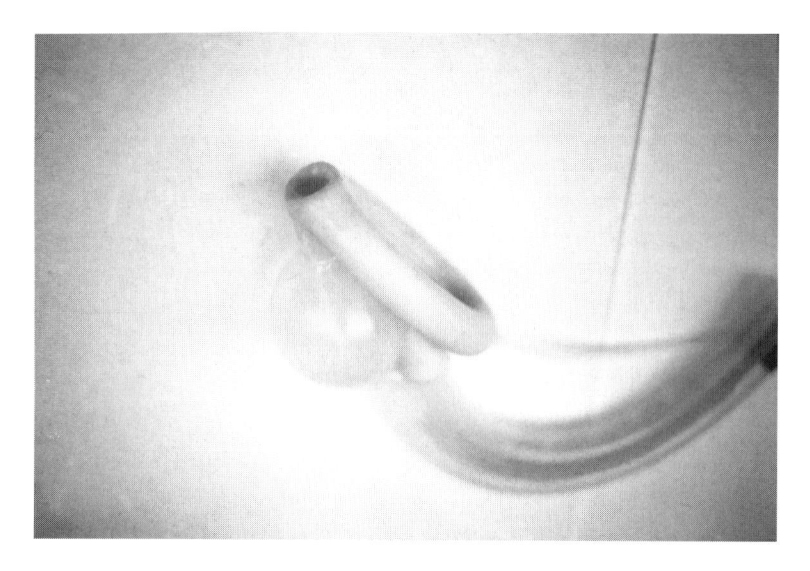

Figure 17.6 Early prototype GLM (1994).

Since the pilot study was conducted, the GLM has been modified to facilitate ease of insertion. The latest design incorporates a collapsible drainage tube of ID 10 mm (size 4) which runs behind the mask within a second posterior cuff and opens into the upper esophageal sphincter region to provide a low pressure route for regurgitation (Figure 17.7). The cuff and the bowl of the mask have been constructed in a softer material than the LMA, which makes the device flexible enough to permit easy insertion, in spite of the large drainage tube, using the standard technique. When the double cuff is inflated, the soft drainage tube is supported on either side by the inflated posterior cuff, preventing its collapse. The drainage tube emerges centrally in the pointed mask tip, but runs obliquely back from the midline of the long axis of the cuff to pass lateral to the airway tube. This arrangement prevents it collapsing at the upper wider end of the mask from pressure against the vertebral column and also ensures it does not become compressed by the teeth where it emerges from the mouth.

The device may be useful for prolonged positive pressure ventilation as in major surgery since it offers a high volume low pressure alternative to the standard device and the presence of the drainage tube should in theory prevent accidental gastric insufflation. It may also prove useful in the intensive care unit permitting more normal function of the larynx and easy access to the gastrointestinal tract while separating the latter from the respiratory tract. It may also have a role in emergency medicine. A disadvantage of the GLM is that leaks may occur if the device is displaced from the hypopharynx. Even a small degree of outward displacement may suffice to detach the mask tip aperture from its sealing contact with the mouth of the upper esophageal sphincter. However, since gases then leak upwards through the drainage tube, this provides a means of detecting such a malposition. Brimacombe reported a case of regurgitation in which a prototype GLM proved effective in protecting the airway[40]. This device is not yet available commercially.

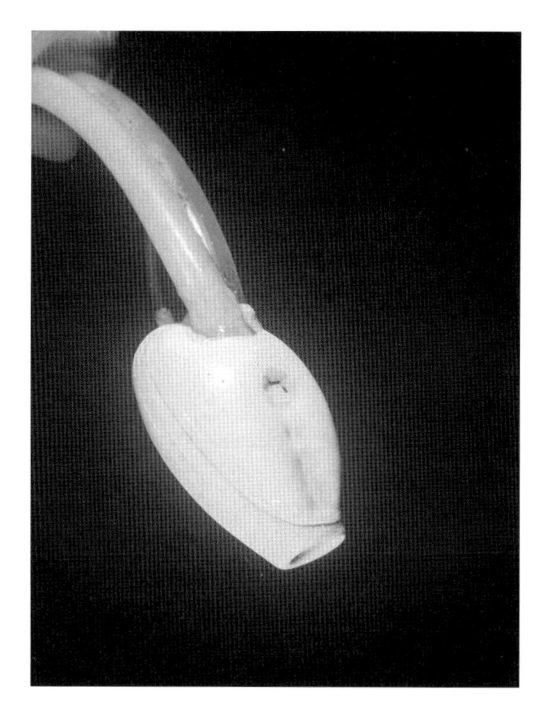

Figure 17.7 Recent prototype GLM (1996).

LMA II

Intended eventually as a replacement for the existing LMA, the LMA II consists of a mask fitted with a gastric drainage tube significantly smaller than that fitted to the GLM, but with a similar additional posteriorly placed cuff (Figure 17.8). The purpose

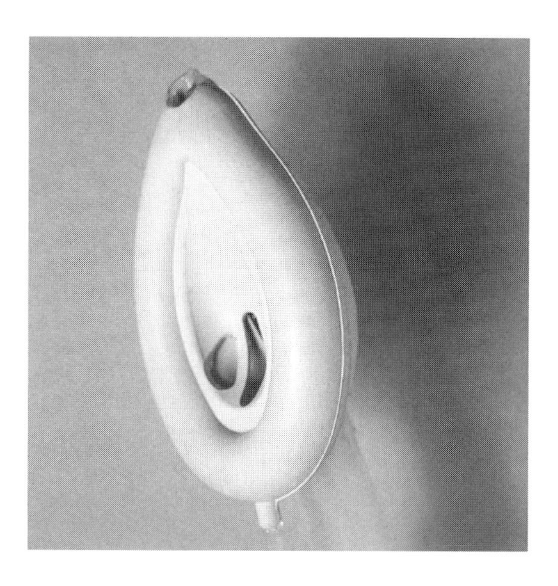

Figure 17.8 LMA II.

is to provide the higher seal capability and an adequate gastric drain to permit blind passage of a 14 FG gastric tube without the higher cost and complexity of the GLM. This device is still undergoing trials.

References

1 Brimacombe J. Analysis of 1500 laryngeal mask uses by one anaesthetist in adults undergoing routine anaesthesia. *Anaesthesia* 1996;**51**:76–80.

2 Brimacombe J, Berry A. A proposed fiber-optic scoring system to standardize the assessment of laryngeal mask airway position. *Anesth Analg* 1993;**76**:457.

3 Asai T. Difficulty in assessing the correct position of the laryngeal mask airway. *Br J Anaesth* 1994;**72**:366.

4 Brimacombe J, Newell S, Swainston R, Thompson J. A potential new technique for awake fibreoptic bronchoscopy – use of the laryngeal mask airway. *Med J Aust* 1992;**156**:876–877.

5 Fujita M, Orima H, Simizu M, Motoyoshi S, Katayama M, Miyasaka K. Use of laryngeal mask airway in small animals. *J Vet Med Sci* 1991;**53**:1081–1082.

6 Brain AIJ. The development of the laryngeal mask – a brief history of the invention, early clinical studies and experimental work from which the laryngeal mask evolved. *Eur J Anaesthesiol* 1991;**4**:5–17.

7 Medda BK, Lang IM, Layman R, Hogan WJ, Dodds WJ, Shaker R. Characterization and quantification of a pharyngo-UES contractile reflex in cats. *Am J Physiol* 1994;**267**:G972–83.

8 George A. Failed cuff inflation of a laryngeal mask. *Anaesthesia* 1994;**49**:80.

9 Newell S, Brimacombe J. A modified tracheal tube mount for sampling gases from the distal shaft of the laryngeal mask airway. *J Clin Anesth* 1995,**7**;444–445.

10 Brimacombe J. The incendiary characteristics of the laryngeal and reinforced laryngeal mask airway to CO_2 laser strike – a comparison with two polyvinyl chloride tracheal tubes. *Anaesth Intens Care* 1994;**22**:694–697.

11 Stevens JE, Burden G. Reinforced laryngeal mask airway and magnetic resonance imaging. *Anaesthesia* 1994;**49**:79–80.

12 Heath ML, Sinnathamby SW. The reinforced laryngeal mask airway for adenotonsillectomy. *Br J Anaesth* 1994;**72**:728–729.

13 Brimacombe J. The use of the laryngeal mask airway in very small neonates. *Anesthesiology* 1994;**81**:1302.

14 Southern DA, Lake APJ, Wadon AJ. The laryngeal mask – a modification in its use and design. *Anaesthesia* 1992;**47**:530.

15 Brimacombe J, Berry A. Insertion of the laryngeal mask airway – not facilitated by cuff inflation. *Anaesthesia* 1993;**48**:79.

16 Brain AIJ. Laryngeal mask misplacement – causes, consequences and solutions. *Anaesthesia* 1992;**47**:531–532.

17 Miura M. Problems during insertion of the laryngeal mask airway and postoperative pharyngalgia. *40th Meeting of the Japanese Society of Anesthesiology, Iwate Prefectual Hall, Japan, 22 April 1993*, pp.2–3. (Abstract).

★ 18 Alexander CA. A modified Intavent laryngeal mask for ENT and dental anaesthesia. *Anaesthesia* 1990;**45**:892–893. *First description of the flexible LMA. Reports its use in 20 patients undergoing molar extraction or tonsillectomy.*

19 Brimacombe J, Johns K. Modified Intavent LMA. *Anaesth Intens Care* 1991;**19**:607.

20 Darling JR, D'Arcy JT, Murray JM. Split laryngeal mask airway as an aid to fibreoptic intubation. *Anaesthesia* 1993;**48**:79–80.

21 Maroof M, Khan RM, Khan H, Stewart J, Mroze C. Evaluation of a modified laryngeal mask airway as an aid to fibre optic intubation (FOI). *Anesthesiology* 1992;**77**:A1062 (Abstract).

22 Brimacombe J. Split laryngeal mask airway. *Anaesthesia* 1993;**48**:639.

23 Maroof M, Siddique MS, Khan RM. Modified laryngeal mask as an aid to fiberoptic endotracheal intubation. *Acta Anaesthesiol Scand* 1993;**37**:124.

24 Darling JR, Keohane M, Murray JM. A split laryngeal mask as an aid to training in fibreoptic tracheal intubation. A comparison with the Berman II intubating airway. *Anaesthesia* 1993;**48**:1079–1082.

25 Maroof M, Khan RM. Ventilatory role of modified laryngeal mask (MLMA) during fiberoptic intubation (FOI). *Anesthesiology* 1994;**81**:A621 (Abstract).

26 Maroof M, Khan RM, Bonsu A, Raza HS. A new solution to fibreoptic intubation in the presence of blood and secretions. *Can J Anaesth* 1995;**42**:177.

27 Murray JM, Renfrew CW. Arterial carbon dioxide tensions during fiberoptic tracheal intubation: a comparison of the split laryngeal mask with the Berman II airway. *Anesth Analg* 1995;**81**:1311–1312.

28 Squires SJ. Identification of laryngeal mask airways. *Anaesthesia* 1992;**47**:533.

29 Akhtar TM. Oesophageal vent-laryngeal mask to prevent aspiration of gastric contents. *Br J Anaesth* 1994;**72**:52–54.

30 Brain AIJ. The oesophageal vent-laryngeal mask. *Br J Anaesth* 1994;**72**:727.

31 Asai T. The oesophageal vent-laryngeal mask. *Br J Anaesth* 1994;**72**:726.

32 Sorooshian SS. The oesophageal vent-laryngeal mask. *Br J Anaesth* 1994;**72**:726.

33 Gajraj NM, Pace NA, Pennant JH. The oesophageal vent-laryngeal mask. *Br J Anaesth* 1994;**72**:726–727.

34 Akhtar T. The oesophageal vent-laryngeal mask. *Br J Anaesth* 1994;**72**:727.

35 Cheam EWS. The use of tracheal tubes as oesophageal obturators. *Anaesthesia* 1994;**49**:734.

36 Lopez-Gil M, Brimacombe J, Brain AIJ, Wenck D, Wilkins H. The double-lumen LMA. *Anesthesiology* 1996;**84**:1263–1264.

37 Brain AI. Three cases of difficult intubation overcome by the laryngeal mask airway. *Anaesthesia* 1985;**40**:353–355.

★ **38** Kapila A, Addy EV, Verghese C, Brain AIJ. Intubating laryngeal mask airway: a preliminary assessment of performance. *Br J Anaesth* 1995;**75**:228P–229P (Abstract).
Pilot study of 78 patients intubated using a prototype intubating LMA. The success rate was 92% within two attempts. This prototype has since been improved.

★ **39** Brain AIJ, Verghese C, Strube P, Brimacombe J. A new laryngeal mask prototype – preliminary evaluation of seal pressures and glottic isolation. *Anaesthesia* 1995;**50**:42–48.
Paper describing new LMA prototype and comparing seal pressure and glottic isolation with the standard device in 20 patients.

40 Brimacombe J. Airway protection with the new laryngeal mask prototype. *Anaesthesia* 1996;**51**:602–603.

18 Progressing along the LMA learning curve

1 GENERAL

Optimal use of the LMA requires the user to appreciate that its placement, the stimulation it provokes, the position it occupies, the precise manner in which it is fixed in place, the way in which it is used with positive pressure ventilation, and the timing and manner of its removal all differ from other current airway devices. Though apparently very easy to use, there are both short-term[1] and long-term[2] learning curves. Careful attention to seemingly unimportant details is likely to shorten this learning process, benefiting patients and clinicians alike.

Before using the device in patients, it is advisable to practice insertion using the modified Ambu dummy available from the distributor. Then start by using it in simple short ASA 1–2 cases, so attention can be focused on learning the technique. For those who do not have access to short cases, note that the LMA can be inserted using the standard technique even when there is a tracheal tube in place (see Chapter 12, *Tracheal tube/LMA exchange*).

2 CHOOSING THE CORRECT SIZE

See also Chapter 5, *Size selection.*

If the mask is too big:

- it tends to displace when inflated
- too much of the tube lies outside the mouth when fully inserted

- obstruction may occur during anesthesia due to the epiglottis lying below the level of the mask aperture (don't confuse with incomplete insertion which also causes obstruction).

If the mask is too small:

- the aperture may be below the level of the glottis, causing obstruction
- the epiglottis may be forced between the aperture bars (possible epiglottic trauma and obstruction[3]
- accidental misplacement is more likely
- overinflation may be needed to obtain a seal

Risks: premature cuff failure, high pressure points against mucosa, possible nerve damage)[4].

The following guidelines should be followed when choosing the LMA size.

1. Size 4 is the normal adult size for male and female subjects.
2. Size 3 is a pediatric size in the population. Use it for children over 30 kg or adults in whom a size 4 will not stay in place when the cuff is inflated to 60 cm H_2O intracuff pressure (do not hold the tube while inflating the cuff). Note that this pressure will rarely equate with the maximum recommended inflation volume.
3. In adults, weight is not a reliable guide to appropriate mask size. Many adults will comfortably take a size 5. Consider changing to a larger size if leaks occur when the lungs are inflated to peak airway pressure <20 cm H_2O. (But check first that this is not due to adequate anesthesia.)
4. When in doubt, it is better to use a large size with small inflation volumes than a small size excessively inflated. The aim should be to achieve an optimum ratio of intracuff pressure to seal pressure.
5. Always have a size larger and smaller immediately available.
6. Start by choosing the largest size you think will fit and inflate with the smallest volume required to obtain an adequate seal. In practice you will find that the larger the size used, the lower the intracuff pressure needed to obtain an adequate seal.

3 INSERTION

The palate and oropharynx above and behind the tongue is curved, but the laryngopharynx into which the mask fits is not (Figure 18.1). It is possible to deflate the mask so that it curls in the same direction as the curved palate behind the tongue[5,6]. In this shape, it will fit well behind the tongue but will tend to become entangled with the glottis or epiglottis when pushed further down. The arytenoid cartilages may be bruised using this technique and the mask may occasionally fold over[7].

Lesson: Avoid deflating the mask so it curls forwards.

The LMA is not designed to be inserted inflated. The bulk of an inflated device may represent a greater stimulus than the correctly deflated device. The mask may not reach its intended destination and the method is unsuitable for patients with restricted mouth opening or who have not been paralyzed. Brimacombe and Berry have shown less success with this method

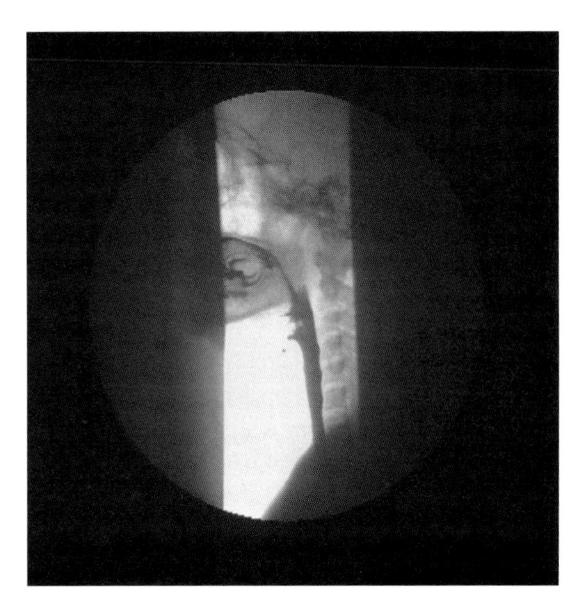

Figure 18.1 The palate and oropharynx above and behind the tongue is curved, but the laryngopharynx into which the mask fits is not (swallowed contrast medium to demonstrate hollow anatomy of pharynx, lateral view).

than with the standard technique[8] though these findings have been contested[9] (see Chapter 6, *Alternative insertion techniques*). In cadavers, the inventor has found inflated insertion tended to force the mask tip anterior to the arytenoids so that it lodged in the glottic vestibule (Figure 18.2), a position first shown radiographically by Nandi et al[7].

Lesson: Do not insert inflated.

Another solution adopted with early prototypes was to rotate the mask round the corner. This technique has a high success rate[8], though the mask may remain partly rotated when in place

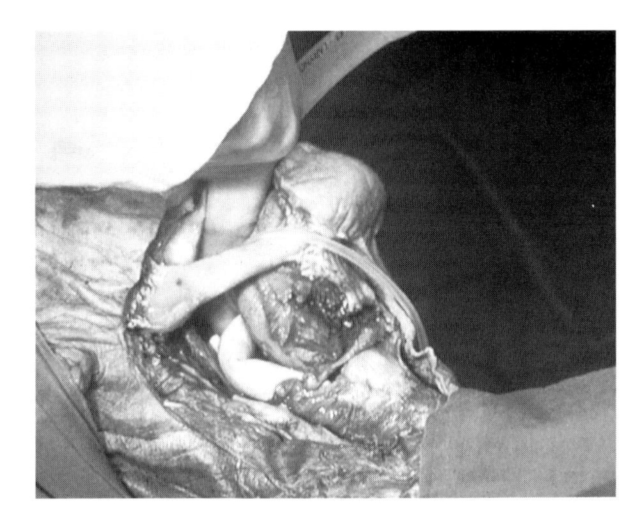

Figure 18.2 Inflated insertion could direct the mask tip into the glottic vestibule.

and is unsuitable for the flexible LMA owing to the flexibility of the tube. Nerve trauma, poor seal or obstruction could result. Excessive shearing force on the tube from rotation might be expected to cause tube fracture, especially if the tube has previously been damaged by biting.

Lesson: Rotational insertion is not the method of choice.

To face the right way when in the hypopharynx, the mask is fixed to the tube at an angle of 30 degrees. This means it points upwards towards the hard palate when passed into the mouth. So if it is simply passed straight back over the tongue, the leading edge tends to curl over, allowing the pointed tip to traumatize the posterior upper pharynx in the region of the uvula[10] (Figure 18.3).

Lesson: Carefully flatten the deflated mask into the palate so the leading edge follows the soft palate as it bridges over the nasopharynx. The soft palate then automatically directs the leading edge downwards, provided the index finger maintains a cranial pressure on the tube.

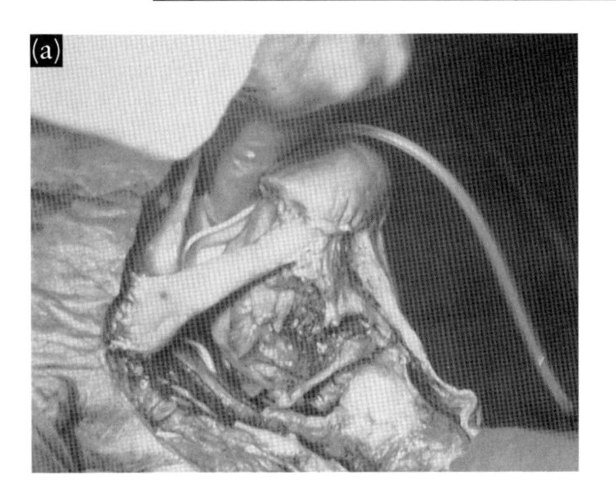

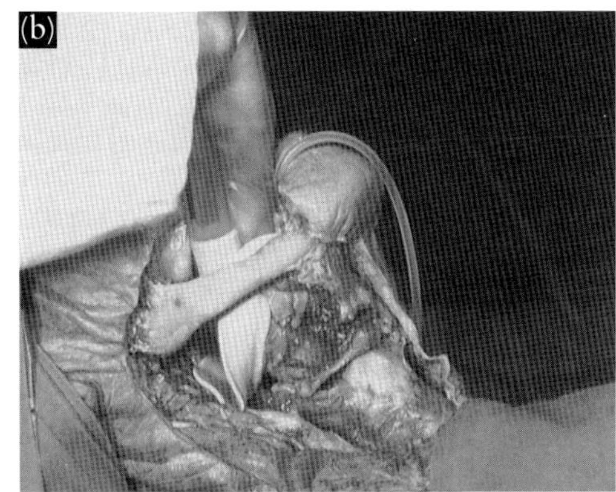

Figure 18.3 The deflated tip must be pressed up into the palate to prevent trauma to the posterior pharyngeal wall. (a) Correct, (b) incorrect.

A thin saucer-shaped leading edge is achieved by deflating the mask to a high vacuum. To retain the collapsed shape, the LMA valve must be competent and the deflating syringe not left attached to the valve. The rim of the saucer shape should curl upwards, so there is slight resistance to flattening out this curled shape when the mask is pressed into the palate. The results are: (1) a redistribution of pressure which prevents the pointed end of the mask from scratching the mucosa of the pharynx; (2) a thin wedge shape is formed which passes easily behind a posteriorly lying epiglottis; and (3) the thin leading edge is firm enough to wedge itself into the hypopharynx, lifting the larynx forwards so as to ensure correct placement in the base of the hypopharynx. This may be important in optimizing placement in the presence of cricoid pressure.

Lesson: Think of the desired deflated form as a 'floppy shovel'. Take care to deflate correctly – use the deflator device when possible. Older or dirty valves may fail to retain complete deflation – check regularly. Avoid inserting with air in the cuff.

LMA placement has a number of parallels with swallowing of food:

- It is difficult to swallow food when the mouth is dry. Lubrication of the mask is equally important, especially when antisialogogues have been given.
- The smaller the food bolus, the easier it is to swallow. The mask should be deflated fully for the same reason.
- The food bolus must be soft so it can be molded by the tongue into an appropriate shape to be swallowed. The mask shape must be appropriately pre-molded by correct deflation.
- A swallowing reflex can be triggered by stimulation of the palate. The mask can be shown to stimulate swallowing when used to massage the palate in neonates. It is preferable to stimulate the swallowing reflex than the vomiting reflex since stimulation of the swallowing reflex may inhibit the vomiting reflex.
- Barium swallow radiography shows that the tongue sweeps the food bolus centrifugally upwards and backwards before swinging it downwards into the hypopharynx. The mask is passed into the hypopharynx using the index finger to perform the function of the tongue.
- Radiographic study shows that slight head extension occurs during swallowing. Extension of the head facilitates passage of the mask behind the tongue. Table 6.1 shows how the LMA insertion technique parallels these features of deglutition.

Lesson: A careful imitation of the swallowing process should permit atraumatic insertion of the LMA in any patient able to swallow food normally.

To imitate the action of the tongue, the index finger must be placed at the junction of the tube and mask in line with the central mask aperture, tucking the finger behind the deflated upper rim of the mask (Figure 18.4). The finger remains in this position until the mask is fully inserted. Take care to avoid getting lubricant on the finger, or it will tend to slip off the tube.

Note: if it is not possible to prevent the finger becoming slippery, an alternative technique is to maintain pressure on the tube to hold it against the hard palate while sliding the tube in over this finger using the other hand.

The reason why neck flexion is so important when inserting the LMA is that when the relatively soft tissues in front of the cervical spine are drawn into a taut line by elevation of the jaw, a space can only be created in the pharynx if the axis of the cervical spine diverges from this line, forming a space behind the stretched laryngeal structures. Merely extending the head will not achieve this because the cervical spine will consequently also tend to be extended, creating a convexity behind the larynx which actually obliterates the pharyngeal space instead of opening it up.

Lesson: Swallowing is a complicated process. Imitating this process requires attention to detail. Obstruction occurring at the back of the tongue is the commonest problem encountered in LMA insertion. It is usually due to inadequate neck flexion but may also be encountered in inadequate anesthesia and incorrect mask preparation. Never try to overcome obstruction with force.

4 HOW TO GET A 'JUST SEAL' VOLUME

1. Initially, use a commercially available manometer such as the Portex Cuff Inflator (Hythe, Kent, UK). Gently squeeze the blue balloon to learn the feel when the intracuff pressure is

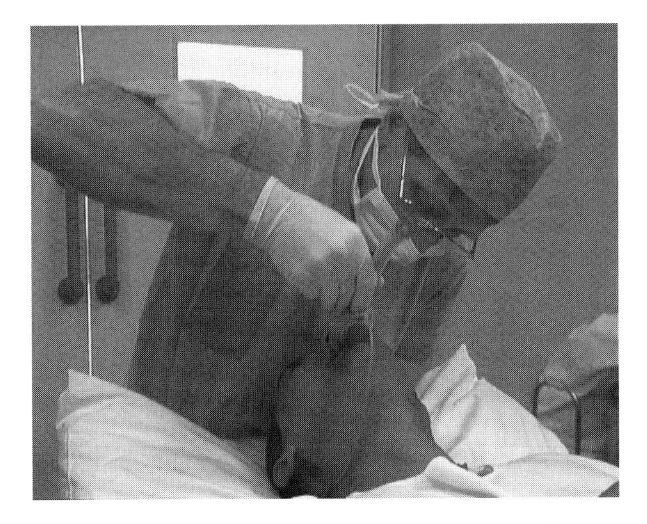

Figure 18.4 The position of the index finger shown here is critical, enabling the tube to be pressed up into the palate as the mask slides inwards.

60 cm H_2O. Subsequently a pressure approximating to this can be verified by manual palpation of the balloon alone.

2. If nitrous oxide is used, cuff pressure will increase and should be reduced by reducing the air volume carefully while gently palpating the blue pilot balloon until the same soft consistency is noted. It has been shown that maintaining pressures of this order reduces sore throat incidence[11].
3. With experience it becomes possible to judge the appropriate volume required, which will be different for every patient. The volume should normally be well within the recommended maximum volume. If more seems necessary, the mask is too small or the patient requires more anesthetic, or the cuff may be leaking.
4. If very little air causes pressure to rise rapidly in the pilot balloon, the mask may have folded over, the pilot balloon tube may have kinked or be caught between teeth, the mask may be misplaced into the laryngeal vestibule, or the patient may simply be squeezing the mask by contracting the constrictor muscles if anesthesia is insufficient.
5. During anesthesia, in the absence of nitrous oxide, an increase in tension in the pilot balloon could only mean an increase in tone of the muscles surrounding the mask, indicating inadequate anesthesia, while a decrease might indicate failure of gas-tightness of the system, reduction in tone or loss of mask position.
6. If lung inflation is difficult after LMA insertion and peak airway pressures are high (>20 cm H_2O), injecting more air into the cuff than the maximum recommended volume is not appropriate.

5 CAUSES AND MANAGEMENT OF LMA PROBLEMS

Problems related to insertion

Inflation of the stomach

Inflation of the stomach may be caused by vigorous or high volume manual bag inflation prior to LMA insertion, especially in small babies. This predisposes to reflux and reduces pulmonary compliance. Difficult face mask ventilation may lead to a degree of gastric insufflation which in turn may result in reflux and aspiration prior to or during LMA insertion.

Hiccup at induction

Hiccup at induction is common with propofol and does not normally make lung inflation more difficult. It may be associated with transient relaxation of the lower esophageal sphincter[12]. Suspect reflux and possible aspiration if lung inflation becomes difficult following hiccup.

Postinsertion problems

Obstructed ventilation

Upper airway obstruction may be confused with bronchospasm when using the LMA unless the side of the neck is auscultated to exclude a laryngeal cause. The mistake is easily made if the patient is asthmatic, for example.

Lesson: Neck auscultation is good practice when using the LMA.

Gastric insufflation

Compared with the tracheal tube, relatively small rises in airways resistance are sufficient to overcome the seal at the mask–larynx junction. If undetected, this may result in progressive gastric insufflation, increasing the potential risk of regurgitation as anesthesia continues. However, there is a relation between adequacy of anesthesia/neuromuscular block and airways resistance, so if such small pressure rises are monitored, anaesthetic depth/ adequacy of paralysis can also be more closely controlled. For this reason the ventilator alarm is preferably set to a pressure just below the measured leak pressure.

Lesson: When using positive pressure ventilation, set the alarm to a pressure just below the measured leak pressure.

Closed larynx

If the larynx closes completely as a response to inadequate anesthesia, there is a danger of rapid gastric insufflation if mechanical ventilation is allowed to continue, especially if the ventilator is of the volume cycling type.

Lesson: Pressure cycling ventilators may be more appropriate when using the LMA for positive pressure ventilation.

6 MANAGEMENT OF ADVERSE EVENTS

Gurgling sounds/bag stops moving

Loud gurgling sounds are suddenly heard (PPV) or the bag suddenly stops moving (SV). This usually means the patient is waking up or needs more muscle relaxant.

Lesson: DO NOT REMOVE THE LMA but instead DEEPEN ANESTHESIA/GIVE MORE RELAXANT as appropriate.

Fluids in LMA tubing during anesthesia

Fluids are suddenly seen emerging through the LMA tube during anesthesia. This is either gastric reflux (often bile-colored) or bronchial secretions. Always assume any fluid seen in the tube to be from the stomach. Litmus paper may be useful in differentiating between the two. The inventor's recommendations are:

1. **Leave the LMA alone.** It is important to limit the rate of reflux. If you take the mask out, this allows reflux to occur more freely. Also, the mask may be difficult to get out of the mouth if the patient is light, because of biting on the tube. If the mask gets trapped in the mouth, this may prevent fluids escaping and make aspiration more likely.
2. **Use gravity** to drain fluids out of the pharynx (Trendelenburg position).
3. **Regain control of the airway** by deepening anesthesia
4. **Use very gentle manual bag-squeezing** to avoid forcing fluids further into the bronchial tree.
5. **Apply suction only when control is regained** preferably using a fiberscope, so the extent of aspiration can be seen directly.
6. **Order a chest X-ray within 2 h of the event.** There is evidence that if radiographic changes suggestive of aspiration cannot be demonstrated within 2 h after the completion of surgery, clinically significant aspiration is unlikely to have occurred[13].

Lesson: The adage 'when in doubt, take it out' does not always apply when problems occur with the LMA.

Factors which would favor removal of the LMA are:

1. It is not possible to maintain an expired tidal volume compatible with normal blood gases (device malfunction likely); or
2. Oxygen saturation/capnography/blood gases indicate a deteriorating trend in spite of acceptable peak airway pressure and inspiratory/expiratory ratio (pulmonary dysfunction is likely). Immediate improvement in expired tidal volume after substituting one airway device for another indicates that there was either obstruction or leak using the first device. However, if after airway substitution the oxygen saturation is not improved from a previous abnormally low figure, this suggests that airways obstruction lies further within the bronchial tree. If peak airway pressure increases after substitution of an LMA with a tracheal tube, this may be due to the narrower diameter of the tracheal tube or broncho-constriction associated with the stimulus of inserting the tube and/or its continued presence, particularly in a patient with known irritable upper airways. A tracheal tube should not be substituted for an LMA when an aspiration is suspected only in order to facilitate fiberoptic bronchoscopy. Introduction of a fiberscope through the LMA has been shown to permit examination and aspiration of the larynx and upper trachea without laryngoscopy[14].

Fluids in LMA tubing during recovery and patient coughing

Fluids are suddenly seen emerging from the LMA tube during recovery and the patient is coughing.

Don't: Paralyze and intubate. This prevents effective coughing.

Note: the cough mechanism is more likely to be an effective bronchial clearing mechanism than the suction catheter.

Do:
- Ensure reversal of neuromuscular blockade is complete
- Assist postural drainage
- Assist inspiration if there is stridor
- Provide oxygen if saturation is below normal
- Remove the LMA when the cough reflex is fully effective.

7 INVESTIGATION OF POSTOPERATIVE PHARYNGEAL MORBIDITY

Was the LMA in the wrong place?

The LMA is designed to form a low pressure ring structure around the glottic aperture by filling up the space made available for the passage of ingested food. When correctly placed, pressure on the mucosa should be evenly distributed about this space. Throat soreness/ nerve damage may be due to a localized area of high pressure corresponding to an incorrectly placed mask or a mask that has become doubled over. Hypoglossal[4], recurrent nerve[15] and lingual nerve damage[16,17] have all been reported, though it is not possible to be sure of the exact mechanism.

Was there too much air in the cuff?

Even when the mask is ideally placed, significant throat soreness may be associated with excess cuff inflation. Unrecognized misplacement may cause leaks and it may be tempting to try to overcome the poor seal by increasing cuff pressure. This is likely to increase the risk of trauma.

Was a nonrecommended chemical used to decontaminate the LMA?

The silicone cuff will absorb many chemicals. Nonrecommended agents may diffuse out of the cuff causing local tissue damage.

Lesson: The LMA is not inherently traumatic. Attention to insertion technique, cuff pressures and device preparation are necessary to avoid trauma.

REFERENCES

1 Lopez-Gil M, Brimacombe J, Cebrian J, Arranz J. The laryngeal mask airway in pediatric practice – a prospective study of skill acquisition by resident anesthesiologists. *Anesthesiology* 1996;**84**:807–811.

2 Brimacombe J. Analysis of 1500 laryngeal mask uses by one anaesthetist in adults undergoing routine anaesthesia. *Anaesthesia* 1996;**51**:76–80.

3 Miller AC, Bickler P. The laryngeal mask airway. An unusual complication. *Anaesthesia* 1991;**46**:659–660.

4 Nagai K, Sakuramoto C, Goto F. Unilateral hypoglossal nerve paralysis following the use of the laryngeal mask airway. *Anaesthesia* 1994;**49**:603–604.

5 Wright E. The laryngeal mask airway. *Today's Anaesthetist* 1990;**5**:223.

6 Brain AIJ, Nunn JF. The laryngeal mask airway – insertion technique. *Today's Anaesthetist* 1991;**6**:18.

7 Nandi PR, Nunn JF, Charlesworth CH, Taylor SJ. Radiological study of the laryngeal mask. *Eur J Anaesthesiol* 1991;**4**:33–39.

8 Brimacombe J, Berry A. Insertion of the laryngeal mask airway – a prospective study of four techniques. *Anaesth Intens Care* 1993;**21**:89–92.

9 Canevet C, Baelen E, Krivosic Horber R. Insertion du masque larynge gonfle. *Conferences d'Actualisation, Congres National d'Anesthesie et Reanimation, Paris, October 1994*;R128 (Abstract).

10 Lee JJ, Brain AIJ. Laryngeal mask and trauma to uvula. *Anaesthesia* 1989;**44**:1014–1015.

11 Burgard G, Mollhoff T, Prien T. The effect of laryngeal mask cuff pressure on postoperative sore throat incidence. *J Clin Anesth* 1996;**8**:198–201.

12 Roberts CJ, Goodman NW. Gastro-oesophageal reflux during elective laparoscopy. *Anaesthesia* 1990;**45**:1009–1011.

13 Warner MA, Warner WE, Webber JG. Clinical significance of pulmonary aspiration during the perioperative period. *Anesthesiology* 1993;**78**:56–62.

14 Du Plessis MC, Marshall Barr A, Verghese C, Lyall JRW. Fibreoptic bronchoscopy under general anaesthesia using the laryngeal mask airway. *Eur J Anaesthesiol* 1993;**10**:363–365.

15 Lloyd Jones FR, Hegab A. Recurrent laryngeal nerve palsy after laryngeal mask airway insertion. *Anaesthesia* 1996;**51**:171–172.

16 Ahmad NS, Yentis SM. Laryngeal mask airway and lingual nerve injury. *Anaesthesia* 1996;**51**:707–708.

17 Laxton CH, Kipling R. Lingual nerve paralysis following the use of the laryngeal mask airway. *Anaesthesia* 1996;**51**:869–870.

Quick reference

TROUBLESHOOTING GUIDE

Problem	Common causes	Solutions
Failure to insert LMA	1. Inadequate anesthesia 2. Suboptimal head/neck position Incorrect mask deflation Failure to press LMA into palatopharyngeal curve during insertion 3. Cricoid pressure (CP) 4. Pathology, e.g. large tonsils	1. Deepen anesthesia 2. Ensure correct insertion technique or try alternative technique 3. Temporarily release CP 4. Try alternative insertion technique; start with diagonal approach
Laryngeal spasm and coughing	1. Inadequate anesthesia 2. Tip impaction against glottis 3. Aspiration	1. Deepen anesthesia 2. Check LMA position. Re-insert if necessary 3. See Table 9.3
Mask leaks, or unable to manually ventilate the lungs	1. Inadequate anesthesia ■ glottic closure ■ low lung compliance 2. Malpositioned mask ■ rotation ■ wrong cuff inflation volume ■ folded back on itself 3. High airway pressure 4. Mask too small	1. Deepen anesthetic 2. Check LMA position. Re-insert if necessary 3. Reduce airway pressure ■ lower tidal volume ■ lower inspiratory flow rate ■ muscle relaxation ■ treat bronchospam if present 4. Insert larger size
High end-tidal carbon dioxide	1. Drug/anesthesia induced hypoventilation	1. Reduce MAC, avoid further opioids. Assist ventilation
Displaced after insertion: ENSURE FIXATION	1. Inadequate anesthetic depth 2. Pulled or twisted tube 3. Mask too big	1. Deepen anesthesia 2. Avoid circuit dragging. Ensure appropriate fixation 3. Use smaller size

Problems during recovery	1. Removal of LMA at inappropriate anesthetic depth	1. Remove LMA when patient opens mouth to command. Only remove with patient deep if no reflexes returned
	2. Oral secretions entering larynx on cuff deflation causing laryngospasm or coughing	2. Deflate LMA only as it is removed, or remove still moderately inflated
	3. Adverse events when patient moved or stimulated	3. Avoid patient stimulation when patient is 'light'
	4. LMA occluded by biting	4. Use bite block throughout recovery period
	5. Regurgitation	5. See Table 9.3

INSERTION PROBLEMS

Inadequate anesthetic depth

May cause an adverse reaction to insertion, such as coughing or breathholding. Anesthesia should be deepened immediately and manual ventilation resumed.

Failure to negotiate the back of the tongue

Often results from a failure to maintain a constant centrifugal force with the index finger against the curve of the hard palate, or from suboptimal positioning of the head and neck. The tip of the LMA may fold on itself or impact on an irregularity or swelling in the posterior pharynx, e.g. hypertrophied tonsils. If the cuff fails to flatten or begins to curl over as it is advanced, it may be necessary to withdraw the mask and re-insert it. If difficulty in insertion persists, an alternative technique is advised.

Warning: to avoid trauma, force should not be used at any time during insertion. Ensure adequate oxygenation prior to insertion.

Inadequate mouth opening

If mouth opening is less than 1.5 cm, it may be difficult to insert the mask into the mouth using the standard technique. Ensure the patient is adequately anesthetized. An assistant can be asked to pull the jaw downwards during insertion into the mouth. Cease jaw pull during passage through the pharynx.

Epiglottic downfolding

Occasionally following placement, gross downfolding of the epiglottis may occur and lead to increased work of breathing and sometimes complete airway obstruction. This is more likely to occur if the LMA is inserted with the cuff semi or fully inflated or if the rim is deflated anteriorly. It is also more likely to occur if the LMA is not pressed into the posterior pharyngeal wall during its passage towards the hypopharynx. For similar reasons the tip of the LMA may collide with the arytenoids or laryngeal inlet resulting in laryngeal spasm or stridor.

Over/under insertion

If the LMA is not inserted far enough, the tip may cause the arytenoid cartilages to infold or enter the larynx and can cause airway obstruction. If the hypopharynx is visible through the fiberoptic scope, the mask is not inserted far enough or folded back on itself. Insertion of too small a mask or using excessive force or holding the LMA tube during inflation may result in penetration of the distal mask into the upper esophageal sphincter or glottic inlet. Inflation of the cuff will result in airway obstruction as the proximal cuff inflates over the laryngeal inlet. Folding of the LMA is possible if excessive force is used, the mask is incorrectly prepared or the cuff is not pressed into the hard palate and posterior pharynx. Torsion of the mask may occur, particularly if the mask is rotated during insertion.

MECHANICAL OBSTRUCTION

1. Observe the position of the LMA tube and particularly the black line. If the latter does not face the upper lip directly, the LMA may be twisted onto its side. (This does not apply to the FLMA.)

2. If the tube has slipped out beyond the point at which it was fixed, push it back into place until resistance is felt. However, if the airway is not immediately cleared, it may be necessary to remove it completely and insert another correctly prepared LMA. This is because the epiglottis may be pushed into a downfolded position if the LMA is pushed past in the inflated state.

3. Respiratory obstruction is most commonly due to light anesthesia. If a patient becomes too light the pharynx may constrict, squeezing a poorly secured LMA upwards out of position. Mechanical obstruction can thus sometimes be secondary to patient reaction. If obstruction is associated with breathholding, coughing or laryngeal spasm, the well-secured LMA usually remains in place. Breathholding is commonly due to a strong surgical stimulus in the inadequately anesthetized patient.

EARLY TRAINING PERIOD

Anesthetic depth

A readjustment of the operator's preconceived sense of anesthetic requirement is necessary when learning to use the LMA as anesthesia is now given for the intensity of surgical stimulus and not for airway tolerance.

Early maintenance

If propofol has been used for insertion the LMA can very often be inserted rapidly and an effective airway immediately achieved with easily inflated lungs. The situation can change quickly as the effect of the propofol wears off if anesthesia has not already been deepened with an adequate concentration of volatile anesthetic.

Anesthetic agents

Standard volatile agents and total intravenous anesthesia with propofol are suitable for use with the LMA.

Mode of ventilation

Surgical and anesthetic requirements will dictate the mode of ventilation and the requirements for muscle relaxation.

Cuff pressure

Cuff pressure should be checked at intervals either by feeling the tension in the pilot balloon or by monitoring changes with a pressure transducer. Volume may then be withdrawn or added to maintain values close to the initial seal pressure.

Time factors

Beginners should confine themselves to brief procedures (<30 min). Use of the LMA for >2 h is controversial.

POSITIVE PRESSURE VENTILATION

Seal/Leak

Make an assessment of seal pressure. Inflate the cuff slowly by closing the circuit popoff valve and note the pressure at which gas first escapes. This is best detected by neck auscultation (leak test). If seal pressures are inadequate even at the maximum recommended cuff volumes, either re-insert or choose a larger LMA. Leaks may disappear after the first two or three breaths and may be less likely with the neck flexed. New leaks developing are usually due to glottic closure secondary to inadequate depth or the relaxant wearing off. Cuff failure is an uncommon causes of leaks.

Ventilatory pattern

Use a ventilatory pattern which provides adequate minute volume, but minimizes peak airway pressures (<20 cm H_2O). Tidal volume should be 8–10 ml kg^{-1}. Inspiratory flow rates may be slowed to lower peak pressure. Adjust minute volume by varying rate. Peak pressure must be maintained below gastric insufflation pressure.

Monitoring

Auscultation of the anterolateral neck and epigastrium and observation of the capnograph trace are useful in assessing leak. Fiberoptic laryngoscopy can differentiate between glottic closure and malposition.

Reversal

Reverse neuromuscular block under a continued level of anesthesia to minimize the risk of laryngeal spasm and/or regurgitation. Allow the patient to commence spontaneous breathing and recover as described in *Post anesthesia care unit guidelines*.

Gastric distension

More common in children and may be managed by passage of a nasogastric tube (NGT). A NGT may be passed pre-emptively in infants. It is possible to pass a NGT blindly behind the partially deflated LMA cuff in children and adults.

POST ANESTHESIA CARE UNIT GUIDELINES

1. The LMA is designed to be removed when the patient is fully awake. However, it may also be removed under deep anesthesia. It must not be removed at a halfway stage or laryngeal spasm, coughing or gagging may result. Awake removal is probably the most common and preferred technique, particularly in adults. The smoothest recovery is probably obtained by reducing the intracuff pressure to the minimum required to maintain an effective seal. The inventor recommends maintaining intracuff pressure at 60 cm H_2O for all sizes.

2. When patients are transferred from the operating table or turned on their side, anesthesia should be maintained deep enough to prevent reflex responses to the stimulus of being moved.

3. Check that the airway is clear as soon as the patient arrives in the PACU. Place the palm of your hand about 1 cm away from the end of the tube to feel the expired breath. A recommended bite block should be in situ (see Chapter 5, *Bite blocks*).

4. Do not stimulate the patient. Apply monitoring equipment immediately upon arrival in the PACU. Active stimulation of the patient (includes cuff overinflation) may cause premature rejection of the LMA or provocation of incomplete and therefore ineffective reflex responses. This may promote laryngeal spasm or regurgitation.

5. Oxygen should be administered during the recovery period, but care must be taken to ensure exhalation is not obstructed by the oxygen delivery system. A clear plastic face mask or T-piece system enables airway patency to be continuously checked by observation of expired breath condensation on the transparent plastic surface. Take care that the T-piece does not cause obstruction to the LMA tube.

6. There is no need to manually support the airway with the LMA in position. Lifting the jaw may result in movement of the mask relative to the larynx, causing laryngeal spasm or malposition.

7. There is no clinical advantage in turning the patient onto the side with an LMA in situ unless there is an urgent indication to do so, such as regurgitation or vomiting. An exception to this rule is patients undergoing oropharyngeal surgery; they should be recovered in the lateral position to allow the continual drainage of blood and secretions from *above* the mask. If the anesthesiologist wishes the patient to be on the side during recovery, this should be done in the operating room under adequate anesthesia before transfer to the PACU, to avoid patient stimulation.

8. Look for the onset of swallowing as a sign of the imminent return of reflex function. However, the interval between swallowing and the ability to open the mouth is variable. Remove the adhesive tape from the face when swallowing begins.

9. Do not deflate the cuff until the LMA is removed. If the cuff is deflated before the return of effective swallowing and coughing reflexes, secretions in the upper pharynx may enter the larynx, causing laryngeal spasm. The cuff is deflated as the LMA is withdrawn from the mouth. The current trend is to remove it still inflated so that pharyngeal secretions are brought out more effectively on the mask surface, taking care to avoid trauma to the cuff from the teeth. However this may constitute quite a strong stimulus if the cuff has been allowed to become overinflated.

10. Do not remove the bite block until the LMA itself is removed.

11. **Only remove the LMA when the patient can open the mouth on command.**

12. Coughing is not necessarily an indication for removal but indicates the presence of secretions in the bronchial tree or larynx. Sputum removal is possible with an LMA in situ.

13. If the patient struggles or is restless during recovery from anesthesia, this is not an indication for removing the LMA. The restlessness may be followed by a quiescent phase during which the patient is still unable to maintain the airway without assistance.

14. It is not necessary to perform oropharyngeal suction before the LMA is removed. The secretions in the upper pharynx do not enter the larynx provided that the cuff is not deflated prior to removal. Oral suction may be performed after removal if necessary. Tracheal suction can be performed through the LMA, although there is danger of provoking laryngeal spasm. An anesthesiologist should therefore be present for such a maneuver.

BLIND INTUBATION VIA THE LMA

1. Blind intubation may be conducted under general or topical (awake) anesthesia.

2. The LMA is inserted in the standard way and the cuff inflated.

3. Holding the LMA tube firmly, the well-lubricated tracheal tube is introduced with the bevel rotated through a 90 degree turn to the left. This enables the bevel to pass through the central aperture in the mask aperture bars (MAB) (see Table 5.7 for tube sizes).

4. Oxygen is administered by positive pressure ventilation, or during spontaneous ventilation if the patient is awake, throughout the intubation procedure. The adequacy of respiration may be monitored by capnography.

5. Once through the MAB, the tracheal tube is rotated anteriorly and the head extended to enable the tube tip to pass anterior to the arytenoids. Push the tracheal tube until resistance is felt at about 3 cm down.

6. Flex the head to free the tube from impaction, permitting further passage of the tracheal tube into the trachea. A variety of head maneuvers may be attempted if this fails.

7. The tracheal tube cuff is now inflated, and the lungs manually ventilated to check correct position by auscultation and capnography.

8. The tracheal tube lies inside the LMA tube which is too long to be removed over the tracheal tube. The LMA is normally left in place after deflation of the cuff.

FIBEROPTIC GUIDED INTUBATION VIA THE LMA

1. Fiberoptic intubation may be conducted under general or topical (awake) anesthesia.

2. The LMA is inserted in the standard way and the cuff inflated.

3. A well-lubricated, fully deflated tracheal tube connected to resealing connector is threaded over the fiberoptic bronchoscope with the rotated bevel 90 degrees to the left (see Table 5.7 for sizes).

4. The tip of the fiberoptic scope is then introduced and passed into the LMA tube.

5. Oxygen is administered by positive pressure ventilation, or during spontaneous ventilation if the patient is awake, throughout the intubation procedure. The adequacy of respiration may be monitored by capnography.

6. Once the vocal cords are visualized, the tip of the fiberoptic scope is passed through them and into the trachea.

7. The tracheal tube is gently threaded downwards into the trachea over the fiberoptic scope. The tip may be rotated anteriorly as it passes through the MAB.

8. The fiberoptic scope is removed.

9. The tracheal tube cuff is now inflated, and the lungs manually ventilated to check correct position by auscultation and capnography.

10. The tracheal tube lies inside the LMA tube which is too long to be removed over the tracheal tube. The LMA is normally left in place but the LMA cuff should be deflated.

ALTERNATIVE TECHNIQUE FOR INTUBATION VIA THE LMA

1. The LMA is loaded with a well lubricated tracheal tube (TT) with the tip just entering the central aperture of the MAB, so that when pushed down it passes smoothly through the middle aperture.

2. The TT is marked where it emerges from the LMA connector and 3 cm above it. The TT cuff is then inflated to stabilize it in place and provide a seal.

3. Insert the loaded LMA normally and inflate the LMA cuff.

4. After deflating the TT cuff, hold the LMA tube firmly and push the TT gently down while simultaneously extending the head, until resistance is felt. If resistance is felt before arriving at the 3 cm mark, epiglottic or arytenoid impaction is likely. Withdraw to the first mark, press the LMA tube downward about 1 cm, and repeat the insertion attempt. If resistance is felt at or beyond the 3 cm mark, impaction of the tube tip against the anterior laryngeal or tracheal wall is likely, and this is confirmed by anterior neck bulging at the point of impaction. Release downward pressure momentarily, flex the head and then gently press down again on the tracheal tube to complete insertion.

   Step 4 can also be accomplished using a fiberoptic scope inserted through a resealing connector, with the advantage that head and neck manipulation may be avoided.

ESOPHAGOSCOPY AND GASTROSCOPY

1. Do not attempt this technique in patients who are at risk of aspiration.

2. Using a flexible gastroscope, flex the neck of the patient slightly and insert the scope slightly flexed, holding it about 15 cm from the tip. It may be necessary to remove some of the air from the LMA cuff to pass the scope behind it. Adequate lubrication is important. It is easier to get the tip of the scope behind the LMA using direct vision rather than looking through the scope itself.

3. Loss of pressure indicates that the tip has entered the cricopharyngeal sphincter and passed into the esophagus. The scope may pass more easily behind the LMA cuff if it is straightened out during passage.

4. Hold the tube of the LMA, or ask an assistant to do so, to prevent dislodgment while getting the scope tip past the cuff. If the scope is flexed excessively, it may pass anterior to the mask and so into the larynx, so care must be taken to avoid this. The well-lubricated gastroscope will usually not dislodge the LMA once it is past the cuff, but can be slid upwards or downwards behind it. The LMA must, of course, be properly secured in place.

FIBEROPTIC LARYNGOSCOPY AND BRONCHOSCOPY

1. A flexible bronchoscope can be passed easily through the LMA tube. This may be performed with general or local anesthesia.

2. Use a tube connector incorporating a rubber seal to permit passage of the fiberscope without loss of seal at the connector. This permits leisurely examination of the bronchial tree without loss of anesthetic gases.

3. Hold the bronchoscope correctly oriented so that the tip flexes anteriorly and posteriorly. Pass through the aperture bars slowly choosing the central aperture. The epiglottis may be resting against the middle of the bars, above them, or sometimes pointing downwards towards the lower part of the aperture. In the last case angle the tip of the scope down to pass under the tip of the epiglottis.

4. The vocal cords will come into view and a full inspection of the larynx and bronchial tree will then be possible.

AWAKE INSERTION (ADULTS)

1. Discuss the procedure with the patient. Warn patient that passage of the device may be a little uncomfortable, but that this will settle once in situ.

2. Ask patient to gargle lidocaine 4% gel, or spray the throat with a metered lidocaine spray. For best results, administer a drying agent such as glycopyrrolate 30 min before the procedure to reduce secretions.

3. Sedate using propofol, midazolam or fentanyl.

4. Administer 4 ml 4% lidocaine via cricothyroid puncture (only if lower airway is being instrumented).

5. Position the head and neck as per tracheal intubation.

6. Introduce the LMA into the mouth, gently stroke the hard palate with dorsal mask tip and ask the patient to swallow as the mask is pushed into the pharynx. Some patients may find the LMA easier to swallow if inflated with 5–10 ml air. It may help to allow the patient to hold the device as they retain a feeling of control and can remove it if it is too uncomfortable.

7. Gently push the LMA into place and then inflate the LMA to about half maximum volume (the awake patient has higher tone so smaller pharyngeal volume).

8. Check position by unobstructed respiration and visibility of vocal cords through the fiberoptic scope.

THUMB INSERTION TECHNIQUE

1. Useful in situations where access to the head end of the patient is difficult, such as during stereotactic neurosurgery or in resuscitation (Figures 19.1 and 19.2a–c).

2. The anesthetist stands to one side or in front of the patient.

3. The thumb replaces the index finger and is placed in the same position.

4. The dorsum of the wrist, instead of facing the patient's feet as in the standard technique, faces in the opposite direction, towards the anesthetist's face.

5. The nondominant hand may be used to obtain the 'sniffing' position, but it is often possible to insert successfully using only one hand.

   Note: The reason insertion using the thumb may not require use of the second hand is that the thumb causes the head to be extended by pressure on the hard palate. Provided the neck is already flexed by a pillow, the 'sniffing' position is achieved automatically.

6. As the thumb pushes the mask upwards and backwards behind the tongue, the four fingers extend straight over the patient's nose and forehead.

7. When the thumb is inserted to its fullest extent, the other hand grasps the end of the tube, again pushing cephalad until resistance is felt, as in the standard technique.

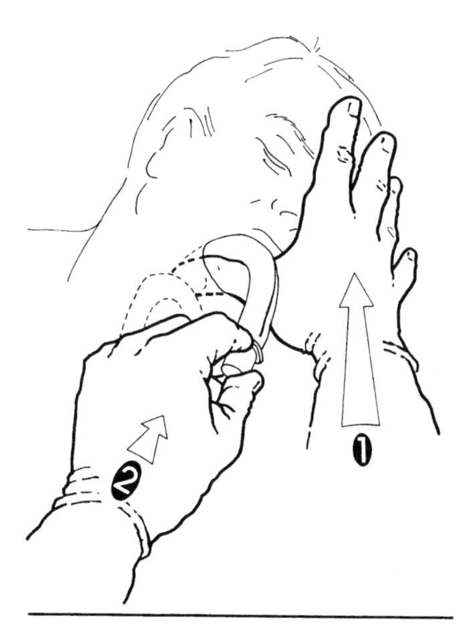

Figure 19.1 Thumb insertion technique.

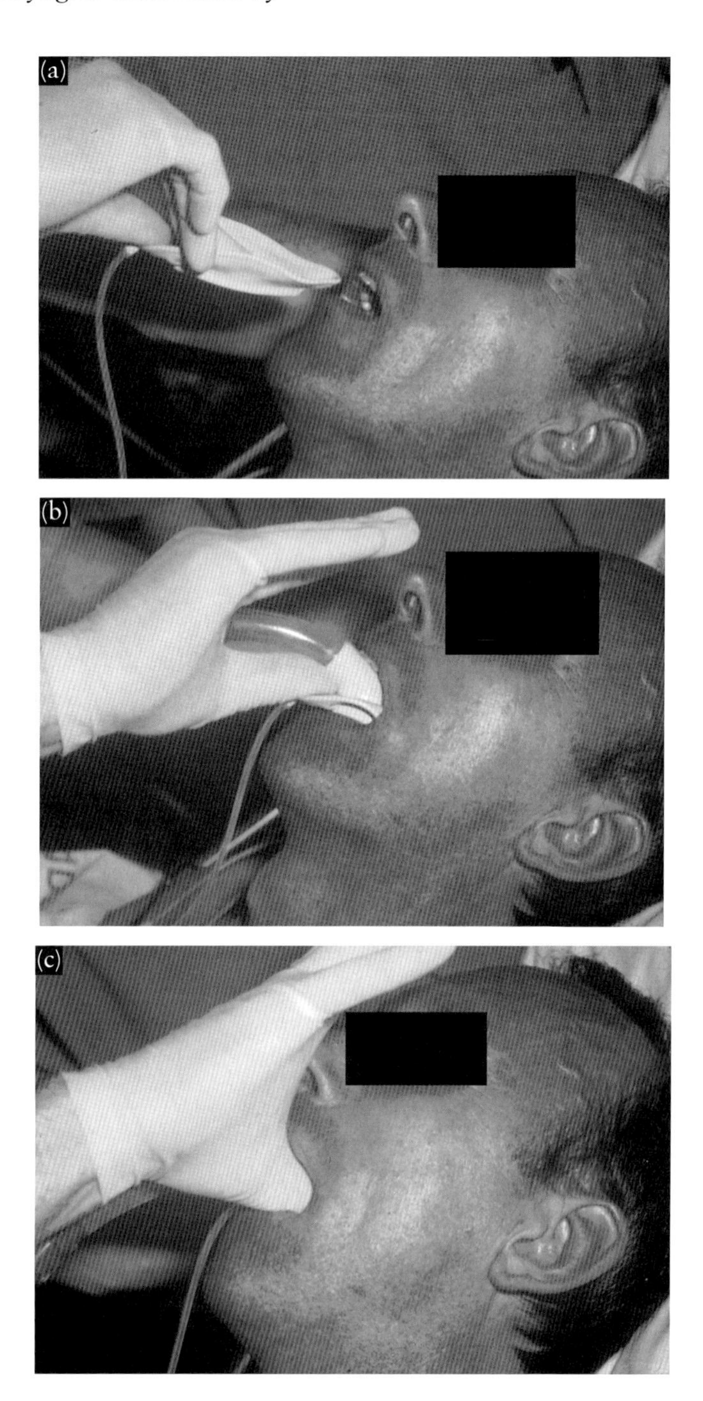

Figure 19.2 The thumb technique – useful when an operator cannot gain access to the head from behind.

EMERGENCY INSERTION TECHNIQUE

1. An alternative to the thumb or index finger techniques when the presence of secretions/blood in the mouth makes it difficult to avoid the finger or thumb slipping off the tube as it is pushed inwards.

2. Insert the mask fully into the mouth using either of the previously described techniques.

3. Now press the LMA tube firmly up against the hard palate by placing a lubricated finger or thumb just inside the mouth under the tube (Figure 19.3).

4. Maintaining firm pressure as in (3), use the other hand to push the tube inwards, aiming in a cephalad direction so that it slides between the finger and palate until resistance is felt. Only release the pressure applied in (3) when resistance indicates the mask is fully inserted.

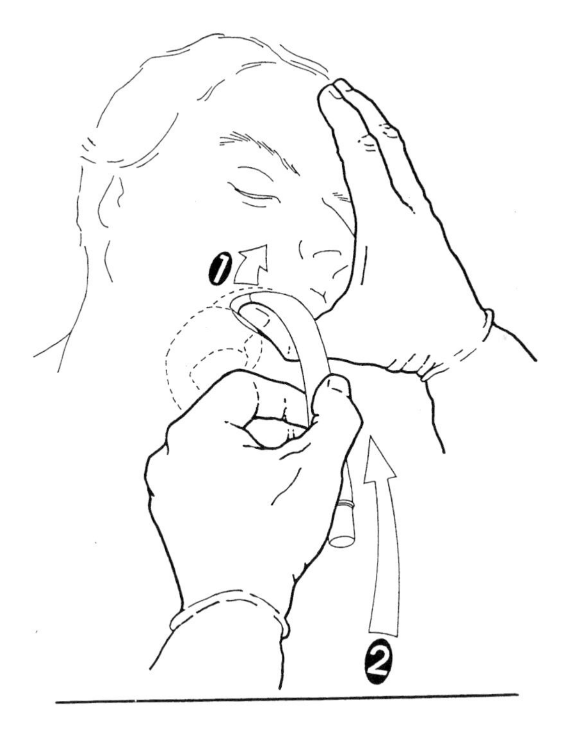

Figure 19.3 Emergency insertion technique.

Index

Page numbers in *italics* refer to illustrations and tables; **bold** page numbers refer to main discussions.